The Social Construction of
Community Care

Also by Anthea Symonds (with Sheila Hunt) and published by Macmillan

THE SOCIAL MEANING OF MIDWIFERY
THE MIDWIFE AND SOCIETY: Perspectives, Policies and Practice

The Social Construction of Community Care

Edited by

Anthea Symonds
and
Anne Kelly

MACMILLAN

First published 1998 by
MACMILLAN PRESS LTD
Houndmills, Basingstoke, Hampshire RG21 6XS
and London
Companies and representatives throughout the world

ISBN 0–333–66298–9

A catalogue record for this book is available from the British Library.

This book is printed on paper suitable for recycling and made from fully
managed and sustained forest sources.

10   9   8   7   6   5   4   3   2   1
07   06   05   04   03   02   01   00   99   98

Printed in Malaysia

To all those who are living in and for the community

Contents

List of figures

List of tables

Foreword

I am pleased to write the Foreword to what is an important contribution to a much used, much discussed, much debated term, community care.

Since at least 1601, when the Elizabethan Poor Law came onto the statute book, the state has formally accepted some responsibility for the poorest, most needy members of the community, when they or their families cannot support them. Yet who deserves help, how it should be provided, how it should be paid for, organised and distributed, and the balance between public and private responsibilities have been questions which have had different answers at different periods of history. Community care has been one way of answering these questions. But historical and sociological research shows that community care is at one and the same time a description of people's everyday experience of life, 'a euphemism for women's labour in the home' and a distinctive range of professional practice (Bornat *et al.* 1993: xi). Whilst carrying the 'rosy glow' of the caring community, it has also been used as a cheaper means of control than institutional care, but equally coercive and excluding in its practice (Thomson 1992). Community care is also shorthand for the legislative framework within which health and social care services have been delivered since 1990. But what it is and what it should be, remains opaque. It has been used by governments of different political persuasions to convey what are often opposite meanings (Baldwin and Hattersley 1991), it is a concept which is overladen with myths, preconceptions and assumptions, and has become in popular discourse a code word for chaos and danger on the streets (Wilkinson, this volume Chapter 15).

Hence the timeliness and significance of this book, a volume which will assist academics, students and practitioners in making sense of great changes in the location of care provision, in the values and practices of care providers and users, and in the whole culture of health and social care which contemporary community care reforms signify. The book's contribution to unravelling the mysteries of community care is not to do the impossible – provide a once and for all definition. Rather, its approach is to examine how, through the building and interweaving of sets of ideas, present community care policy and practice have been constructed.

In the four chapters which constitute Section One of the book Anthea Symonds sheds light on a much neglected area, the history of community care. Showing a rare mastery of developments in both health and social care she demonstrates that the apparently inexorable march towards the present community care framework has in fact been comprised of a patchwork of contradictory impulses and motives. The present reality, she demonstrates, is full of promise and full of problems: the promise of 'empowerment' for 'citizen consumers'; the problems of containing aspirations in a system already under administrative and financial strain.

The community care policies of the 1990s were not a fresh start, but imposed on long established and apparently powerful groups of professions, semi-professions and voluntary organisations. Hence some of the struggles over competing definitions of community care, what it should mean, what it does mean, and how it should be managed and organised. The impact of community care on these groups, and their responses to it are the subject of Section 2 of the book. Alongside rather depressing analyses of the constraints imposed by public sector management strategies and financial stringency, the reality behind the rhetoric of empowerment, come some grounds for optimism. Professionals, on the whole, recognise it as their duty to provide care, despite the constraints. Some are finding ways of combatting the often divisive individualism implicit in the community care reforms through developing working alliances with communities they are trying to serve. There remains a place for the positive ideals of professionalism, altruism, an ethic of care and a sense of justice within the changed and changing culture.

Community care is not just about policies, or about paid workers, it is also about people in need. A watch word of the third section of the book is diversity. The community care reforms were about creating diversity – of providers, of provision, of practice. A diverse population, it was argued, needed, not monolithic unresponsive and hidebound services, but choice, consumer power, autonomy. The metaphor for this cultural shift in the terminology of the New Right, was the market. A market could deliver where the welfare state had failed – efficiency, economy and effectiveness. But, like community care itself, the market is a metaphor. Completely free and untrammelled markets are no less a figment of the imagination than true equality. More than most, the market in community care is constrained. The aim is not to stimulate demand, but to contain it. The customers are not the end users, but the purchasers. Many of the intended beneficiaries of the market are amongst the most powerless and least informed members of society. They are also, overwhelmingly poor. It is against this background that the contributors to the third Section of the book write. They raise important questions about the viability of community care when communities are themselves impoverished, the conceptual language available to conceptualise their situations is limited, and the services which are intended to support them are under-resourced.

Sadly, it seems probable that the higher ideals of community care, the aspiration to give people who need care dignity, autonomy and choice, are unlikely to be realised for many in the immediate future. But this book will be an inspiration and an illumination to those involved in the struggle to realise those ideals in the testing times ahead.

JAN WALMSLEY

Preface

The 1990s have seen a revolution in the provision of health and social care in Britain; a system of beliefs, practices and expectations which has been in existence for over fifty years has been turned upside down. The basic premise of this book is that the concept of placing care for certain groups of people within the location of a 'community' is one which is loaded with contradictions and complexities for both professional health and social care providers and for people in receipt of such care.

The book is in three parts; Part I sets out the social construction of the provision of care delivery social policies; Part II focuses upon the professional, managerial and informal and voluntary sector responses to changing policy direction; Part III concentrates on the underlying demands of a truly needs-led service.

The idea of community care is far more than merely a change in the site and location of care provision; it signals a change in values, occupational practices and assumptions. Whole traditions of professional beliefs and practices must be altered, and so must the expectations and realities of users of services. It is above all a *cultural* change.

Running through all three parts in the recurring theme of the all-embracing nature of this change. Part I looks at the historical development of health and social care provision via social policies and also attempts to pose a sociological understanding of the structures and processes of British society within which these policies were enacted. Part II looks specifically at the present and future roles of health and social care professionals and the voluntary sector in the delivery of community services within a mixed economy of care. Part III addresses the underlying needs of vulnerable groups of users in the 'community' and the necessity for professionals to develop new ways of working with those living in poverty and need.

Overall this book seeks to 'push' practitioners and students into questioning their preconceptions and into constructing new and effective means of practising real care for the community.

ANTHEA SYMONDS
ANNE KELLY

Note: the editors and publishers are grateful to *The Independent* newspaper for permission to use the illustration on page 212.

Notes on the Contributors

Ken Blakemore has written extensively on race relations, the ageing of Britain's black and Asian communities, and on other policy issues closely related to community care. He has recently co-authored a study of equal opportunity policies and is currently collaborating with Anthea Symonds to prepare a book on the sociology of health and illness for nurses.

Bill Bytheway is Lecturer in Sociology at the University of Wales Swansea. He edits the journal *Ageing and Society* and is a research fellow at the School of Health and Social Welfare at the Open University.

Stephen Clarke is Lecturer in Applied Social Studies at the University of Wales Swansea. He has practised and taught community development for many years in Britain and in southern Africa. He is the author of *Social Work as Community Development*.

Matthew Colton is Senior Lecturer in Applied Social Studies at the University of Wales Swansea. He has published widely and is a member of the Executive Committee of the European Scientific Association on Residential and Foster *Community Alternatives: International Journal of Family Care and the International Journal of Child Welfare*.

Pat Davies works as a research nurse in mid-Wales. She is qualified as a psychiatric nurse and has worked as a lecturer in nursing. Currently she is studying for a PhD, and is specifically interested in the effect of prescribed courses on nurse education.

Robert F. Drake is Lecturer in Social Policy at the University of Wales Swansea, Associate Lecturer with The Open University, and Honorary Research Fellow at the University of Wales Cardiff. He has published widely and is currently engaged in writing a book on contemporary disability policies.

Mark Drakeford works at the School for Social and Administrative Studies at the University of Wales Cardiff. He teaches social policy and social work, having particular interest in poverty and social exclusion. He has previously worked as a probation officer and community development worker on the Ely estate in Cardiff.

Charlotte Drury is a researcher at the Department of Social Policy and Applied Social Studies, University of Wales Swansea. Her main interests lie in evaluative and research studies in the field of child care, and working with adult survivors of child sexual abuse. She is co-author of *Children in Need* and *Staying Together*.

Nancy Harding teaches health management at the Nuffield Institute for Health at the University of Leeds. She is the co-author of the forthcoming book, *Confused Professionals: The Social Construction of Dementia*, and is currently working on another, *The Social Construction of Management*.

Julia Johnson is Lecturer at the School of Health and Social Welfare at the Open University. She is also co-editor of *Ageing and Later Life*.

Anne Kelly is Lecturer in Health and Community Services Management at the University of Wales Swansea, where she previously had substantial experience as Director of the Community Health Nursing Course. She has been a member of the Health Visitors' Joint Committee of the United Kingdom Central Council, for Nursing, Midwifery and Health Visiting, the Welsh National Board for Nursing, Midwifery and Health Visiting, and the Professional and General Purpose Committee of the Health Visitors' Association.

Gaynor Mabbett fulfilled a clinician role in general medical wards and coronary care before pracctising as a district nurse. Her career in nurse education began in 1986. Since 1993 she has had a lead role in the district nursing component of the Diploma in Community Health Studies course at the University of Wales Swansea.

David Rea teaches at the Institute of Health Care Studies, University Wales Swansea. He has previously taught at the Universities of Plymouth, Huddersfield and Brighton. His research interests include the behavioural aspects of financial management in health care organisations and the development of social markets.

Tim Stainton is Lecturer in Social Policy and Applied Social Studies at the University of Wales Swansea. He has worked in the practice, policy and research areas of community care with a particular interest in learning disability and disability rights. His book *Autonomy and Social Policy* sets out a theory of rights-based policy for community care.

Anthea Symonds is Lecturer in Social Policy at the Department of Social Policy, University of Wales Swansea. She has written extensively on the female professions of midwifery and health visiting She is currently researching the effects of policy changes on community-based practice and the potential of anti-poverty strategies to improve health care services.

Renata Thomé has a background in general nursing, children's nursing and health visiting. She was appointed as Lecturer with the University of Wales Swansea in 1991. Since then she has pursued interests in primary care and community nursing developments through working as course coordinator for the first Nurse Practitioner Diploma course to be set up in Wales.

Irene Webber is Lecturer in Nursing at the School of Nursing Studies, University of Wales College of Medicine, Cardiff. Her particular interests are children's nursing, child family health care, primary health care and ethical issues in nursing.

John Wilkinson wrote his contribution to this book while he was Staff Development and Training Officer for the West Glamorgan Mental Health Strategy, which was a joint health, social services, voluntary sector and academic post funded by the Welsh Office. He is currently Mental Health Commissioner in the Department of Public Health, East London and the City Health Authority.

Margaret Williams is Assistant Professor, Faculty of Social Work, University of Calgary. Her major interest lies in evaluative and research studies in the field of child care. She has published widely and is co-author of *Children in Need* and *Staying Together*.

PART I

The social construction of the reality of community care

Introduction

Part I of this book sets out to deconstruct and analyse the concept of community care. Care in, by and for the community has always existed – it did not come into being in 1990 – but before we can proceed with this exercise we must first attempt to hold down a workable definition of 'community'. The concept of community is an ambiguous one, but it is this very ambiguity which lends it strength as an all-encompassing ideology.

Community as a site of delivery of care does not exist; this is at the same time its problem and its power. The concept of the community as a place where care can be received does not exist either in the concrete world of everyday practice or in the ideological world of people's lived reality. Try a simple test: ask for a delivery of supplies to be made to 'the community' and the first question will be, 'Where?' This will then lead you to name a specific and *fixed* site which will be another description; that of a hospital, a private home, an institution, a clinic, a community centre, but the phrase 'community' will be revealed as an empty and non-existent site.

Likewise the idea of community as a place for the receipt of care is not held in the individual consciousness. It is people's homes that they think of as the alternative to a fixed site of care. People express a wish to 'die at home', 'have a baby at home' care for a sick or dying relative 'at home', or 'remain in their own home', *not* 'in the community'.

Community in this sense of the delivery and receipt of care does not and cannot exist. Nevertheless it does exist; in Britain today health policies have been reconstructed and aimed at providing 'care in and by the community'. It is a *social reality* not only for the providers but also for the recipients.

■ Defining community care

There are three main ways in which 'community care' can be defined:

- Care *in* the community.
- Care *by* the community.
- Care *for* the community.

In this first part these are further defined as follows:

3

☐ Care *in* the community

This means care which is geographically placed within a locality with close proximity to the people living there and is a part of their local culture and everyday life – hospitals would fit into this category. Hospitals will be seen as a production plant within a locality – they are for emergencies which cannot be coped with outside, and their purpose is to make 'productive' again those who are temporarily 'unproductive'. These categories of 'unproductive' and 'productive' will reoccur throughout this part and are based upon a definition of distinctive groups of recipients. The 'productive' in this sense are seen as those people who are the bulk of hospital patients – the temporarily ill and curable. They are also potentially productive economically: wage earners, mothers, children.

In the nineteenth and early twentieth centuries, institutions such as asylums or long-stay mental hospitals and homes for the elderly, together with orphanages and children's homes, functioned to protect both the inmates and the surrounding population. They were built within close proximity to a community and occupied the dual role of 'threat' and 'sanctuary'. They were used to threaten with incarceration and punishment those who transgressed the 'normal'; for, ironically, institutions which separated out the 'deviant' were often called 'homes'. A commonly heard threat to an elderly relative or an unruly child was that 'they will put you in a home' – a curious reversal of the accepted idea of a home as a place of warmth and comfort. In one respect, however, institutions *were* like homes in that they offered a measure of protection and sanctuary from the outside world to those for whom the surrounding community was not a friendly or supportive place. Such sites are 'fixed' and immobile, and within them the inhabitants or inmates are also fixed and immobile – separated from the outside community socially although visible physically.

There is also the other form of care *in* the community, which is almost akin to the new enlightened type of zoo. This is where the potential 'patient' population is free and mobile but is serviced within this framework by state professionals such as GPs, community nurses, health visitors, and social and community workers. Sometimes these services are delivered in, for example, a clinic, a drop-in centre or a community centre – fixed sites, albeit somewhat loosely connected. But the most common form of care *in* the community is care within the home. Whether this care is formal or informal, the home is the predominant site of its provision. Like an institution, this is often a private place to which open and public access is difficult, but, unlike an institution, it 'belongs' in some measure to the inhabitant, the recipient of the care.

☐ Care by the community

This also has two distinct meanings. One is care by state professionals, trained personnel who take a formalised system of care into people's homes or to the loosely connected sites. These workers may be a mixture of paid and voluntary workers from the private or public sector, but they are part of an organised network. The other form of care in this sector is provided by individual family members, neighbours and friends, and by voluntary helpers both with and without formal management.

☐ Care for the community

This is a wider provision. It requires a distinct definition of who constitutes 'the community'. It can take the form of a universal system of public health, welfare benefits, social security, which covers all the population, or it can take the form of distinguishing distinct groups within the population as either needing or requiring care. The concept of 'productive' and 'unproductive' is used to distinguish these groups, but it must be remembered that these categories are not fixed.

■ Mapping community care

Table I.1 may help to clarify the analysis to be used.

Table 1.1 Care in, by and for the community – past provision

| *Home* | Care in the community – where? Sites of care | | |
	Clinics	*Hospitals*	*Institutions*
	Health centres		
	Community centres		
	GP practices		
	Resource centres		

| *Families* | Care by the community – who cares? Providers of care |
	State professionals
Neighbours	Community nurses
Friends	Health visitors
Volunteers	Social/Community workers
	Domicilliary services
	Voluntary sector
	Private sector

| Care for the community – who is cared for? Recipients of care | |
Universal provision	*Targetted provision*
Social and welfare benefits	Vulnerable groups
Public health	Productive/Unproductive
Free access to services	groups cared for
Unproductive/Productive groups	
protected and cared for	

The main argument to be pursued in Part I is that in the nineteenth century and up until 1945, then from 1945 to 1979, and finally from 1979 to the present, these definitions of community care changed and were connected and disconnected.

During the nineteenth century and until the foundation of the centralised, state-organised NHS in 1945, care was provided firstly by family and the voluntary sector, joined increasingly by state professionalisation and more and more sites of care and separation of groups.

During the period from 1945 to 1979, care for the community was stressed, care being concentrated on sites and universal access to professionalised care.

During the period from 1979 to the present, care in and by the community was stressed, but with emphasis on the home as the site of community work care not hospitals and other institutions, and on management of informal care by professionals, with a targeted rather than universal delivery.

This part addresses three main themes in the social construction of the reality of community care in the 1990s. In Chapter 1, the whole concept of a social construction is unpacked and the sociological implications traced of the usage of the concept of community in delivering care. Chapters 2 and 3 are concerned with the social construction via policies of the practices, practitioners and sites of care which developed and alternated throughout the period from the nineteenth century until the present. Chapter 4 looks at the recipients of care and at how they too have been constructed via social policies into differing identities.

Chapter 1

Social construction and the concept of 'community'

Anthea Symonds

■ Introduction

This chapter continues the theme of the concrete unreality of a place called the community which nevertheless has achieved an identity and a social reality of its own. For it is one thing for sociologists (such as myself) to argue for the non-existence of community, when groups of professional workers are expected to deliver care to groups of recipients in precisely such a site!

First, in this chapter the concept of the construction of a social reality is examined; second, we look at the construction of the concept of community as an ideal in our culture before moving on to examine the social implications of such a concept for the delivery of care.

■ The social construction of reality

It is first necessary that the way in which the term 'social construction' is used in this book be carefully defined. We have used this term to describe the building of a set of ideas through which a system of practices has been implemented. The idea of the 'social construction of reality' is a familiar one in sociology. Sociologists have argued that the reality of our world and life experiences are in fact constructed via ideologies and that individuals are then socialised into a system of beliefs, norms of behaviour and institutions which reflect and reinforce that reality. Berger and Luckmann (1984) presented the view that 'everything we know' is in fact the product of socialisation and the consistent reinforcement of learned definitions of reality. But humans exist in many realities; the example of waking from a dream which appeared real to face 'reality' is given by these authors as an illustration of the way in which we can move from one reality to another, both of them equally 'real' at the time of experience. The transition can be a shock, but we somehow make this shift. However, 'the reality par excellence ... is the reality of everyday life' (Berger and Luckmann 1984 : 35). But this everyday life has been constructed by human agency. We are all born into a world which is 'already there'; we had no hand in its creation and our early years are a journey of discovery and negotiation. We learn what is 'real', we learn what behaviour is appropriate for our gender, class, family and society. This pattern of socialisation into the values, norms and beliefs of the surrounding society is a common experience to us all. It is an ongoing process throughout our lives: the primary socialisation agency of the family is followed by our peer group, education, work, the media and our entire cultural millieu.

However, this does not mean that ideas and patterns of behaviour cannot undergo change; they are not set for ever. The socialisation agencies are just channels by which the transmission of 'everything we know' takes place. But realities themselves change. What causes or prompts change? Why and how does a 'truth' of one era become a 'falsity' of another? Most of us can point to one belief with which we grew up and which constructed our behaviour and 'reality', the belief for instance that certain foods were good for you which have now been 'revealed' to be a health hazard.

The agents of change can be defined as a greater store of knowledge, a change in the political priorities, or advances in technology, but whatever the reasons it is obvious that what we perceive as an unarguable reality can be altered. What then is 'the truth'?

■ The production of 'the truth'

Within the sociology of knowledge, the concept of ideology is a fundamental one. Different schools of sociological thought have utilised this concept in one way or another. There are two basic questions to be answered in this sociological debate: Is there such a thing as 'the truth'? Is knowledge neutral or does it serve the purpose of powerful groups in society?

In recent years the work of Michel Foucault has become widely used and quoted especially in sociological analyses of health care. Foucault's description of the development of institutionalised treatment for madness (1967) and his argument that modern societies have utilised more sophisticated means of surveillance and control over 'deviant' groups have rendered his work of special interest to those working in nursing and social work education.

Foucault's main tenet is that societies produce 'regimes of the truth'. This means that every society at specific historical periods produces an all-enveloping 'truth' to which people in that society adhere (Foucault 1980b). This is their 'reality', but it has been constructed and produced by people in that society themselves. The 'truth' therefore is not a universal or everlasting entity; it is a *product.*

Foucault than goes on to describe the transmission of this truth through a variety of *discourses*. A discourse is a set of ideas, practices and beliefs which coalesce to produce an over-arching picture of reality. In the eighteenth century, religion was the dominant discourse in European societies through which a 'truth' was constructed. But with increasing industrialisation and technological advance, modern societies developed other more powerful discourses: science and medicine. These discourses, with another set of practices, beliefs and sites of operation, produced a new regime of 'the truth'. Technologies were developed which reinforced this new 'truth', and these technologies also brought into existence 'new' populations or groups which could be defined as being 'different' (Foucault 1973). The development of definitions of insanity meant that whole populations of 'the mad' were created to be incarcerated in mental institutions and treated by professional 'experts'. The human body became the site of medical and scientific practice and specially designated 'experts' developed the 'clinical gaze' with which they viewed and defined human physical properties. The discourse of medical science defined what was 'healthy' and this definition was then applied to human behaviour and sexuality. The concept of 'good' or 'evil' which was dominant in the religious discourse was replaced by concepts of 'normality' and 'disease'. People in industrialised nineteenth-century European societies inhabited a different regime of the truth from that which had existed previously – it was a different reality. It was a reality based upon science and rationality, upon increasing mechanisation, urbanism and secularisation and it defined the modernity of the world in which we live.

■ Knowledge and power

Is knowledge neutral? Or does it 'belong' in some way to the groups in society which possess social and economic power? This is the question with which the sociology of knowledge has long debated. We 'know' what we know because we have been taught that reality through socialisation from childhood. But what of the *content* of this knowledge? Does it in fact reinforce power structures within society, so that we accept that men should have power over women, white men should have power over black men, professionals over the lay public, adults over children, the 'healthy' over the 'ill'? These everyday sets of power relations go largely unchallenged because they are our reality. Very often these interactions have taken on the appearance of being 'natural' and therefore are not perceived as being the exercising of power at all. For Foucault, power is exercised in such a way, it is diffuse and diverse, and power relations are everywhere and to be found in all social interaction. Relationships of power permeate and are reinforced by all social relations. Power is not imposed from above, there is no *one* centre of power. This is, for many, the weakness of the Foucault position, the vague absence of a centre of power. But his view that power relations take place all the time and everywhere is, I think a useful one. Where there is power, writes Foucault, there is resistance. This can be a very valuable insight into the everyday relations of power which all experience. For example, in their everyday practice many health and social workers experience a resistance by clients to their position as holders of legitimate authority and often offer resistance themselves to authority being exercised over them by other professionals. Resistance to authority can take many forms, from overt defiance to covert techniques which involve the failure to pass on messages, the 'losing' of documents or the communication to others that they are just 'obeying orders'. For instance, health visitors often experience resistance from the grandmothers of families they visit who challenge their professional expertise with reference to their own lived experience of mothering. The challenge to the acquired knowledge gained through formal education, which is the basis of professional power, is often articulated with reference to the gaining of experiential and non-formal knowledge gained through 'living'. This is the basis of the opposition to formal education as existing in an 'ivory tower' and remote from 'real life'.

But it is the role of knowledge in the possession of macro-power which interests Marxist writers. The classical Marxist view saw power as stemming from the economic base, in other words, whoever had power in the economic sphere had power in all other structures of society. For Marx 'the ruling ideas in every epoch are those of the ruling class', which clearly sets out the argument that ideas have a *class*-belongingness (Marx and Engels 1970).

A school of neo-Marxist writers such as Antonio Gramsci, however, saw power as being legitimated through the ideological structure of society. Power to organise the culture of a society into transmitting an all-enveloping view of the world which appeared as 'common-sense', was, Gramsci argued, the true power of an ideology (Gramsci 1971). He argued that a set of ideas gains *hegemony* and becomes articulated by a social class faction in alliance with others. When an idea has gained hegemony it dominates all social and political discourses and all debates have to be conducted within its parameters. An example of this could be the consensus to a system of state welfarism which dominated in Britain after 1945 which was transmitted or carried by many discourses in politics, the media, and 'common-sense', social policies were based upon it and a whole generation's working lives were constructed within this hegemonic idea.

Today another set of ideas has hegemony, those of the values of a market-based system, of value for money and of the necessity for people to fend for themselves rather than to rely upon the state for their security and care. This discourse is carried by the media, in education and in political debate, and is reflected in everyday conversation and has become legitimised. But this is not to say that there is a universal consensus to a hegemony of ideas; as we understand from the work of Foucault, the exercise of power creates resistances. Access to education, and especially a more analytical form of academic education, can prompt a counter-hegemony to be created. Most academic disciplines are essentially discursive and offer alternative interpretations of an accepted 'truth'. This is why many people find the study of social sciences to be conflictual; an analytical approach forces people to view taken for granted assumptions in a new and, sometimes, oppositional way.

The perspective which sees knowledge as something which is not a concrete entity, separate and neutral, but which is a construct of a society at a specific historical time, can be both liberating and confusing. It can be liberating in the sense that it allows us to analyse and really *understand* the world around us – our reality. But it can be conflicting in that we could see people (ourselves included) as empty robots who are brainwashed into believing anything at any time. This would be great misreading of this sociological perspective, as it must be remembered that discourses and sets of ideas have to make 'sense' of social reality as it is experienced by people. Ideologies or sets of ideas allow us to make sense of the world around us they are a 'lived' reality. But realities change over time, what was real for people living in the eighteenth century is no longer real for us.

■ How does reality change?

But why should realities and truths change over time? Is it just that the old truths can no longer be trusted to give reassurance or are not adequate in their explanations of a changed environment? Thomas Kuhn's theory of paradigmatic change is one which can most usefully be applied to explain changes in the body of knowledge and practice of professionals. Using the example of change in scientific practice and beliefs, Kuhn (1970) argued that paradigms (models of practice and beliefs used to solve problems) which had been accepted by the scientific 'community' for generations could be rendered inadequate when they fail to address increasing anomalies which appeared. In other words, when the existing beliefs and practices cannot fully explain or solve problems then the time is ripe for a 'scientific revolution', a change of paradigm. This theory of Kuhn's sees supposedly 'objective' and 'neutral' science as a practice which is open to change but which is also subject to the reluctance of many people to adopt new ways of thinking or practising. Change of paradigm comes not from *inside* the established scientific community but from *outsiders* who have not been socialised into the existing and, by now, inadequate paradigms. Change does not take place either immediately or without opposition. The established order is reluctant to alter and outsiders may not 'belong' in the status hierarchy of the society.

Kuhn's definition of scientific practice was based upon the view that scientific enquiry was dominanted by one paradigm at any given time; thus Newton's theory of gravity was replaced by Einstein's theory of relativity − a new time, a new reality.

The practices of medicine, nursing and social work have been subject to paradigmatic change. In medicine there have been succeeding paradigms within which medical practice was conducted. Theories and practices based upon beliefs of disease causation have changed from those which saw disease as a result of 'humours', or body fluids, requiring bleeding or sweating, to those which saw disease as caused by 'miasmas' which affected certain places, to the germ theory, to lifestyle theories; all these paradigms have dominated medical practice at different historical periods. At the same time, of course, none of them have really disappeared; they all continue to exist within the framework of both medical and popular beliefs and practices.

The *provision* of health and social care has also undergone great paradigmatic change since the nineteenth century. If we use the concept of a paradigm to describe an overarching 'truth' which constructs sets of practices, beliefs and realities, then we can see how the provision of health and social care is enveloped within the dominant economic, social and political paradigms or 'truths'.

It was stated earlier in the Introduction that care in, by and for the community has always existed in reality, but it was not until this century that the phrase 'community', to denote a place for care delivery, became a public discourse. The word itself became an organising principle for policies and practice, and gained a hold on everyday common sense because it already existed within our cultural framework; but what does it mean?

■ Unpacking 'community'

The concept of 'community' occupies two parallel realities. One is the 'social lived reality' within which we work and live, that of localities which to some degree have a recognisable value system or culture which consists of 'knowing' the various people, the deviant and the conforming, the sets of rules of behaviour which govern everyday life within a specific space and time. Within this reality, we recognise that conflicts exist, that the neighbours and social networks are not always supportive or friendly, that closeness may only relate to actual physical proximity but does not extend to social relationships.

But there is another very powerful reality which also exists, namely the 'dream' world of community life. This world is a structural part of our everyday mental framework; it is what Raymond Williams (1983) described as one of the 'keywords' or cornerstones of our culture. This dream world is a very different place from the lived reality of our experience of 'real' communities. This community 'in the mind' is always warm, supportive, safe and secure. This picture has been transmitted culturally through literature, certain historical 'readings', sociology, and in television soap operas. Interestingly the place of this dream community tends to be a small area inhabited by people who share the same culture, characteristics, history, language and understanding of their world. It is genenerally sited in a rural village or an urban village such as the East End of London or an industrial area in the northern England. These are places of 'knowable communities' in Raymond Williams' (1973) memorable phrase. They consist of a set of social relations between people living in close proximity with a high degree of everyday face-to-face contact – the relationships are transparent. Williams applies a Marxist analysis to the traditional division made in the English culture between the 'corrupt' city and the 'innocent' country and argues that the village was a social construction of agricultural capitalism, so that the picture of rural peace camouflages a deeply unequal and repressive society. Likewise, the tightly knit working-class enclaves of the new industrial towns were socially constructed to serve the production process; there was nothing organic or 'natural' about them as communities. Women, men and children were forced into the close, back-to-back houses or the slum 'rookeries' and developed cultures as responses and forms of resistance to the appalling deprivation.

Despite this element of initial coercion, a picture of a so-called 'traditional' working-class life, especially in an undefined period of the past, has taken root in our collective cultural imagination and has come to stand for a lost golden age. This picture has been the subject of many autobiographies (Hoggart 1957; Roberts 1973) and has been further constructed by sepia photographs of a picturesque world which is far away but not quite out of reach. This constructed world of the past has become the basis of historical theme parks, of folk museums, and is prominent in advertising and styles of interior decoration and design which emphasise the purity and simplicity of this world in comparison with the decay of the present. It is a world which is transmitted on television every day through popular 'soaps' such as Eastenders and Coronation Street.

But what was the basis of this lost world of working-class community which occupies this place .in our dream? It was surely the collective response and 'resistance' of people in the same locality and social position to the ever-present threat and reality of poverty; what the sociologist Norman Dennis (1968) has called the 'mutuality of the oppressed'. Close proximity produced a tight network of social relationships based upon this shared experience. The culture which was produced was a means of negotiation with a social reality which made the poor vulnerable to destitution and disease and thrown upon their own resources for protection.

Oral histories and personal remembrances often stress the quality of the support given by people to each other against the common threat of poverty; John Langley recalls that 'There was a marvellous neighbourly spirit in those years. If you were ill the whole street was concerned and wanted to do something about it and they did' (Langley 1976 : 11). But who 'belonged' in this world and who did not? Anna Davin's powerful history of home and street life in London before 1914 points to the conflicts and racism which existed. This illustrates a parallel reality: 'we had no Jews or foreigners living among us. They would have had a rough reception and their life made a misery had they attempted to live in "our" street' (Davin 1996 : 37). The main mode of construction of both of these realities was the external world of social and economic policies. These localities were constructed then and since by structures beyond the control of people and to which they could only respond or resist. During the 1950s and 1960s housing policies and increasing affluence removed the worst of the effects of past poverty. But they were also instrumental in breaking up extended families; there was a high degree of mobility, and the building of new towns and estates meant that 'old traditional' communities were split up. It was at this moment of disintegration that famous sociological studies of the vanishing world were conducted (Willmott and Young 1957; Dennis *et al.* 1969) to catch this world and preserve it in our consciousness. In the sociological tradition the disintegration tended to be defined as a 'loss' not just historically but more importantly culturally and emotionally. This 'reading' is very much influenced by the classic work on the impact of the modern world on pre-existing forms of society by the nineteenth-century writer Ferdinand Tönnies (1957). He defined the change with industrialisation as that from a world based upon close-knit ties and kinship (*Gemeinschaft*) to one based upon contract and acquaintance (*Gesellschaft*). This very influential work dominated much of sociological studies of community in the following years. In many of these studies (Wirth 1938) it was urbanism and modernisation which were seen as a 'problem' and destructive of rural-based community values. Other studies, such as that of Pahl (1965) and Newby (1977), point to the impact which urban-based wealth and affluence have had on the pre-existing way of life. With wealth and affluence have come a different set of values which are not based upon 'mutuality' or collectivity but upon individualism and materialism.

When writing of the move of the previously impoverished working class to the new estates in the 1960s, Dennis had warned that such a move could not be accompanied by the same set of values. The foundation for the much-praised working-class support and mutuality – the collective experience of poverty – had disappeared under increased affluence, consumerism and materialism. The impact of external cultural, social and economic change is regarded by Beatrix Campbell (1993) as the foundation for the change which we see around us in the new and 'dangerous places' in Britain in the 1990s. Estates where young men terrorise the streets and young women have babies without male support, she argues, are the result of employment and social policies which have destroyed any other alternatives. We must always remember that the 'reality' of the past, which is sometimes hidden, is that these places have always existed, marginal, peripheral and outside social control.

But is this dream community then a constructed ideology? Kumar (1978) has argued that the 'decline of community' view which has permeated much of nineteenth-and twentieth-century thinking has been used in a reactionary way to support right-wing political philosophies. The appeal to a vision of a lost golden age which existed *before*, when women and black people 'knew their place', men were in charge of work and play and 'masters in their own home', women were self-sacrificing and in their 'place', children were seen and not heard, he argues, is the powerful theme which underpins much of the dream of community.

The problem, of course, is that this dream place is the one in which 'care' is to be delivered, not the reality, which is care in different sites, mainly the home, and by families, mainly women. For the dream community, like the reality, is of course, essentially a gendered place.

■ Community – a woman's place

As Beatrix Campbell (1995) has illustrated, it is *women* who have created what is thought of as a 'community'. The community is not the factory or the mine but the streets and houses – female territory. All the fond reminiscences of 'helping each other' were based upon a female network. Community spirit is connected to caring for others, chatting to neighbours, knowing other peoples' business, helping out with children and elderly people, babysitting, cooking meals for the ill and disabled – traditional female territory. The epitome of the community spirit in

British popular memory is that of the Blitz, a time, of course, of almost exclusive female occupation of towns, streets and communities. In the early post-war 'lost' golden age of community values when the male breadwinner was not seen from early in the morning until the evening, he was not expected or able to partake in the everyday life of the community. When he ceased work, he often became the recipient of community networks of care, especially if he was single or widowed, but rarely was he the provider of hands-on care to others. Women were absent from the public world of communities based upon an occupation such as mining; theirs was the 'hidden' community of homes and families and the provision of care.

The recent decline in the male occupational base has been one of dramatic significance for our understanding of a 'community'. In many areas today in the late 1990s, many 'communities' are once again based upon women, but with a difference: there is no male breadwinner whose arrival is awaited in the evening or 'after the war'. It is of course these very communities which have been castigated by right-wing politicians and sociologists (Dennis and Erdos 1993; Murray 1990) as embodying the values of an 'underclass' which is out of control.

The ideal dream community is a place where women are and where they stay and provide care and support to those around them, men are absent for most of the time, but their financial contribution enables them to provide a distant and reliable authority which can be drawn upon in times of need. It was the fear that a policy of community care would attempt to reconstruct this ideal that prompted much feminist criticism.

■ Care – a woman's role in the community?

Caring for elderly people, children, and the sick has long been taken up by families and specifically by women. This work of caring was, of course, unpaid. This was far more than a mere ideological vision; it was the social reality for the majority of married women this century. This invisible, unpaid and private world of informal and unpaid care attracted the attention of feminist writers by the 1980s (Graham 1983; Henwood and Wicks 1984; Lewis 1988). Bill Bytheway and Julia Johnson pursue this feminist critique and its significance for policies on carers in their Chapter 18 in Part III.

The policy moves towards an actual system of care *by* the community, which was mooted by 1986, prompted further concerns that it was women who would be exploited by these moves. As Janet Finch and Dulcie Groves put it, 'in practice community care means care by the family, and in practice care by the family equals care by women' (Finch and Groves 1980 : 494). In her studies of carers Clare Ungerson (1988) illustrated the different realities of female and male carers. Women tended to care for elderly relatives often not their own, while men tended to care for wives. The primary reason given by women for their undertaking this role was 'duty' while for men it was 'love'. There have been many studies which have shown that male carers actually receive better formal support in their caring role than do women (Finch and Groves 1980).

Gillian Dalley (1988), arguing against the policy of community care because of its demands upon women, advocated more 'collective' solutions rather than the focusing upon individual families. 'Women', she maintained, 'have a right *not* to care'. But as Hilary Land and Hilary Rose (1985) have argued, women very often do not have this freedom, being subject, rather, to a 'compulsory altruism'. The social construction of caring as a predominantly female role is one which has permeated our culture and social policies and is a 'social reality'.

In recent years this 'reality' has been challenged by another; that of the right of a woman to work and to create a more autonomous life. The impact of a political and social philosophy based upon the individual and the primacy of self-fulfilment has in fact eroded the old ideal of female self-sacrifice. The rise in divorce and single-parent families has also meant that many of the old patterns of family responsibilities and obligations are being eradicated. Recent studies have shown that the numbers of male carers (especially for elderly people) have been underestimated (Family Policies Study Centre 1989); nevertheless both informal and, importantly, formal community care are still delivered predominantly by women (Finch 1984).

■ Summary

How then can we understand this social construction which is now a lived reality? This chapter has attempted to trace the complexities of the concept of the social construction of reality and also to unpack the concept of 'community'.

It has been argued that the very phrase 'community' evokes a set of meanings and images which can be not only misleading but, for some people, a dangerous negation of reality. The almost deceptive cosiness of the word 'community' can in fact disguise a social reality in which people are left in isolation and poverty. The reality is that the provision of social and health care has now, in effect, been placed into what many would regard as an ambiguous and meaningless concept.

The social policy theorist Richard Titmuss's warned against this move from rhetoric to reality in the provision of 'community care', when he described the *cultural* place that the phrase 'community' occupies. He spoke of the idea of community care as embodying the 'everlasting cottage garden' and asked: 'Does it not conjure up a sense of warmth and human kindness, essentially personal and comforting?' (Titmuss 1979).

This chapter has attempted to peel away the layers of ideological covering which have surrounded the concept of a 'community' and to reveal the contradictions it contains. The social and cultural construction of the concept of 'community' must be seen against the economic and social structures which have in fact created *locations* in which people of similiar social and ethnic identities live out their lives. But to confuse the two is to confuse an ideology with a reality; a further complication is that not everyone experiences a reality in the same way.

Men and women, old and young, black and white, ill and healthy, affluent and poor: these variables will be paramount in ordering different experiences of the reality of a community. Communities have always been fragmented in this way, familiar territories to some and alienating to others. But it was the ideology of community which pervaded the policy shift to place care into a location of community. There has been a paradigm shift from the dominance of centralised and institutionalised care into a decentralised and fragmented system which has left many feeling that they are indeed 'foreigners' in a once familiar country. In the late 1990s, the move from the public provision of social and health care to this personal and private sphere has become the lived reality for both social and health care practitioners and groups of users living and working in the 'community'. But we now need to map out the development of this reality; in the next chapter we look at the construction of another reality – that of the centralised state provision of health and social care which existed prior to the 1980s.

Chapter 2

The social construction of public care: from community care to care by the state

Anthea Symonds

■ Introduction

This chapter traces the shift in a set of discourses concerning the necessity for a publicly funded and state centralised system of provision of health and social care from a position of marginality in the nineteenth century to one of centrality and hegemony in 1945. This represented a paradigm change of massive cultural and political significance and set the scene for the development of policies we are presently addressing. How and why did it happen? In order to answer these questions we will be looking at the discourses surrounding the initial moves towards a state interventionist role in the nineteenth century when the first professionalisation of care by the community took place. This professionalisation was an answer to the existing system of care in and by the community which was operated by both charities and individual philathropy and performed by voluntary workers, and which was increasingly seen as inadequate. The inter-war years saw an increase in both the interventionist role by the state and also the debates and political discourses which sought to further this role. This was the period when Fordism both as a method of manufacturing and in the provision of care was initiated. The ideas which fermented during this period came to maturity and hegemony during the Second World War and formed the basis of thinking, policies and practices in the thirty years which followed.

This is not a complete history of social policies on health and social care provision, but it is important that these policies are noted and understood. This chapter, however, traces the development of a hegemonic idea, that of the dominance of state welfarism which gained a consensus as part of the post-war reconstruction ideal. Before looking at this development it is important to note that the provision of care has historically always been undertaken by four main agencies:

- *The public sector* – which includes all state institutions including local government and health authorities.

- *The voluntary sector* – including charities and non-profit-making organisations.
- *The family* – including neighbours and all informal unpaid care.
- *The market* – all private purchasing and provision.

These providers represent the supply side of care in, by and for the community, and can be said to represent the existence of a 'mixed economy', which has always existed in some form or another (Wistow *et al.* 1994). All four agencies are constantly present, but the emphasis on a single one or on an alliance between two or more will be emphasised above the rest. During the period with which we are concerned here, we will see the emphasis changing from one which stressed the pre-eminence of the voluntary sector and the family within a market system to one which stressed the position of the state as the main provider. As we will see, care in, by and for the 'community' changed its definition in these years.

■ Charity, philanthropy and self-help

The nineteenth century is often regarded as the golden age of charitable and philanthropic activity and influence (Davis Smith 1995). But two important factors have to be borne in mind; that this influential position was gained against a backdrop of the repressive but non-supportive role of the state, and that motivation and objectives differed within the voluntary movement itself.

The predominance of charity work and voluntary provision was the result of the hegemony of the philosophy of *laissez-faire*. This meant that any state intervention in the form of provision of welfare was opposed by legislators on political and moral grounds. Undoubtedly the guiding principle of much charitable work was a religious belief in the possibility of redemption and concern over the moral welfare of the poor. Nevertheless it must not be forgotten that there also existed a strong belief among many of the wealthy from both the upper and the middle classes, that possession of wealth carried a responsibility to others. Those on whom wealth and privilege had been bestowed often felt that they owed it to God or society, whence their wealth was derived, to 'put something back'. This ethic of public service dominated the work of many famous philanthropists such as Dr Barnardo, Thomas Stephenson (founder of the National Children's Homes), Octavia Hill the housing reformer and countless others. In a later generation this ethic of service very often filtered into the state professional sphere or into party politics.

It was the passing of the Poor Law Amendment Act 1834 which acted as the spur to much of the work of the voluntary sector; it meant that a tripartite system of provision of social and health care was created: institutionalisation in the workhouse, relief by charitable organisations, and self-help. Although for many the workhouse replaced the receiving of outdoor relief, it was the principle of 'less eligibility' contained within the Act which prompted the increase in inspection and policing of welfare recipients. This principle meant that relief always had to be paid at a lower rate than could have been earned in work. Central to this tenet was the division in the definition of the poor into the 'undeserving' or the pauper class and the 'deserving' – the respectable working class. Jane Lewis (1993) has recently argued that this division was more accurately understood as that between the 'unhelpable' and the 'helpable'. This division dominates all accounts of the life of the poor in poverty studies. It was the increase in pauperisation, the reliance on benefits rather than wages, which concerned most social reformers and social investigators and which prompted a change in the direction of traditional charity 'visiting'.

It had always been the practice of the wealthy, especially 'ladies', to visit the poor with gifts of food or clothing, but this visiting took on a more inspectoral quality with the advent of poor law relief. The founding of the Charity Organisation Society (COS) in 1869 to coordinate the work among the poor led to a closer interconnection with the state and eventually to the professionalisation of social work. It is from this early practice of family visiting that the subsequent dominance of casework-based practice was derived (Clarke 1993).

There was another objective and practice of voluntary charitable effort, namely that of reforming and educating the poor by example. This mode of social action found its place in the Settlement movement, which is credited with being the embryo of community work (Seed 1973). The movement came about simply because the social classes occupied totally separate realities. For the rich undergraduates to go and live among the poor was the contemporary equivalent of the white explorer 'going native' and this was precisely the motivation of the founder, Canon Barnett, who argued that 'the best for the worst' was the only way in which the poor and uneducated could be redeemed and brought into mainstream society (Young and Ashton 1956 : 226). Thus was the social worker identified as a missionary rather than policeman or judge, to 'help the poor to help themselves' – but the poor already had strategies of their own to do just that. Both the 'respectable' and the paupers resented the intrusion of charity visitors into their lives and homes and often preferred to fend for themselves if they could.

Such self-help took two main forms, the collective strategies for countering poverty and disease and the purchasing of insurance policies against contingencies and the buying of patent medicines and drugs on the market. This market-based activity is not often defined as self-help, but it is the essence of the poor as consumers.

For the 'respectable' working-class, self-help meant 'saving for a rainy day', by providing for themeselves and dependants without recourse to either charity or the poor law. Belonging to a friendly society was a mark of respectability in itself, and social researchers showed how this contribution was regarded as one of the most important items of expenditure even within budgets which did not allow for sufficient food to be bought (Pember-Reeves (1979). As David Vincent chronicles, by 1914 door-to-door salesmen were administering 46 million policies a year, 'many paid for at the expense of food on the table or pennies in the gas meter' (Vincent 1991 : 17).

It is important to realise that aid either from the poor law or from charities was to replace the wage of the breadwinner in times of crisis such as death, unemployment or sickness. The actual provision of health care services took two forms: first, medical and nursing care in voluntary charity hospitals or 'on the district', both of which were funded by charitable donations, and second the wide availability on the market of patent medicines and drugs which had huge sales (Webster 1993).

This tripartite system was fragmented and chaotic; it may have fulfilled the requirements of a social and economic philosophy which was based upon the primacy of the individual, but by the latter decades of the century it was proving woefully inadequate.

■ Discourses of poverty, imperialism and national efficiency

The discourse of the *management* of poverty has been well documented as one of the major dynamics behind the development of nursing and public health (Dean and Bolton 1980). Poverty was predominantly seen as a *cultural* deficiency, not as a structural part of a capitalist economic system. This was, of course, to be the basis of the Marxist critique of charity and social work among the poor which first became articulated in the 1880s. The poor became blamed for their own poverty; they were poor because they were lazy, feckless or ignorant. Education of the poor therefore became a keypoint of the strategies of the management of poverty because it was here that intervention could be made. The poor had to be taught to change their behaviour, culture and values. But why had poverty become a problem? One of the main reasons was that it had become so obvious and public; the migration from agricultural areas to the new urban areas grew rapidly, especially with the onset of the agricultural depression in the 1870s. In the cities and towns poverty was public and apparent, and the spread of infectious diseases and overcrowding added to the feeling that this deprivation was linked to depravity and moral decline and was widespread and out of control.

The discourses of imperialism and motherhood, eugenics and national efficiency were all linked to this need to manage and administer the poor. One of the overriding connections between them was that at the same time as Britain was expanding its overseas empire, at home the birth rate was decreasing and infant mortality was high (154 deaths per 1000 in 1900). The decline in the birth rate was seen as of great symbolic importance because it was among the most 'fit', the educated middle classes, that the decline was most significant. The state of health among the groups who were 'over-reproducing' and suffering the highest rates of mortality, therefore became of great importance. Sons were needed for the Empire as soldiers, for industry as workers, daughters were needed to be mothers of the next generation. At the same time, eugenicist concerns grew over the *quality* of the population and this fed into the discourses on imperialism and the importance of good motherhood.

Politically, the need to gain control of the situation resulted in the growing intervention of the state. A series of Public Health Acts designed to clean up the surrounding environment were passed during the 1870s and a national education system was also developed during this period, while the institutionalisation of the 'unfit' in asylums increased in all large urban areas. But the advent of the Boer War in 1899 focused attention on the appalling state of health of the young male population, and this set in motion demands for increased state intervention and the provision of welfare in a more direct way. The poor state of health of recruits to the war shocked the military; of the 20 000 volunteers only 14 000 were considered 'fit' enough for service and, in the case of Manchester, which was the leading industrial centre, out of 11 000 volunteers only 1200 were accepted as fit. The imperial army was short, emaciated and tubercular, and had bad teeth. The daughters of the empire fared no better; although the state of health of women and girls could not be examined in such a public way, the high rate of maternal mortality and morbidity was the subject of Government reports and studies. The paradigm of *laissez-faire* appeared to be inadequate to cope with this situation and a new paradigm began to be sought for. It appeared within the discourse of national efficiency.

The Fabian Society presented its manifesto on national efficiency in 1901; it put forward a programme of social reform based upon the primacy of state control and administration. The Fabians, acting as an advance guard of intellectual change, championed efficiency in all spheres of public administration, business, social welfare and economic life as the organising principle of state activity (Mackenzie and Mackenzie 1979). It was a programme which attracted support across the political spectrum, but it eventually found its home within the Labour Party, which was founded shortly afterwards (Searle 1971). It was inherent in the drive for national efficiency that the social evils of an unregulated society could only be eradicated by the secularisation and professionalisation of social welfare. This was the articulation of an alternative paradigm, of a collectivist rather than an individualist view, however, it was based not upon skills and knowledge becoming democratised within the 'community' but rather upon their direction by experts and professionals.

■ The professionalisation of care

The discourses of poverty, eugenics, imperialism and motherhood together formed a new 'truth'. This was that society could no longer continue to function in a fragmented and *laissez-faire* mode; a measure of state intervention and responsibility was essential for the future of national prosperity. The goverment set up the Committee on Physical Deterioration in (Hmso 1904) and the Committee on medical Federation and the Feeling of Children attending Elementary School (HMSO, 1906) their findings were used to increase the demands for more state action, especially in the care of children.

The intervention by the state took three main forms: public health for all the community, professionalisation of care provision to and in the community, and finally a measure of welfare provision and access to professional health care to certain groups. The initiating measures spanned the period from the end of the nineteenth century until the inter-war years.

Public health provision included the whole sanitarian movement which focussed upon cleaner water, air and a reaction against the public squalor and pollution in the public arena. It also included a range of activities which operated more in the private arena of the home such as the creation of health visitors, district nurses and social workers.

The creation of cleaner public spaces involved not only the building of parks and civic buildings but also the sweeping away out of sight of the morally 'corrupt' and 'degenerate' (Busfield 1986; Dingwall *et al.* 1988). The institutionalised 'unfit' included not only people who were mentally and physically handicapped or mentally ill, but also orphaned children, runaways, girls who were suspected of immoral behaviour and unmarried mothers. We look in more detail at this social construction of the 'cared for' in Chapter 4. However, the increase in institutionalisation constructed a new and definable 'community' who could be cared for in their own homes and so saved from incarceration.

Health visiting, which rapidly became professionalised in the early years of the twentieth century, had as its main task the education of working-class mothers. Within the discourses of poverty and motherhood the person of the working-class mother was seen as both the *cause* of the family's ill health and poverty and at the same time as the *solution* to the problem. Histories of health visiting in this period (Davin 1978; Symonds 1991; Lewis 1980) all illustrate that it was the growing relationship between the family (especially women and children) and the state at this time which framed the role of this state profession.

The focusing upon children's health led to the provision of school dinners and to the setting up of the school medical service, which in turn created the professional school nurse. The Midwives Act 1902 meant that midwifery became officially recognised as a legitimate and specialised occupation requiring training and education. District nursing too was becoming professionalised and undertaking work which was allocated by local authorities as well as voluntary agencies. Monica Baly (1986) describes the growing resentment felt by the newly qualified and trained district nurse graduates from the Queens Institute (known as Queen's Nurses) towards the authority exercised by local charitable 'ladies'. The focus remained that of nursing of the 'sick poor' in their own homes, but after 1908 the payment of old age pensions meant that more elderly people were remaining out of the workhouse.

The growing move towards professionalisation was also reflected in the scientific studies of poverty which were carried out at this time and of the growth in the idea of a social science training for social work. Descriptions of the lives of the poor had often been published and had achieved a wide readership, but the study by Charles Booth (1889) into the conditions in London marked a new direction for reporting of this type. This was the first such study to be carried out in a scientific and systematic way and claimed a measure of objectivity and professional neutrality. A later study by Rowntree in York (1901) followed in this tradition, and both studies pointed to the main cause of poverty as being low wages. These studies, which set the pattern for empirical social research in Britain, had a two-fold effect: first they cemented the idea of a scientific and objective appraisal of social problems, and second, they pinpointed the economic rather than the cultural causes of poverty. The Rowntree Foundation, established in 1904, had as its objective to seek out the causes of social evil. This marks a distinct shift in the activities of philanthropic organisations from the supplying of help to the poor to the supplying of research-based information to the public and government in the hope of initiating change in the system.

The influence of a scientific approach can be seen in the moves towards the training and professionalisation of social work. Social work was being moved from the hands of well-meaning and sincere 'do-gooders' into the hands of educated and trained providers. It was the economic causes of poverty which the state began to recognise and to address.

The National Health Insurance Act 1911 is often regarded as the real beginning of the welfare state. It did mark a milestone in the responsibility of the state for the health care of certain groups but it was also an example of the continued existence of a *laissez-faire* belief in individual self-help. It was contributory and was to provide a measure of short-term support for certain low-paid breadwinners (almost exclusively men) and a limited access to medical care. The years from the middle of the nineteenth century until the outbreak of war in 1914 had seen the hegemonic philosophy of *laissez-faire* challenged by a competing paradigm of state intervention and responsibility. The war was to shift these ideas still more to the centre.

■ Change and reconstruction

The overwhelming picture of the inter-war years is one of social and economic contradictions and uneven development. In many ways, British society was greatly changed; women had gained a measure of autonomy, new methods of industrial production were introduced, and though there was comparative affluence in the some of the areas of new industrial development this was countered by deprivation and increased poverty in the distressed areas of high unemployment. The divisions between rich and poor remained and were added to by increasing divisions within the working and middle classes. The health of the nation improved overall but with alarming increases in illness and disease among the unemployed and the poor (Webster 1982).

The inter-war years saw the increasing role of the state in types of welfare provision against a background of continuing concern over poverty within a society greatly changed by experience of war and unemployment and the emergence of a discourse which set the framework for the post-war system, namely that of planning.

The war had increased the intervention by the state into people's lives in ways which were unknown previously – from the first ever state imposition of compulsory conscription, to the payment of widows' benefits, tax allowances for dependants, public assistance systems, disability benefits; these measures, both coercive and supportive, made the presence of the state felt.

The reconstruction programme which followed the war laid great stress on the care of the community, with special attention paid to the building of 'homes fit for heroes' and officially recognised the connection between poverty and ill health. The state provision of public housing which increased with succeeding Housing Acts from 1919 to 1930 prompted the growth of large council estates, the creation of new 'communities'.

But the problem of poverty remained and after 1929 the spread of mass unemployment and increased deprivation caused care for the community by the state to be stretched to its limits. For the unemployed and the poor, self-help remained the only way to avoid the stigmatisation of poor law relief. Benefits still centred around replacement income for the loss of a working wage and the 'less eligibility' principle still operated within the means test which was enacted in 1931.

■ State provision – a move from the margins

This was the era of what Seed (1973) has termed the 'household state', which eclipsed social work as a vocation and social movement. The heyday of philanthropy was passed, and total state provision was not yet an all-embracing social policy, but the voluntary sector was moving into a new era. Charities and voluntary workers still provided care to and in the community to the poor, but a closer relationship with the state had been formed. This sector still sponsored the education and training of social workers as well as employing them and began to move to a much closer relationship with the state. The Fabian view (Webb and Webb 1912) had been that the state and the voluntary sector could be likened to a set of parallel bars both providing a means to an end and having the same objective, but remaining strictly separated. By the middle of the 1930s however the bars were becoming connected.

Elizabeth MacAdam (1934) has called this the era of the 'new philanthropy', in which the voluntary sector remained an important provider of social services which were however state-funded. By 1934, 37 per cent of the total income of registered charities was received as payment from contracts with the state via local authorities. The voluntary sector, through the organisation of National Council of Social Services (founded in 1919), worked with local authorities and sponsored training centres and recreational facilities in deprived areas, set up clinics and nursery schools, ran soup kitchens and organised 'treats' for children.

In fact, by 1939, half of all nursery schools, a quarter of all child clinics and all of the family planning clinics were provided by voluntary organisations. But unlike fifty years before, this provision was now in conjunction with the state.

Many in the working class and the middle classes still purchased health care through the market system. Wives and children were not covered by National Health Insurance and medical and midwifery care had to be purchased. This was proving an increasing drain on low incomes, even among the lower middle classes. Much of the day-to-day care of elderly, disabled and terminally ill people was still shouldered by families, and for many the conditions under which this care was given had not changed since the previous century.

But care by the state and professionals continued with the implementation of the registration of nurses in 1919, the expansion of health visiting and the setting up of the home help service which followed the Maternal and Child Welfare Act 1918. The Midwives Act 1936 made midwives employees of the state and finally ended their independence and autonomy of practice. Although not yet free and universal, health care was being provided on a wider scale by professionalising workers. This latter trend was given a boost when in 1929 the responsibility for the old poor law infirmaries passed to local authorities. Many of these, especially those controlled the Labour Party, saw this as an opportunity to increase the access to hospital care for those who were in greatest need. Hospitalisation became a political project, with the number of beds in the public sector increasing faster than those in voluntary hospitals (Abel-Smith 1964). The voluntary hospitals were in increasing financial difficulties, unable to raise sufficient funds owing to the economic depression and the increasing demand for their services.

This then was a transitional stage in the construction of state provision; there was a feeling of crisis as state provision increased but so also did the demands for health and social care; the acceptance of a measure of state responsibility had been largely achieved but there were now demands that this should be further increased and that state responsibility should become centralised control.

■ Discourses of public health, planning and Fordism

As in the nineteenth century, there was a set of linking discourses which produced a social 'truth' and which accompanied policies of increased state intervention.

As in the previous century, it was a decreasing birth rate which underpinned many of the eugenicist concerns in public health in the 1920s and 1930s, but unlike the previous era it was a high maternal mortality rate which was focused upon. The birth rate in Britain had declined faster than any other European country. It had fallen from 23.6 per 1000 in 1906 to 19.9 in 1925 and in 1935 it was 15.0 per thousand – a decline of almost 80 per cent from the beginning of the century – but at the same time the maternal mortality rate rose by 22 per cent between 1923 and 1933. The loss of male lives during the war, coupled with the vast number of disabled men, the 'broken dolls' (Bourke 1996) to whom war pensions were still being paid, added to the concern over the 'missing mothers'. The lost war generation was not being replaced. Women, it was increasingly argued by government spokesmen and in articles in the Press, were not bearing children because of the fear of childbirth and its attendant dangers. The problem of maternal mortality had been the subject of government reports from 1924, where it had been described as 'this burden of avoidable suffering' (Ministry of Health 1924 : 5). By 1937 this 'deep and continuous stream of mortality' (Ministry of Health 1937 : 51), had become a political issue. The campaign to 'save the mothers' involved the government, the aspiring professional group of obstetricians, health professionals, women's organisations and the popular Press and became one of the public health discourses of the inter-war years (Hunt and Symonds 1995; Symonds 1996).

Connected to this focus upon maternal mortality was the concern over the health of the poor as a whole and especially the unemployed. As Charles Webster has argued (Webster 1982), the poor health of the latter specific group was rendered even more obvious by the comparative rise in living and health standards among the rest of the population. The increasing focus in public health matters on the health of specific groups was the result of a change in the direction of public health organisation. Public health was now the remit of the Ministry of Health, which brought many doctors into contact with a population they had not previously seen close at hand. The result was that it was the state professionals such as local medical officers of health who pointed to poverty as the main cause of ill-health and mortality (Jones 1994). A much-publicised study of diet and nutrition among the unemployed by the scientist John Boyd Orr (1936) illustrated the appalling effect of poverty caused by the inadequacy of state benefits. The effect of slum housing on health was largely accepted, but despite the fact that there had been an extensive programme of housebuilding and slum clearance since 1918 the legacy of slums and overcrowding continued to plague Britain. A report by two public health doctors in Stockton (M'Gonigle and Kirby 1936) showed that even when families were removed from the slums to the new estates the increased rents caused greater hardship and their health (especially that of mothers) actually deteriorated. The strength of such findings was based upon the fact that they were made by experts and professionals. They had a scientific validity which had been the power of the social researches decades before and which had prompted governmental reforms. This application of a scientific methodology to social problems dovetailed into the dominant discourse of the 1930s – planning.

Like the discourse of national efficiency of which it was in many ways a descendant, the appeal of 'planning' cut across political party lines and became the organising principle for many groups and interests. By the middle of the 1930s, the concept of planning as a solution to the economic crisis had gained wide support (Marwick 1964; Wood 1955; Macmillan 1933). The belief in the necessity for a more rational economic and social system planned along scientific lines and embodying both industrial development and social welfare became the hegemonic idea of the pre-war period. Many disparate groups organised on the principle of planning as a solution to the crisis and as a tool for future development; they included the social research group Political and Economic Planning (PEP) and the interventionist-capitalist Next Five Years Group formed by the radical Tory Harold Macmillan in 1935. But it was a significant and highly visible group of socialist scientists who formed the Social Division of Science group within the British Association, and who argued tirelessly and amid great publicity for a social use to be made of science and technology, who gave the planning movement its focus (Werskey 1978). The application of science was held to be the neutral and apolitical solution to the problems of unemployment, disease and ill health.

Planning and the rational reorganisation of society on scientific lines extended into sections of medicine and health care. The Socialist Medical Association (SMA) campaigned for a planned national health system, a national maternity service and a salaried service for doctors working from large health centres. The research group PEP published its plan for a British Health Service in 1937 which attracted great publicity. For many in these years the Peckham Health Centre embodied a large part of the philosophies and beliefs of the health planners, based as it was upon a concept of treating the health of a whole 'community' in a holistic way which incorporated not only health care but education, leisure and social life (Pearce and Crocker 1943).

One effect of this belief in the supremacy of a scientific and technological application in health care was evidenced by the steep rise in hospitalisation of two specific 'new' patient populations: pregnant women and the mentally ill. The changing site of childbirth from the home to hospital was prompted by the belief that this was 'safer' because of the ready availability of new pain relief techniques and drugs which combated the main cause of mortality, puerperal infection. The debate over whether in fact this was a retrograde step for mothers is well known (Oakley 1984, Tew 1995), but it was nevertheless a process which became unstoppable and, by 1945, 45 per cent of births took place in hospital. The move to hospitalisation was also seen in the treatment of mental illness and handicap. In the Mental Treatment Act 1930 they were categorised separately for the first time and this led to an increase in hospital-based treatment both inpatient as well as outpatient. The development of psychiatry and the importation from America of curative techniques led, in 1939, to the use of electro-convulsive treatment in mental hospitals. Hospitals were becoming seen not as dark places full of dread but as factories for the production of the fit.

This ideal of a scientific state which was based upon technical rationality and which offered a measure of security, equality and release from poverty, had two main sources. Firstly, there was the existing Fabian belief in the necessity for a centralised state and secondly, there was the political and cultural appeal which the Soviet Union as a 'model' of this type of state made to a generation of scientists and intellectuals in the interwar years. This concept embraced the essence of modernism. In the modernist world which was coming into being in Britain in the 1930s there were new architectural designs of public buildings and factories which were large, open and light. These were in direct contrast to the old cityscapes of cramped, dark and closed-in buildings. The new buildings epitomised a new culture; the new estates and factories were large and homo-genised, and efficiency was the prime objective. The workforces of the new industries based upon new production methods and placed in the new towns of

Oxford (Cowley) and Dagenham were 'different' in that they were concentrated in new communities based upon employment but also embodying the new consumer entertainments like the cinema and the dance-halls. New working-class communities were being constructed. The new methods of production were efficient and large-scale, the assembly-line was the mode of the future. This methodology, known as Fordism after its pioneer Henry Ford, became synonomous in the inter-war period with large-scale car production but also became the mode for the supplying of care services. The Fordist social service state was in its initial stage of construction. Charles Mowat (1955) has stated that by 1939 Britain had constructed a 'welfare state in scaffolding'; it had also become a modernist society. This modernity was uneven in its development, however; the design of factories, housing estates, cinemas and shops illustrative of this trend were mostly to be found in the areas of the south and east of England where the economic depression had not reached and where a new type of economy based upon mass production was already in place.

■ The people's war

The Second World War was to further consolidate this process. This, unlike the First, was to be a 'total war', which involved everyone and which finally put the state in the position of dominance in the provision of health and social care. Many historians have chronicled the effect of the war on the practice and ideas surrounding the role of the state (Addison 1994; Calder 1971). Many of the measures adopted during the war – the Emergency Medical Service, the evacuation programme, provision of free school milk and meals, provision of nursery schools – set the pattern for the post-war welfare state. The low standards of health and living of the poor became increasingly obvious during evacuation and the blitz and the intervention of government into all areas of social life became the norm.

In 1942, at a particularly low ebb in Allied progress, the Beveridge Report (HMSO, 1942) was published. This famous programme for post-war welfarism, which became referred to as the 'Beveridge Plan' with its promise to slay the 'Five Giants' of want, squalor, disease, idleness and ignorance, was the culmination of almost a hundred years of slow development towards the state as provider from 'cradle to grave'.

■ Summary

In this chapter we have traced the development of the state in the provision of health and social care and as the engine of the professionalisation of the providers, and also the growing connection between the state and the voluntary sector, in the period preceding 1945. During this period, the state became increasingly involved in the provision of housing for the less well off and in the monitoring of children's health and well-being. This was paralleled by an increasing emphasis on the professional nature of health and social surveillance and with it the growing collaboration between the state and the voluntary and charity organisations. Tables 2.1 to 2.3 offer a guide to some of the most significant developments in these areas.

By 1945 under the impact of two major wars there had been a radical change in the perception of the role of the state in the provision of health and social care. The discourses of national efficiency and planning had played a part in the construction of a hegemonic view that it was the responsibility of government to safeguard and protect the health and well-being of its citizens. In the following chapter we look at this commitment and its consolidation in policies until the next great paradigmatic change after 1979.

Table 2.1   Important landmarks of state measures and concern before 1945

1834	POOR LAW AMENDMENT ACT. Curtailed outdoor relief; workhouses set up and principle of 'less eligibility' institutionalised.
1848	PUBLIC HEALTH ACT. Set up local boards of health in areas of high mortality.
1872	PUBLIC HEALTH ACT. Sanitary authorities set up nationwide.
1875	PUBLIC HEALTH ACT. Enabled local authorities to set up hospitals, sewage collection and supply clean water on rates.
1890	HOUSING (WORKING CLASSES) ACT. Beginning of local authority provision of public housing.
1904	Inter-Departmental Government Committee on Physical Deterioration set up to investigate the state of the nation's health.
1906	EDUCATION (PROVISION OF MEALS) ACT. Allows local authorities to supply meals for 'needy' children.
1907	School Medical Service set up.
1907	REGISTRATION OF BIRTHS ACT. Enabled health visitors to monitor new births. Collection of data on infant mortality.
1911	NATIONAL INSURANCE ACT. Contributory; did not include 'dependants'; available to certain groups of workers earning less than £160 per year; paid sick pay, limited medical benefits; 90% of married women and all children excluded.
1918	MATERNAL AND CHILD WELFARE ACT. Development of local authority clinics, home help service and health visiting.
1919	ADDISON ACT. Local authorities given responsibility and subsidies to assess housing need and to build houses.
1924	WHEATLEY ACT. Increased state subsidies for public housing; large council estates begin to develop.
1929	LOCAL GOVERNMENT ACT. Local authorities take over old Poor Law infirmaries; public assistance committees replaced boards of guardians.
1930	GREENWOOD ACT. Subsidies for programmes of slum clearance.
1931	Means Test introduced.
1935	Publication of Ministry of Health Maternal Mortality Report – showed rise in mortality rates.
1936	Agricultural workers included in National Insurance scheme.
1938	Domestic servants included in scheme.
1938	Barlow Commission – to set up national plan of housing development.
1940	Emergency Medical Service – nationalisation of hospitals.
1942	Publication of Beveridge Report – blueprint for welfare state.

Table 2.2 Important milestones in voluntary provision before 1945

1862	Peabody Trust formed – one of the largest housing charities to provide 'model housing for the working classes'.
1865	Octavia Hill buys first houses, which begins the philanthropic housing movement based upon management of existing rented properties.
1869	Charity Organisation Society (COS) formed – sets pattern for casework and home visiting. Function of monitoring those in receipt of poor relief.
1870	Dr Barnardo founds first 'Home' for 'destitute lads'.
1871	Wesleyan Movement Founds National Children's Homes.
1884	Settlement Movement found in East End at Toynbee Hall by Canon Barnett.
1904	Rowntree Foundation set up to investigate the causes of social distress and poverty.
1905–9	Royal Commission on Poor Law – supports the continued dominance of voluntary and charitable provision in Majority Report.
1914–18	Red Cross and St John's Ambulance have high profile in hospital service provision – funded by central government.
1919	National Council for Social Services founded – now Council for Voluntary Organisations.
1938	Women's Voluntary Service (WVS) founded.
1939	Citizen's Advice Bureau formed.
1940s	WVS develops 'meals on wheels' service to victims of Blitz.
1944	Age Concern founded.

Table 2.3 Professionalisation of health and social care to the community before 1945

1867	Manchester and Salford Ladies Sanitary Association employs the first 'mission woman' – the beginning of health visiting.
1889	Queens Institute founded for the training of 'skilled nursing of the sick in their own homes'.
1895	First paid hospital almoner employed by the Royal Free Hospital.
1896	Medico-Psychological Association (MPA) course instituted for the training and qualifying of asylum nurses.
1902	MIDWIVES ACT. Register for qualified midwives only.
1903	Charity Organisation Society (COS) launches first social work education programme to rid social work of its 'philanthropic and Lady Bountiful' image.
1904	Some universities – Birmingham, Southwark and LSE – offer courses in social science and social work.
1907	Following the Registration of Births Act, local authorities require health visitors to be qualified. London colleges offer a two-year course.
1914–18	Welfare workers attached to munitions factories. Children's officers visit homes of children 'in need'. Moral welfare officers appointed by religious groups and charities to monitor families in deprived circumstances.
1919	NURSES REGISTRATION ACT. Men admitted on register for the first time. Supplementary register for mental nurses.
1920	MPA qualification accepted by General Medical Council for mental nurses registration.
1921	Registration of dentists.
1936	MIDWIVES ACT. Midwives became salaried employees of local authorities. End of 'independent practitioner'.
1936	British Medical Association sets up Board of Registration of medical auxiliaries – physiotherapy, radiography, chiropody all registered.
1940	Pacifist Service Units set up to help families made homeless by the Blitz – beginning of family casework.

Chapter 3

The social reconstruction of care: from the state to the 'community'

Anthea Symonds

■ Introduction

The period from 1945 to 1996 has seen the social reconstruction of forms of care in and by the community. But as in all reconstructions the form of community care in the 1990s is vastly different from that which appertained before 1945. Yet the society within which this reconstruction has taken place bears some similarities to that which has existed since the nineteenth century. This chapter reviews the passage of this reconstruction over the past fifty years from the high noon of state-centred care provision to the slowly developing move towards the fragmented supply of care within the mixed economy. The shift towards a different method of supply of care did not just 'happen' in 1990; it was slow but perceptible from the 1950s onwards. It was a move which was accompanied by discourses on social equality and democracy in a 'civilised' society, followed in the 1980s by an individualistic dedication to 'roll back the state'. Within all these discourses there was a different identification of the concept of 'community'. It was argued in the previous chapter that by the outbreak of war in 1939 many areas of British industrial production and organisation had become Fordist in orientation. This process will be seen to have accelerated during the war and to have become dominant in the post-war period. The move away from Fordism was remarked upon by writers during the 1980s (Murray 1989), and by the 1990s the new concept of post-Fordism was being applied to descriptions of the change in the supply of services and goods. The main differences between these two processes may be made clearer by Table 3.1.

Such a move may have taken place in our social reality of the supply of care services, but we need to look more closely at this change. It may be a change in the method of supply, but the agencies of care provision we pinpointed in Chapter 2 – the state, the voluntary sector, the market and the informal networks of family and friends – remain the same. Therefore we have a situation of continuity within change. This has provoked contradictions and tensions as the emphasis in supply has alternated between the various agencies. It has also meant a *cultural* change as the post-Fordist method of supply has been accompanied by discourses which focus upon market values and individualism which may have produced a new 'regime of the truth' but which can be contradictory and confusing. Likewise the previous mode of supply, the Fordist model, was increasingly accompanied in the 1950s and 1960s by discourses which stressed social justice and individual liberties, which also set up anomalies.

This chapter seeks to chronicle these changes and the effect they have had on the various agencies which supply health and social care.

Table 3.1 Fordism and post-Fordism

Fordism	Post-Fordism
Standardised and undiversified product	Diversified, specialised product
Mass consumption	Niche group consumption
Vertical hierarchical management	Horizontal matrix management
Centralised bureaucracy	Decentralised organisation
Professional demarcation	Skill-mix 'flexibility'
Collective philosophy	Individualist philosophy

■ The 'New Jerusalem'

The landslide victory of the Labour Party in the 1945 general election was seen by supporters and opponents alike as heralding a new type of society (Fyrth 1995). The war had in many ways promoted a consensus to the interventionist state. Many of the trends present in the inter-war period – such as a belief in planning, increased national efficiency – now become intertwined with a commitment to a more egalitarian society. The Beveridge Report, published amid great interest during the war, had become the blueprint for the post-war world. In many respects the Fabian belief in a 'national minimum' standard of housing, income and welfare, first articulated in the nineteenth century, now became public policy. From 1946 onwards the policies aimed at achieving the destruction of want, ignorance, idleness, squalor and disease succeeded each other in a gathering momentum. Nationalisation policies in the economy, which saw the public ownership of the mines, railways, electricity, gas and transport, also saw the nationalisation of health and social care. In both spheres the concept of the public as owners is an ambiguous one. The public 'owned' in a very loosely defined way; in the nationalised industries the motivation was not one of private profit but of subsidised service, and the same went for the health and social welfare systems. But the 'public' were at the same time the users of the services; they paid (even if subsidised) for transport, coal and utilities and indirectly (subsidised) for health care. Social and health care to the community was placed in sites in the community, but who provided this care?

The nationalisation of the hospitals which had been a part of the wartime contingencies set the pattern for the post-war settlement in health care delivery.

Much has been written of the 'battle with the doctors' (Honigsbaum 1979, Webster 1991) which preceded the implementation of the National Health Service in 1948, but following this negotiated settlement a specific system was set up. This service was essentially focused upon the *curing* of ill-health and disease. The primary site of the curing process was to be hospitals, and access to the professional expertise of the growing medical and nursing specialities was to be through the GP. The *curing* of social problems such as juvenile delinquency, dysfunctional families and anti-social behaviour was to be placed within the newly professionalising social work departments. Within both spheres, the supply of cure-care was to be dominated by the qualified state professions. The state also took on the responsibility of caring for the community by applying both universalist and particularist measures to ensure social support and security. The universal benefits of family allowances and old age pensions were accompanied by the particularistic ones of national assistance, unemployment and sick pay. The policies on social security and social support were aimed, as they had always been, at replacing the male breadwinner wage during times of temporary hardship or crisis. Unlike the previous National Health Insurance policies, the 'dependents' of the male worker were now given equal access to health care services, indeed they were often the focus of services.

■ Social citizenship and motherhood

The welfare state which was based upon the Beveridge proposals forged a specific relationship between state services, responsibilities and 'the family', particularly women. As in the nineteenth century, there was a renewed concern in the 1940s about the decreasing birth rate. In fact, there was later shown to have been a 'baby bulge' by the end of the war due to an increase in illegitimate births. But at the time it was argued by Beveridge and others that all social policies must be seen as an encouragement to women to stay at home and breed, and that there must be a 'premium on marriage' (Timmins 1996 : 54). Consequently, many of the post-war policies can be seen to be pro-natalist in objective. In housing policies, for example, it was assumed that after the war family life would need to be reinforced and supported, and this was reflected in both the allocation and design of houses. Many of the eugenicist concerns which had always been present within discourses on the organisation of social life emerged strongly during the planning of housing estates (Mumford 1945; Roberts 1991). Houses were designed for the nuclear family with female economic dependency as a built-in structure; this was the 'Beveridge model' family, which has been the subject of much feminist criticism (Van Every 1992; Gittins 1985).

In defining the role of the family as suppliers of care, Beveridge laid great stress upon the 'contract' between the married woman and the state: 'During marriage most women will not be gainfully employed . . . (she has a vital service) in ensuring the continuance of the British race and British ideals in the world' (Beveridge 1942 : 50). As has been argued (Wilson 1977, Pascall 1986), this ideology of the family placed women firmly in the role of unpaid care-givers in and for the community. But the parallel reality was that more women were in fact going into paid work than ever before. By 1943, two out of five married women were at work and between 1951 and 1971 2,500,000 more married women entered the labour market. Nevertheless, in the years which followed it was the social construction of a particular type of family which predominated in proposals to place more care 'in the community', which meant away from other sites such as hospitals and institutions and into the home.

In both health and social care, the role of motherhood became once again the focus of attention by state professionals. This return of the person of the mother to centre stage was the product of many discourses from psychology, criminology and social citizenship. As the state had become the provider of the basic minimum of support, bypassing the husband and father, so mothers were now called upon to perform their role in social citizenship. While men gained this identity through work and their contributions to the social system, women were to be allowed access to benefits through their contribution – that of care in the community.

There was a renewed emphasis on the importance of mothering from the much publicised work of the social psychologist John Bowlby (1951, 1953). His work on the theory of 'maternal deprivation' was taken up with alacrity by the expanding state professions of health visiting and social work (Riley 1984, Sapsford 1993).

In the post-war climate of universalism and growing social equality, it was no longer structural poverty which was seen as the main enemy, but dysfunctional socialisation, and this was not confined to the poor or the lower classes. In social work, the theories of Cyril Burt (1925) began to have an influence in the analysis and treatment of delinquency. This approach argued for the application of psychology to the 'treatment' of young offenders and the concept of the 'emotionally defective' child emerged. It was argued that it was poverty of affection which caused children to offend (Summer 1981). There was an increase in health visiting to all families, and for the first time many middle-class mothers were 'visited'. Thus within a universalist system, the 'individualising' of social problems became the dominant practice. Both casework and family visiting at home concentrated on working with individuals and families and not with 'the community' (Abbot and Sapsford 1990).

This then was one of the contradictions which emerged during the dominance of state provision: The other was the expansion of the voluntary sector as both provider and campaigner for those who had been left behind in homes – the so-called 'Cinderella services'.

■ The voluntary sector as fairy godmother

By the beginning of the twentieth century, the relationship between the state and the voluntary sector in the provision of services was undergoing change. During the inter-war years, as we have seen, the voluntary sector developed a much closer financial relationship with the state. With the creation of the welfare state after 1945 it was assumed by some both in and outside the voluntary sector itself that the new dominance of state provision would leave it without a purposive role. But as Nicholas Deakin (1995) illustrates, the voluntary sector continued to play an important part in the field of social care even during the period of greatest state welfarism and public-sector provision. It was during this period of the dominance of state provision that the voluntary sector itself took on a more open politicising role. Groups were formed to campaign on issues which it was felt the state was performing inadequately. From the inception of the NHS concern was voiced that there were 'Cinderella services' that had not been invited to the ball, in other words that the services for the elderly, mentally and physically handicapped and the mentally ill were being neglected in the move to increased hospitalisation and the emphasis on *cure* of the sick.

This prompted many interested groups to set up to campaign for recognition of special needs and also to take on service provision themselves. Most notable were MIND, MenCap and Age Concern, which all came into being in the same year as the NHS. Care and concern for the elderly following the deprivations caused by the war and the growth of poverty among pensioners led to the founding of both Age Concern and, later, of Help the Aged. The institutionalisa- tion of people with both mental handicap and mental illness continued despite the 1930 Act which had encouraged outpatient treatment. MIND is a good illustration of the new role which the voluntary sector carved out for itself within the welfare state. As well as a programme of public education, it ran services including residential homes, training schemes for health professionals and employment projects. It was during the 1940s and 1950s that the voluntary sector took on the role in which it has now become firmly established – the concern with and provision for groups with 'special needs' rather than the management of the poor. The concern with groups who had been left behind in the general increase in private affluence and public welfare provision became a major political and popular campaigning issue in the 1960s.

■ The rediscovery of poverty – the 'civilised' discourse

Amid the affluence and economic growth in consumerism during the 1960s, poverty in the community was rediscovered and seen as an affront not only to the values of the welfare state but to a civilised nation. But why were there still people who were poor, and who were they?

First, the actual structure of the benefit system as it had been implemented in 1946 had been inadequate. Because it was based upon the old principle of 'less eligibility', the base taken was the minimum subsistence level, rather than, as in the post-war states in continental Europe, a level of earnings-related payments (Timmins 1996). The result was that those on especially low *universalist* payments, namely retired pensioners, the sick and disabled, single women with children and any unemployed persons who were not entitled to National Insurance benefit, used the National Assistance scheme as a 'top-up' from the very beginning. Consequently the numbers of those in receipt of supplementary benefit and dependants almost doubled from 3 per cent of the population in 1948 to over 5 per cent by 1961 (Lister 1975 : 9). This growing cost was the subject of a great divide in political opinion between those (on the Right) who argued for an end to universalism and a move towards more means-tested and targeted payments, and those (on the Left) who argued for an extension and an increase in universal payments (Lowe 1993). This debate was fuelled by the publication of a report in 1965 entitled *The Poor and the Poorest* (Abel-Smith and Townsend 1965). This report, published on Christmas Eve, showed that the number of people living in poverty, far from decreasing with the welfare state, had actually increased from 600,000 in 1953–4 to 2 million in 1963–4. But who were these people whom the welfare state had failed? They were defined and identified using a new definition of poverty, that of 'relative' poverty (Townsend 1979); this meant that poverty was now judged against the standards of the surrounding 'community' and not by some static economic formula. Phrases such as the 'poverty trap' and 'generational poverty' became used by politicians and policy-makers. This was a new discourse of poverty, based upon the ethical need to extend the benefits of the welfare state and booming economy to the excluded. Most of the poor, as the report showed, were families with more than three children, elderly pensioners (who had been too old to make enough contributions under the National Insurance scheme in 1946), and an increasing number of divorced mothers with dependent children. In the cultural context of the 1960s concern for the poor was focused upon the inadequacies of the system rather than, as before, on the personal inadequacy of the poor themselves. Following the report, the Child Poverty Action Group was formed in 1965, as was the more miltant Claimants' Union, which became very vocal in its critique of the system of social security.

In November 1966 the TV play *Cathy Come Home*, written by left-wing writer Jeremy Sandford, and directed by Ken Loach, created a sensation with its portrayal of homelessness and the ease with which the 'ordinary' working-class family could fall into poverty and destitution. This was shown only days before the public launching of Shelter, the pressure group which was to campaign on behalf of the homeless in the decades to come. At the same time, housing associations in 'blackspot' urban areas began to pressure the Wilson government for action on the housing crisis, with, it was estimated 3 million families in Britain living 'in the slums, near slums or in grossly overcrowded conditions' (Timmins 1996 : 258).

This new discourse of social consciousness was directed, ironically, against a Labour government which had come to power promising to 'modernise' Britain. The continued existence of poverty and homelessness seemed to be an anachronism in a country struggling to come to terms with the 'new scientific revolution'. The numbers of self-help and pressure groups exploded during the latter years of the 1960s; Gingerbread (for single parents), the Low Pay Unit, the Disablement Income Group, the Pre-School Playgroups Association, all bearing witness to the belief that people could make a difference to services, practice and policies by organising themselves. It was a measure of the self-confidence which had been constructed during the years of security and affluence.

The concept of the freedom of the individual was placed against that of the state and its restrictions. But the 'individual' in this concept was identified as one who was 'disadvantaged' and needed support and legislation to construct a 'belongingness' to mainstream society, to bring outsiders into the 'community'. This was evident in the legislation which legalised both male homosexuality and abortion in 1967, and abolished theatre and literary censorship. These measures signalled a willingness to extend the concept of civil liberties to acts of personal behaviour. The Divorce Reform Act 1969 removed the concept of 'guilt' from divorce and opened up the right to divorce to all those whose marriage had 'unretrievably broken down'. In all these measures one can see a reconstruction of the relationship between the individual and civil society (a point to which we return in the next chapter). The concern over those who were separated and marginalised by the 'community' was transposed to health policies, where the idea of actually transferring care from the sites of hospitals and institutions and into the community took hold.

■ Moving care into the community

There were actually two different but connected agendas in the moves to transfer care for certain groups out into the community. First, there was the problem of escalating costs in the supplying of hospitalised and medical care; second, there was growing articulated concern about the ethics and practice of institutionalisation for certain forms of mental illness. Among the elderly, the dread of 'being put into a home' had always existed, and revelations about the standards in nursing homes and geriatric institutions added to this fear, but the pressure groups representing elderly people did not make the same level of demands that care should be deinstitutionalised.

The problem of escalating costs had always plagued the Health Service since its inception, but what made the situation different by the mid-1960s was the development of new drugs and technologies. As Rudolf Klein (1989) has argued, the period from 1960 to 1975 can be characterised as 'the heyday of technocratic politics'. It was a time in which governments of both parties attempted to control expenditure while at the same time maintaining services in the light of changing circumstances. The values of efficiency, organisational reform and planning were evoked to cope with the growing supply crisis.

Why was there this crisis in a period of economic affluence and growth? The Labour Health Minister Richard Crossman summed it up in 1969 when he diagnosed it as 'the pressure of demography, the pressure of technology, the pressure of democratic equalisation' (Crossman 1969).

The demographic pressure was that of an ageing population, due to the very success of the social and health service post-war reforms; in 1951 there had been under 7 million people of retirement age, in 1961 this had risen to over $7\frac{1}{2}$ million, and by 1971 it topped 9 million. Moreover there had been a growth in the population aged over 75 who were more likely to be in need of services.

New techniques and drugs had also potentially revolutionised the site of treatment of certain illnesses. It was hoped by many that drug therapy especially would help in the treatment of mental illness. During the 1960s there had been a series of scandals on the conditions in long-stay mental hospitals; these had prompted the government to fund the pressure group MIND, who were set on exposing hospital conditions. On the surface it seems perverse to officially fund a group bent on criticising health service provision, but it 'fitted' with the overall objective of government, which was to move care out of hospitals and into the community.

Despite the fact that all governments since 1950s had been engaged upon the building of hospitals and had been competing with each other to build the most, the placing of certain chronic, long-term conditions in hospitals was losing its appeal. In 1953 the Guillebaud Committee, which had been set up to monitor costs in the NHS, had recommended that 'care in the community' be adopted for the treatment of certain groups, mainly by the mental health services. In 1961, the Conservative Health Minister, Enoch Powell, stunned a meeting of the National Association of Mental Health when he described the existing mental institutions as 'rising unmistakable and daunting out of the countryside – the asylums which our fore-fathers built with such immense solidity' (Timmins 1996 : 211). He then went on to say that these 'doomed institutions' must be destroyed by 'setting a torch to the funeral pyre'.

The conditions remained the same however in the late 1960s when Richard Crossman, then the Labour Health Secretary, said to a friend after a visit to Friern Hospital 'I am responsible for the worst kind of Dickensian, Victorian loony-bin' (quoted in Timmins:259). Following this commitment to improve mental health services, the Hospital Advisory Service was set up by Crossman to monitor conditions in all long-stay hospitals. But despite this disenchantment with existing mental hospitals, both parties remained wedded to the idea of building bigger and more technologically advanced hospitals for other conditions. The medical profession, of course, had a vested interest in this expansion because it increased its members status and public profile. Glamorous surgery such as heart transplants attracted popular media attention and the idea of the 'big hospital' staffed by experts and containing the latest technology was one which appealed to the medical profession, politicians and the public. In many ways it was the universal access to this site which was the essence of the post-war social democracy. Hospitals, especially the new Fordist district general hospitals, epitomised for many the achievements of the NHS. They brought medical expertise and modern scientific progress to the masses; this was what Crossman meant by 'democratisation'.

At the same time as the moves to place care for mental illness and the elderly in to the community were being made, the actual hospital population of the curable or the 'well' was increasing. For it was during this period that the hospitalisation of childbirth became the almost hundred-per-cent norm. So how can we make sense of this apparent disjunction between a move away from hospitals on the one hand and towards hospitalisation for others? To answer this question we need to look at the status and place in the social hierarchy both of the groups whose care was being moved into the community and of the professionals who were delivering that care. We will discuss this in depth in the following chapter, but it is clear that the mentally ill, the mentally handicapped and the elderly were 'Cinderellas' and that within the medical profession itself people with the lowest status (due to either ethnicity or gender) or speciality (psychiatry or geriatric care) were placed together in the backroom of policy-making.

■ Fordist organisation for efficiency

There are many examples of the way in which contradictions ebbed and flowed during the period up to 1979. At the same time as community care for some was being proposed, so the majority of the community were being served by massive, reorganised structures which represented planning and Fordist delivery.

In social services, the Seebohm Report of 1968 had set in motion the restructuring and expansion of social work and the creation of the generic social worker. The idea behind the recommendations was to lessen the intraprofessional rivalries within social work and to offer a universalised service, 'a door on which any one can knock' (Timmins 1996: 231). Social work expanded as it became a popular career choice for the increasing numbers of social science graduates from the new universities and polytechnics which had been created by the expansion of higher education during the 1960s. A reorganisation of social security also took place at this time with the creation of Family Income Supplement, Child Benefit and increased tax allowances in a further attempt to combat static rates of poverty. The main objective behind this reorganisation was the more efficient use of resources by the means of targeting those in most need. The changes to the social security system throughout this period were aimed at replacing support for all to support for some, with the emphasis being placed upon the working poor.

In the NHS a reorganisation was also seen as essential if it was to be in line with the new social services. After 1974, the reforms meant that the bureaucratic levels were increased and that the new devolved management thought necessary to increase efficiency began to expand. There was an attempt to make these two huge structures work in unison through Joint Consultative Committees but, as Timmins writes, the whole structure was too huge and unwieldy. The emphasis on 'consensus management' was in tune with the times but was also proving to be static and indeterminate.

In housing, the 1960s and 1970s also saw a massive expansion. The 'mixed economy' was firmly established, with the increase in council housing and especially the building of high-rise flats matched by the increase in home ownership. Subsidies for mortgages were allowed by local authorities and the sale of council houses was begun. By 1970, half the households in England and Wales were owner-occupied for the first time. But on the other hand, homelessness was becoming a political issue and in 1977 local authorities became responsible for housing homeless people in their area.

Following 1945, the idea that the centralised state should take on the main responsibility for provision of social and health care had gained and retained hegemony. Despite the moves to place care for some outside of the state organ-isations, this hegemony meant that the organisational structure of care provision grew larger and more bureaucratised. But it was also a period of more or less undiminished economic growth and affluence. However, not all of the community had shared in this increase in living standards: poverty still existed and so did the inequality of access to resources and services. By the late 1970s this economic boom faltered and stopped. Recession and the three-day-week followed the oil crisis and the miners' strike. The Labour–Liberal pact, which held on to office through the 'Social Contract' with public-service unions, nevertheless presided over cuts in public spending and the 'winter of discontent' in 1979 was just the final culmination of a growing crisis in the paradigm of state provision.

■ Individualism and market values

The Conservative governments elected in 1979 and in the three subsequent elections of 1983, 1987 and 1992 were very different from others of the post-war years in philosophy, vision and intent. The consensus to the hegemonic view of the primacy of the state as the most efficient provider of services was broken and the importance of the market as the dynamo of change and future provision was instituted. The philosophy of the New Right as the proponents of this view were called was in some ways a return to nineteenth century free market *laissez-faire* and in other ways an embracing of American-influenced values of the economic 'independence' of the market. Within this view, the individual was placed at the centre of concerns and policies and the existing economic and social problems were directly blamed on the post-war reliance on the state. This philosophy had been articulated by many writers since the 1940s (Hayek 1943) but it gained in power during the 1970s. In many ways, we can see its evolution from the criticisms of state provision which were aimed at the Labour adminis-trations of the 1960s and 1970s; however, it was with the election of Margaret Thatcher in 1979 that the discourse of rampant 'individualism' really began to construct policies and practices. Individual social mobility was placed in direct opposition to social equality, which had been the dominant discourse in the post-war world. Margaret Thatcher put it clearly:

> What lessons can be learnt from the last thirty years? First, the pursuit of equality is a mirage. Far more desirable and practicable is the pursuit of the equality of opportunity. Opportunity means nothing unless it includes the right to be unequal.... Let our children grow tall, and some grow taller than others, if they have it in them to do so. (Thatcher 1975)

This negation of the notion of egalitarianism was wedded to a dislike and opposition to the centralised state. Keith Joseph summed up this feeling when he argued that

> the blind unplanned, uncoordinated wisdom of the market.... is overwhelmingly superior to the well-researched, rational, systematic, well-meaning, cooperative, science-based, forward-looking, statistically respectable plans of government. (Joseph 1976)

The primacy of the individual and the move away from the state as the main provider, underpinned by an adherence to the values of the market, were the twin organising principles of the social policies on health and social care which were to follow over the next decade.

This move can be seen in many fields. It was one of the first acts of the incoming administration in 1980 to accelerate the move to home ownership by the selling of council house stock at a discounted price, thus constructing tenants as individual owners. In the education system, the opportunity arose for schools to 'opt out' of local authority control and also to include the 'consumers' on boards of governors. In transport, policies to 'deregulate' public transport were enacted and there was a renewed concentration on the construction of roads to encourage private transport. But it was in health and social care delivery that the most significant market-based and post-Fordist moves took place.

Although private and individual consumption was the target of the housing and transport reforms, this was more difficult to apply to health and social care. Therefore it was the values of the market rather than the actual *practice* of the market which were applied to the NHS after the early 1980s. Following the Griffiths Management Inquiry of 1983, the concept of managerialism entered into the rhetoric surrounding the move to 'marketise' the NHS (Newman and Clarke 1994). This new emphasis on management as a means to administer the objectives of efficiency and value for money revolutionised the status hierarchy in health care (we will look at this in more depth in the following chapter). What came into being following the reforms of 1983, 1989 and 1990 was a 'quasi-market' (LeGrand 1990; Harrison and Pollitt 1994), which was based upon essential contradictions and oppositions to a 'real' market, as illustrated in Table 3.2.

As can be seen, the values and practice of the market exist in a very uneasy juxtaposition within the quasi-market. Users are not really consumers, managers are not owners, goods are not produced and profits in the commercial market sense, are not made. But what was really of great significance was the change in the culture and sets of ideas which emanated from the market discourse.

One of the greatest changes was in the role of the state. From being the sole or main provider of health and social care, the state was to become an 'enabler' (Wistow *et al.* 1994). The division between purchasing and provision meant that in some ways the state retained power within a reconstituted system. The social

Table 3.2 Characteristics of markets and quasi-markets

Market	Quasi-market
Profit	Efficiency
Price	Contracts
Many suppliers	Few suppliers
Individual personal consumer demand	Purchasers demand for users
Unplanned – responsive to changing demand	Planned – set provision and demand
Production of goods	Setting of targets
Owners, shareholders, boards of directors	Managers, trusts, quangos
Private investment	Public expenditure

services in particular gained a new position as the lead agency of the administration of community care.

At the same time, there was a renewed emphasis on the *individual's* responsibility for their own health and well-being. The moves towards a preventive health policy had begun in 1976, but during the 1980s this gathered momentum within the individualist discourse. The Health Education Authority actively pursued the objective of getting people to look after themselves with an almost total emphasis on 'lifestyle' concerns. The move away from health care as a universal service to one which was seen as the responsibility of individuals to implement for themselves was of great significance; it has been criticised by sociologists as forming an ideology of 'healthism' (Nettleton and Bunton 1995). Nevertheless, it fundamentally altered the practice of GPs, community nurses and health visitors, who were encouraged to give advice and to 'help' people make the 'right choices' over diet, exercise, smoking and alcohol consumption as well as other forms of private and sexual behaviour. This individualisation in preventive health care was matched by the increase in the subscriptions to private health insurance companies during the 1980s (around 10 per cent of the population covered) (Webster 1993 : 129). The nineteenth-century strategy of self-help via the purchase of private insurance was reconstructed. The focus on the individual also in some circumstances reconstructed the nineteenth-century view of the cause of poverty, and the causes of certain diseases came to be defined as the fault of the person themselves. This 'victim-blaming' approach (Ashton and Seymour 1990; Davison *et al.* 1991) negated the external factors of unemployment, poverty, pollution and bad housing. In *The Health of the Nation* (DOH 1992) poverty as a cause of ill-health was rendered invisible. Although there were various reports which connected ill health to poverty and inequality (Townsend *et al.* 1988), the overwhelming health message was that of the responsibility of the individual for their own salvation.

But the responsibility of the state to protect individual children remained a fundamental issue. The interests of *the* child were placed at the centre of the Children Act 1989. This firmly asserted the centrality of 'the family', which was to be supported, and it also reinforced the gendered relationship between the state and parents, especially mothers (David, 1991). This relationship was also put into relief by the Child Support Act 1992, in which the state sought to replace the dependence of single mothers on state benefits by a reconstruction of dependence on individual men (Millar 1995). Throughout the 1980s the social security system was radically altered to target the most needy and to shift the payment of benefits from the unemployed to the working poor.

The discourse of individualism was not new to the British culture but it was the placing of it at the centre of policies which marked out the 1980s and 1990s as a specifically different period of time. It was there that the reconstruction of a social reality took place. For many who had been born, educated and socialised within a previous reality, it was a profound and radical cultural change. But alongside this centrality of the individual and the adherence to the values of the free market, the concept of 'community' was also evoked to accompany massive changes in policy.

■ Care by the community

As we have seen, moves to place care for certain groups with the outside 'community' and away from hospitals and institutions has a long history. But it was not until after 1992 with the implementation of the NHS and Community Care Act that these became a social reality. From 1985 onwards a series of reports and White Papers advocated a move to a more fragmented and mixed economy of care provision which placed the main responsibilty for care on to the community. But who were the community who were to provide this care?

The mixed economy was to be made up, as always, of the four main agencies: the state, the voluntary sector, the market and the informal grouping of families and friends. But the emphasis was firmly away from the state as a provider and upon the state as an enabler and purchaser. However, within the discourse of individualism and indeed central to it, the role of the volunteer and the voluntary sector grew in importance. We have seen how the period up until the 1980s was a time of professionalisation, and by the end of the 1970s the relationship between the voluntary sector and the more militant trade unions was cool. But volunteering became very high on the agenda of the New Right, as Margaret Thatcher stated:

> The volunteer movement is at the heart of all our social welfare provision
> ... The willingness of men and women to give service is one of freedom's
> greatest safeguards. It leaves men and women indepenedent enough to meet
> needs as they see them and not only as the state provides. (Thatcher 1981 in a
> speech to WRVS)

As Jos Sheard argues (1995), volunteering has been used to perform different roles at different crises: in the 1970s to oppose union power, and in the 1980s to protect from unemployment. (Sheard 1995). In the 1990s, with unemployment falling, the focus turned to the promotion of community values and caring and the engendering of 'active citizenship'. An appeal to disaffected youth to spend time in voluntary activity was made by Prince Charles in 1996.

According to research (Hedley and Davis Smith 1992), about 50 per cent of the population engage in some form of voluntary activity. On average volunteers spend a total of 62 million hours a week. However, volunteering remains as predominantly female, middle-aged and middle-class activity. However, we should not confuse volunteering with the voluntary sector itself, for the relationship between this and the new 'enabling' state has become far more close and yet more complex.

The institution of the 'contract culture' in the organisation of the NHS has led to a new and contradictory relationship with the state. The reduction in the role of provider has meant that social service departments may have reduced their official cooperation with the voluntary sector and replaced this with a contract relationship. This in turn has meant that many organisations have now 'professionalised' themselves and employed paid staff in administrative posts. As Diana Leat (1995) has shown, the increased role and funding which has been given to the voluntary sector by the government does not come without strings attached. The funding of organisations can come from many different sources and this fragmentation can produce a 'resource dependency' which can mitigate against the autonomous 'giving' of services. Market values have infiltrated the formerly accepted 'altruistic' world of volunteering, and evidence suggests that this is having a profound effect on the provision of services (Mocroft and Thomason 1993). The raising of funds from the public also presents problems for voluntary organisations, for their administrative costs rise the more active in fund raising they become. Therefore, by the 1990s, the charitable and voluntary sector is in a fragmented and contradictory position, involved with the market and yet outside it, relying on volunteers and yet professionalising, a service provider but within an enabling state (this is explored in depth by Robert Drake in Chapter 13); the need to manage this new type of organisation presents even more problems (Handy 1988), but in its fragmentation and contradictions the voluntary sector is indicative of the whole trend of post-Fordism.

■ Fragmentation and contradiction

The picture of the provision of health and social care to the community is rather like a child's kaleidoscope, a constantly shifting pattern of contrasting elements which are brought into close contact by a vigorous upheaval. Almost every element in the organisation and provision of care has its opposite, which is both in direct contention and at the same time operating in parallel. These oppositional elements are shown in Table 3.3.

Many of these contradictions are obvious: the discourse of individualism which posits care in the 'community', the dropping of 'National' from 'Health Service',

Table 3.3 Elements in opposition and in coexistence

Individual	Community
National	Local
Health	Social
Purchaser	Provider
Policy	Practice
Public	Private
User	Consumer
Professional autonomy	Managerial dictate
Volunteer	Paid worker
Employee	Advocate

the imposition of local pay agreements and arrangements, the splitting of health and social care within the work practice, the divisions between purchaser and provider, the new power of managers and 'consumers' in the direction of services, the contradictions within the voluntary sector. But there are contradictions also which health and social care practitioners meet in their everyday working practice: the split between official policies and actual practice, the clash of loyalties between the needs of the 'patient' and that of the employing trust or health authority, between the role of employee and autonomous professional. This is the social reality of a post-Fordist arrangement (Burrow and Corder 1994).

■ Summary

In this chapter we have followed the rise and fall of the state as the main source of provision of health and social care and also the fading of a hegemonic idea – that of welfarism. The enormity of the change of direction in policies can be seen from Tables 3.4 and 3.5, which chart the changes of greatest significance before and after the change of political administration which occurred in 1979. The increasing role of the voluntary organisations in the provision of care and as representatives of groups of users was another phenomenon of the years following 1945, as Table 3.6 illustrates.

The theoretical framework which has been used to provide an analytical understanding of these changes has been that of a post-Fordist organisation (a point to which Anne Kelly returns in Chapter 5). This shifting of care provision in the community from the site of the hospital or institution into the site of the home has also held great significance for the target of provision – those being cared for. In the next chapter we turn our attention to the groups receiving community care within a set of conditions and structures of the surrounding society.

Table 3.4 Landmarks in state provision and concern, 1945–79

1945 FAMILY ALLOWANCE ACT. Allowance for every second and subsequent child under age of 16, paid directly to mother.

1946 NATIONAL INSURANCE ACT. Contributory national insurance scheme extended to include unemployment benefit, sickness, maternity, retirement pension, widow's pension. Married women entitled to some benefits through husband's contribution.

1946 NATIONAL HEALTH SERVICE ACT. Free and universal access to medical care at point of need. Organised under three national services: general practice, local health authorities (district nurses, health visitors), hospital services. Mental Welfare departments for the education and training and supervision of mentally ill and handicapped people in residential homes.

1948 NATIONAL ASSISTANCE ACT. Complementary provision for those not adequately covered by National Insurance. Means-tested benefits to 'top up' universal provision.

1949 HOUSING ACT. Local authority housing provision for all those in need.

1953 Guillebaud Report – investigates increasing costs of NHS and recommends more 'care in the community'.

1954 Bradbeer Report – highlights conflict between professional groups in NHS as 'detrimental' to efficiency.

1962 Local authorities develop meals-on-wheels service.

1964 Housing Corporation founded to fund and monitor housing associations.

1965 RENT ACT. Principle of 'fair rent' for private tenancies introduced with claimants able to take case to rent tribunals.

1968 Seebohm Report – recommends setting up of social services departments – amalgamation of all previous services to specific groups.

1970 LOCAL AUTHORITY SOCIAL SERVICES ACT. Creates social services departments. Home help service moves into social services.

1970 DIVORCE REFORM ACT. 'Liberalises' divorce by eradicating the concept of 'guilt' and substituting the 'irretrievable breakdown of marriage'. Divorce rate doubles in first year.

1971 SOCIAL SECURITY ACT. Introduction of Family Income Supplement (FIS) to target low-paid working families.

1974 NATIONAL HEALTH SERVICE REORGANISATION ACT. Creates regional health authorities, area health authorities and district Management teams. District nursing and health visiting sited in general practices. Medical-social workers transferred to social services. Community health councils set up.

1977 HOUSING (HOMELESS PERSONS) ACT. Defines statutory homelessness and gives priority to vulnerable groups and those with dependent children. Local authorities have responsibility to provide for homeless in area.

1979 Royal Commission on NHS – rejects feasibility of transferring responsibility from central to local government. Endorsement of existing system of hospital-based care.

1979 The Black Report on health inequalities commissioned.

Table 3.5 Landmarks in voluntary provision, 1945–96

1946	Help the Aged founded.
1946	Mencap founded.
1946	Mind founded.
1951	National Council for Civil Liberties. To campaign on behalf of people 'wrongfully detained' in mental institutions.
1955	Spastics Society founded – renamed SCOPE in 1994.
1959	National Council for Single Women and Elderly Dependants founded.
1964	Shelter founded to campaign for the homeless.
1965	Child Poverty Action Group founded.
1972	National Schizophrenic Fellowship founded.
1972	'Our Life' – the first National Conference for people with learning difficulties held.
1973	National Council for One-Parent Families (formerly Council for Unmarried Mother and Child).
1974	Disability Alliance founded.
1975	Cancer Relief – builds first of its own cancer units. First MacMillan nursing teams established to deliver care in patents' own homes.
1977	Wolfenden Report on the future of the voluntary sector.
1981	'Opportunities for Volunteering' administered by the DHSS and a 'Voluntary Projects' programme administered by Manpower Commission.
1986	SANE founded – following concern over release of 'ill and dangerous schizophrenia sufferers' and publicised incidents. Campaigns for extension of hospital beds.
1986	Survivors Speak Out – organisation formed by people who have been recipients of mental health treatment.
1988	National Association of Carers (formerly National Council for Single Women and Elderly Dependants).
1992	Home Office Paper – *The Individual and the Community – The Role of the Voluntary Sector*; recommends the encouragement to be given to volunteering.
1992	Home Office Paper – *Efficiency and Scrutiny of Government Funding of the Voluntary Sector*; recommends that contracts be awarded to those organisations which use volunteers.
1993	Rowntree Foundation convenes a nationwide 'Inquiry into Income and Wealth'; recommends changes in policies and practice to combat increasing poverty.
1993	Rowntree Foundation publishes *Life on a Low Income*, a report on the extent and causes of poverty in Britain; one-third of population is estimated to be living below poverty line.

Table 3.6 Landmarks in state provision, 1979–96

1980	HOUSING ACT. 'Right to Buy' legislation. Statutory duty of local authorities to sell council houses to tenants at discounted prices.
1982	NATIONAL HEALTH SERVICE ACT. District health authorities replace area health authorities – less representation from local authorities. Hospital 'hotel' services to be offered to competitive contract tendering.
1983	NHS Management Inquiry – led by Sir Roy Griffths who recommends a new style of management – that of general manager – to replace teams.
1985	Large-scale voluntary transfer – allows housing departments of local authorities to transfer responsibility for social housing to housing associations.
1985	Select Committee Report *Community Care* calls for government action to move care away from local authority provision and hospitals to be placed 'in the community'.
1986	SOCIAL SECURITY ACT. Supplementary Benefit replaced by Income Support. Social Fund created with loans in place of grants. Benefits removed from 16–18-year-olds living at home.
1986	Audit Commission Report – *Making A Reality of Community Care*.
1988	*Community Care – An Agenda For Action* (Griffiths Report) – recommends a leading role for local authorities in the arrangement and funding of community care.
1988	Acheson Report – reformed role for public health medicine. Public health doctors to be the 'objective advisers' on needs of localities to potential purchasers.
1989	*Working for Patients* – split between purchasing and providing functions. Setting up of trusts and GP fundholding.
1990	NHS AND COMMUNITY CARE ACT. Local authorities to have responsibility to manage care but not to provide it – a purchasing role. Formal mixed economy of care of statutory voluntary private and informal care. Implementation to be over 3 years. No extra funds available.
1990	CHILD SUPPORT ACT. The 'absent parent' to be reassessed for contribution to maintenance of children from previous marriage or relationship. Collected by Child Support Agency – retrospective and payments go to offset Treasury expenditure.
1992	First plans for community care published. Many do not include housing. Nearly all new social housing now built by housing associations.
1992	*Health of the Nation* – stresses importance of individual responsibility for health. Sets 'health gain targets' to be achieved by health care practitioners.
1992	Patient's Charter – sets guidelines for waiting times, referrals and access to GP of choice.
1994	Audit Commission Report, *Taking Stock – Progress with Community Care*, states that resources are stretched and some local authorities are running out of funds.
1995	CARERS RECOGNITION AND SERVICES ACT. Entitles those providing in excess of 20 hours a week care to an assessment of need.
1995	Housing Benefit reduced for single people living alone.

Chapter 4

Care for the community: inmates, patients, consumers and citizens

Anthea Symonds

■ Introduction

This chapter is concerned with an analysis of the social construction and changing relationship between the state and providers of care and the groups who are the 'cared-for' in and by the community. We began this part with a model of the sites of provision of care (see Introduction), and within this model the identity of those who comprise the 'cared-for' was suggested as being that of either the 'unproductive' or the 'productive'. This definition will now be looked at in more depth. The delivery of community care to defined groups takes place within a set of cultural beliefs, an economic structure and a changing society.

Table 4.1 Social reality and delivery of community care

Social reality			
Macro-structures			
	Economy		Culture
Micro-structures			
Employment	Housing	Families	Poverty
Delivery of community care			
Provision			
Health/Social care			
Receipt			
Unproductive/Productive groups			
Objective of care			
Reactive/Preventive			
Assessment			
Needs/Finance			

The social reality of community care is that it is delivered into a society which is fragmented by class and ethnicity, wealth and poverty, age and gender, health and illness, ability and disability. The taken-for-granted assumptions on the structure of families, on security of employment, access to housing and education, rights to health and social care are all being challenged. This fragmentation has led to the creation of many 'communities' within the same locality and the divisions within society are probably wider now than at any time since the last century.

Within this framework, people's ideas and beliefs have also been challenged and changed, and the relationship between the dependent groups and the providers of care has been reconstituted. The individualistic nature of policies from the 1980s has meant that the focus has been turned away from 'community' and onto individual consumers or 'citizens'. The difficulty of perceiving this shift has been further exacerbated by the constant *use* of phrases like 'community' and 'citizen', when the reality is that the very foundations which produce real community or citizenship have been eroded.

In order to really get to grips with this contradiction we need to trace the social construction of dependency of the targeted populations and then to place the delivery of care within the social reality of Britain today. Next, we address the social reality of community care as it is perceived within our culture and within the everyday practice of delivery and administration. Finally, we will look at the nature of the changing relationship between the recipients of care and the providers and at the contradictions within which practitioners are attempting to deliver care.

■ Social construction of dependency

In order to understand this concept we need to differentiate between types of dependency – economic, physical and mental – and also to look at how this dependent relationship has been constructed by society itself. If we take as the main target groups for community care those who are in some way or another 'dependent' upon others for support – children in need, the frail elderly, people with mental illness, or those with physical or mental difficulties – we can see a connection between economic and physical dependence. All of these groups are likely contain a majority of those who are also poor. The very categories of 'at risk' or 'vulnerable' carry with them connotations of economic dependency. All of these groups are also excluded from the productive labour force through either age or disability. The economic circumstances of people deemed to be 'in need' are of course taken into consideration when assessments for the delivery of care packages are conducted. Increasingly, those not economically dependent upon the state for income are expected to purchase care on the market; this is especially true of many older people with property and savings. The recourse to forms of institutional care as an alternative to family-based care was a feature of the 1980s, when the private residential and nursing home sector proliferated especially for the 'frail elderly'. Much of this was funded by the state, although the actual provision was undertaken by the market.

Historically, however, the construction of physical dependency upon one or more of the other agencies of provision (the state, family, voluntary organisations) for specific groups of children, older people, those with mental or physical ill health or handicap has been based upon their poverty. Orphaned children of the rich were not institutionalised, the wealthy 'mad' or disabled were either treated privately or cared for by servants, wealthy older people gained power and influence through the dispensation of their money to relatives. The institutionalisation of groups of people in the nineteenth century was based upon their economic powerlessness.

But this solution was practised only when care by the family had, in some sense, failed or did not exist. Initially it was orphaned children who could not be cared for by their families who received the intervention of the state. The care of elderly frail and 'unproductive' people was seen by legislators as the responsibility of sons and daughters; there were no pensions paid until 1905, no concept of retirement; if a family could not care for them then institutionalisation was the only recourse. Workhouses and asylums remained under local lay control and began to grow at an alarming rate from the middle of the century as more and more people became 'eligible' for entry.

Family care is, of course, a subject which is 'hidden' from empirical research. The numbers of people being cared for by their family has always been unknown. The private world of home and family as the site of care is only revealed by oral histories and personal biography. It is when this care is not available or is seen as unsuitable or inadequate that either charity workers or the newly formed state providers have intervened. In other words it was the 'absence' of informal care which constructed the 'presence' of formal and quasi-formal mechanisms.

The two extremes of the age continuum, childhood and old age, have been the most common reasons for dependency, with other anomalies such as mental illness and disability occurring in far smaller numbers. But children and older people are only classified as dependent either economically or physically if family care is not available or is inadequate. John Baldock (1993) has perceptively argued that the way in which old age is now seen by policy-makers is a mirror image of the way in which children became a focus of attention a hundred years ago. Then in a period of a declining birth rate and high infant mortality, it was the period of childhood which was being extended. Today it is old age which is extended with the population as a whole becoming older. The protection of children and the care of the elderly are both results of a negotiation between the state and the family. The dependency of either group is at the same time a social construct and a social reality. Children are relatively dependent upon adults both economically and physically and the dependence of older people is a mirror image. But the degree of dependence of both groups has been the result of social policies and social divisions. The length and degree of childhood dependency has grown during the last hundred years and is currently undergoing even more change.

■ Children and dependency

Many writers (Aries 1962; Donzelot 1980) have chronicled the historical change in the way in which children have been regarded by society and the role of the state in child surveillance and protection. 'Childhood' in the sense of being identified with a specific length of time, of a set of expectations of behaviour and even of dress and appearance, has always been a social construct. The legal system has defined the actual age of 'adult responsibility' and this has changed over the past hundred years. Education Acts and employment regulations, as well as the legal setting of the 'coming of age', have had the effect of lengthening the official time of childhood. Although to many people today children may appear 'precocious' in their dress, interests and behaviour, compared with nineteenth-century children (especially those of the working class) children today are remarkably 'free' from adult responsibilities and duties but at the same time have become more 'dependent' upon adult care and protection. They are not expected to earn their own living or to keep themselves before the age of 18, but this also means that they are not eligible for benefits or adult wages either. By contrast, as Anna Davin (1996) has illustrated, children in the last century were 'little workers or 'little mothers' by the time they were eight years old. The twin concerns of the care and protection of children have become a prime concern of the state in the twentieth century.

As we have seen, for most of the nineteenth century, the social care of children was met by voluntary organisations such as Barnardo's and National Children's Homes, both of which were founded during the latter decades of the century. The welfare of pauper children however came under the auspices of the state from the Poor Law in 1834. Children were placed into workhouses with other groups and their education, like that of the working class generally, was fragmented and dependent upon the vagaries of local boards of guardians. As the eugenicist concerns grew, so did the focus upon the state's responsibility for such children.

What happened during this period was that the state began to forge a direct relationship with children as objects of care. Total parental authority had been progressively weakened by legislation regarding the care and protection of children. But it was the care and responsibility for 'state' children without families which was the basis of both charitable and public concern. It was this concern which prompted home inspections of 'boarded out' children, fostered children and then working-class homes. The eugenicist concern over 'quality' led to a focusing not just on orphaned children but on 'deprived' ones too. The nineteenth-century concern over the individual responsibility for one's own destiny, however, mitigated against the state taking a direct role in the care and protection of children, because this was seen as a 'private' responsibility of individual families. It could be argued that children as potentially productive citizens were most likely to be defined as 'deserving' and therefore in need of beneficial state intervention.

The protection of children became a concern of the state from the end of the nineteenth century. Children, it was deemed, needed protection from both themselves and their own natures and also from predatory adults. The abuse of children began to be a public issue from the end of the nineteenth century and Gordon (1989) argues that it is at periods when feminism is strongest (1890s, 1960s, 1980s) that concern over the abuse of children is placed on the political agenda.

The directing of state provision towards the young continued throughout the inter-war years. The health of schoolchildren was monitored via regular school inspections, and the provision of school meals for the 'needy' increased. It was, of course, mainly the working-class family, and especially the mother, who was the subject of reconstruction via education, middle-class families and mothers were not seen as a 'problem' (it must be remembered that health visitors did not visit universally until after 1945: they did not enter workhouses, or apply for charity or benefits, and they remained separate from state and voluntary supply except as suppliers themselves. Access to medical and nursing care was purchased on a market basis, as was education, housing and services.

In Britain in 1996, with a falling birth rate, children have become the focus of legislation and policies, and of media concerns. Children are now relatively rare and as such occupy a high value in society. But this value contains contradictions; children are seen at the same time both as prized possessions and (also as innocent and potential victims) and as the source of disorder and their behaviour as evidence of declining standards.

The care and protection of children by the state is initially undertaken via the parents and family. Child surveillance by health professionals is carried out with the nominal cooperation of parents ('good' parents have their children immunised), and the responsibility to detect and help 'children in need' within their families is one of the basic tenets of the Children Act (see Chapter 17 by Colton *et al.*). It is when this family structure breaks down or is seen as inadequate that children become overtly dependent upon the state, rather in the manner of elderly people. The current emphasis on keeping a child within the family whenever possible, which is an objective of the Children Act, is strongly reminiscent of the community care objective of enabling older people to remain in their own homes: in both cases the dependency of both children and older people is counteracted by a policy objective of giving them a nominal independence from the fixed site of institutional care. For both groups also, the site of such care because of its hidden and private nature can be a source of danger and abuse, as recent exposures on some children's homes have illustrated. In a sense, both children and older people are perceived as being 'outsiders' to mainstream society – they are special in that they are not 'productive', but they either are seen to have the potential to be so or else are deemed to have 'earned' their place by past productive activity.

■ Older people's dependency

Chris Phillipson (1982) has argued that 'old age' (like childhood) is itself a construct, and that within a capitalist economy becoming old means that a person becomes economically redundant and poorer. The idea of retirement is of course a relatively modern one; even before the Second World War it was relatively unknown for many to retire. The average life expectancy of a man in 1930 was less than 60 years, and for a woman less than 65 years. But increasing longevity has meant for some, especially for many women and working-class people, increasing poverty. Alan Walker (1980) has argued that it was the result of social policies which artificially removed people from the work force after a certain age and which consequently constructed their dependence. As we have seen, the post-war welfare state provided a subsistence level of income for older people in retirement, but this provision was enacted within existing 'social divisions of welfare' (Titmuss 1963). In other words, all the social and economic inequalities which exist in childhood and throughout one's working life persist into old age. 'The elderly' are no more a homogeneous mass than are children or any other group. The poor at any age are more vulnerable to ill health and disability, and the inequalities experienced by women and ethnic minorities will still be present in old age.

Women are more likely to be represented among the 'frail elderly poor' because they have a longer life expectancy but more likelihood of morbidity, they are less likely to have occupational pensions or private health insurance and they are more likely to be widowed and live alone. The likelihood of living alone increases with age, and of those over 80 the highest proportion will be women living alone. As we have seen from earlier chapters, women's economic dependency has also been constructed via social policies and unpaid family commitments and has been accompanied by exclusion from the full-time, well-paid labour force. The exclusion of many people in ethnic minorities has also followed this pattern and is continued into old age (Blakemore and Boneham 1994; see also Ken Blakemore's Chapter 20). This 'structured' dependency has meant that old age or retirement for men and for women is often a very different experience. Many women do not retire from paid work, but continue to perform unpaid work within the home until a very old age. The role of grandmothers in child care, for instance, is one which has grown in recent years as more younger mothers go out to work (Martin and Roberts 1984). The social networks which men and women have built up during their lives will also have an effect on the experience of ageing. When men stop work they often lose their identity together with their workmates and indeed their whole way of life, and can feel a sense of alienation within the unfamiliar setting of the home.

Not *all* older people are 'dependent' either physically or economically, however. Writers such as Peter Laslett (1989) have drawn a much more optimistic and positive picture of the 'third age' as one of freedom and opportunity. Chris Hamnett (1991) has described the increase in power which many older people experience on the basis of their economic wealth derived from house ownership and investments, though this ownership of property can lead to a situation of being 'house rich and cash poor'. There are whole new markets opening to cater for the wealthy retired – specialist travel operations, holidays, housing complexes, leisure activities and even fashion and cosmetic retailing. Many voluntary organisations rely on the contribution of older people to provide services – often for other older people. A recent study of EU countries showed that on average two out of three older people are 'active citizens' engaged in voluntary and caring work, with only 5 per cent requiring residential care (Family Policies Studies Centre 1993). Nevertheless, the extension of the period of old age has increased the likelihood that more health and social care will be required for some, though, as we will discuss later in this chapter, the cultural attitude of the future elderly may be very different from that of previous generations.

■ The outsiders – dependency and fear

However, the group of people who have always been the subject of care in and by the community have been those with mental health problems or with a mental or physical handicap. It was this group, who used to be referred to as 'idiots', 'imbeciles', 'cretins' or 'mentally defectives', who first initiated the response of institutionalisation. Foucault (1967) has argued that the 'mad' have always been the subject of fear and have often undergone horrendous suffering. But it was not until the early nineteenth century that the actual definition of 'madness' as a disease which could be cured in the right setting and with treatment gained a measure of support. The first asylums were set up for two purposes: to protect society from the mad and to protect the mad from society. The classification of madness into two main forms, melancholia and brain fever, originated with Hippocrates in ancient Greece and much of the original classification remains in that used by the accepted diagnostic standard with added variations.

Sociologists and social pyschologists have been concerned with not only the treatment of mental illness but also how it is diagnosed and the nature of its social meaning. The 'social constructionist' view of mental illness has been vividly articulated by Thomas Szasz (1970). He argues that mental illness is a 'myth' and that people labelled mentally ill are those whose behaviour does not conform to the norms of mainstream society. Institutionalisation, he maintains, merely makes their condition worse and is a violation of human rights. Other writers such as R. D. Laing (1971) have argued that mental illness can be seen as a response to societal pressures which are brought to bear on individuals. These pressures are most notable within a family, and indeed, argues Laing, it is the modern form of claustrophobic nuclear family which has prompted many to 'opt' out and into mental illness as a form of escape.

The person of the 'deviant' has been viewed by sociologists such as Durkheim to be essential to the maintenance of social order. When society can identify and isolate those who are 'outside', then the norms and values of mainstream society can be preserved. The function of asylums, it has been argued, was not to 'cure' the mad but to present them as an example to the 'sane'. The building of asylums in the late nineteenth century seemed to serve this purpose – they were sited just outside a town, usually on a hill and were not easily accessible. Thus they stood above the population as a warning and a threat (compare Enoch Powell's description, quoted in the previous chapter). Joan Busfield has argued that the asylums were for the purpose of incarceration or 'warehousing' rather than treatment (Busfield 1986).

The other topic of interest to sociologists has been: who are most likely to be diagnosed as mentally ill, and why? In some societies political opposition has been defined as evidence of mental illness. When we look at the social facts of mental illness there are some striking factors. The mentally ill person is more likely to be female if white and male if black. Apart from greater male vulnerability to drug and alcohol dependency and schizophrenia, most forms of mental illness, especially depression, are far more prevalent in women. Many more women than men are hospitalised and although the higher numbers of elderly women in the population and the incidence of post-natal depression must have some effect on the figures they do not wholly explain why women seem more prone to mental illness than men. There have been many sociological explanations offered; Pilgrim and Rogers (1993) argue that women are more likely to consult a doctor because of emotional stress, and feminist writers (Ehrenreich and English 1973; Chesler 1972; Busfield 1992) put forward the view that women are more likely to labelled as mentally unstable by a patriarchal male psychiatric establishment.

These perspectives are also applied to explanations of the greater reported incidence of hospital admissions for mental illness among the 'black' ethnic groups. Even after allowing for inadequacies in data collection, the overwhelming picture is one of the over-representation of Afro-Caribbean and South Asian people, especially males, in hospitalisation. Afro-Carribean males are five times more likely and Asian males three times more likely to be diagnosed as schizophrenic than are whites (Bhat *et al.* 1988). Afro-Caribbeans are also more likely to be labelled aggressive and to be subject to a sectioning order (ibid.). The division in sociological debate to explain these phenomena turns on whether the identification of mental illness among women and ethnic minorities is a social construction by male white professionals or whether these groups do in fact suffer more mental health problems because of the discrimination they face in their lives. Both explanations however are based upon societal and not individual causes. For instance, the mental health problems of older people have long been accepted, so that 'going a bit funny' and 'getting forgetful' were common expressions, but in recent years the classification of Alzheimer's disease has become much more used and misused.

How can we explain this increase in rates of mental illness? Talking of the growing crisis in the services for mentally ill people, the Department of Health revealed that in the five years from 1990 to 1995 the number of those formally admitted to mental hospitals rose by 55 per cent and the number of informal admissions rose by 29 per cent. Is mental illness on the increase or has the classification of what constitutes mental illness become wider so that more and more people are diagnosed? MIND recently published figures on the growth in mental distress, with six times as many people being referred to specialist psychiatric services than fifty years ago, a 65 per cent increase in 'first-time' admissions, and with men and young people increasing in hospital admissions (MIND 1996). Interestingly, MIND suggests that social issues such as unemployment, homelessness and loneliness are correlated with this increase. In other words, mental illness is a social construct but very much a reality.

The difference between mental illness and mental handicap was not officially recognised in either legislation or services until the twentieth century (1913 Act). Even then, many people who had physical handicaps such as deafness or blindness were designated as 'mentally handicapped'. Conditions such as cerebral palsy and Down's syndrome have in recent years undergone a more positive and sympathetic description. The previous stigmatising in labels such as 'spastic' and 'mongol' have virtually disappeared from medical language, if not entirely from public use.

Learning difficulty (as it is now rather euphemistically termed) attracts much more public sympathy, especially in children, than do mental distress and illness. In a sense, these conditions are now seen as 'undeserved' and therefore do not attract blame or fear as mental illness among adults does. This was not always so, for often a child who was born with a genetic condition was seen as 'evidence' of parental sin such as incest or venereal disease. To a sociologist, even conditions such as Down's syndrome and spina bifida have social class connotations. Down's syndrome, for example, tends to be more prevalent among the wealthier middle classes, possibly because the mothers are older (although there is current theory initiated by the geneticist Steve Jones that it is the age of the father which is most significant), while spina bifida is more associated with working-class babies due to its connection with the inadequate diet of a mother during pregnancy. So although learning difficulty may appear to be a random phenomenon which is manifest at birth among a small proportion, a sociological perspective would seek to dispel the randomness and to look for social reasons for its occurrence among specific groups.

People with physical disabilities have in recent years become much more assertive and demanding of full citizenship rights. The marginalisation of disabled people which took place has been recognised by many writers as the result not of the disability itself but of the disabling nature of society (Oliver 1990, 1996; Drake 1996). Their argument is that it is the restricting nature of society in employment policies, buildings and the environment which has rendered people with disabilities 'disabled'. This is another example of a social construction – the response of majority groups to the situation of a minority. The physical condition may not have been caused by society directly but the resulting disability experienced is a result of society's actions.

I have argued so far that those groups which are the subject of care in and by the community have been socially constructed, though this is not to deny or negate the actual reality of some infirmities in older age, the vulnerability of children or the actuality of mental illness or disability, but to place such phenomena within a societal context. A social construction is still a social reality. Before industrialisation, not only children and elderly people but also those with mental illness and disabilities lived in their families or communities, and worked or fulfilled roles as their capabilities allowed. The establishment of asylums and workhouses in the nineteenth century progressively removed whole groups from the mainstream of society. The increase in the intervention of the state, especially in the care and protection of children, meant that being removed and placed 'in care' was the most common solution to children in need. In the 1990s, the decanting of the institutions and long-stay hospitals has meant that once more they are placed in the community. But 'community care' in this respect cannot be construed as a return to traditional values. The whole nature of late-twentieth-century society is different; the role of women has undergone a transformation in both the private world of the family and the public world of work, the basis of the economy is different, the expectations of children and elderly people have expanded, and the nature of the labour market means that disabled people are more marginalised. But there is one aspect of modern Britain which the early Victorians would recognise; the extent of poverty and the preponderance of these groups among the poor.

■ Poverty and the 'underclass' debate

It is significant that during the 1980s two discourses ran in parallel: the dependent underclass debate and community care. For at the same time as health policies shifted towards the placing of care into the 'community' so the very nature of the community itself was the subject of a moral panic about the reality of a dependency culture and the creation of an urban underclass. Based upon the writings of the American social scientist, Charles Murray (1990), the concept of an amoral and feral underclass created by the benefit system and inhabiting 'no-go' areas of inner cities entered into the political arena.

During the 1980s, various riots on forgotten and deprived estates, the use of many of the roads on such estates as racetracks for stolen cars and battles with the police, the preponderance of young single mothers, aggressive beggars and the sight of the homeless camped out on the streets, drug wars, and the publicity surrounding the horrific murder of James Bulger in Liverpool all seemed to coalesce in an apocalyptic vision of decay.

The breakdown of the 'traditional' family and the connection between single mothers and the delinquency of their children brought up without a father as role model also attracted the attention of sociologists (Dennis and Erdos 1993). The crisis of the inner cities, which had suffered increasing unemployment, lack of investment and deprivation, became a metaphor for 'Britain in crisis'. Ironically, it was into this Britain that care in the community was to be placed; the desire of people to 'remain in their own homes' was set against the reality that 'home' for many had became an unpleasant and threatening place. Poverty has increased and the division between the relatively affluent and the poor is as wide in 1997 as it was a hundred years ago, though the actual picture of poverty is a more complex one.

Primarily, it must be remembered that 'the poor' are not an underclass. In the debate the underclass has tended to be identified in *cultural* terms. The members of the underclass are seen primarily as lacking the values and beliefs of mainstream society – they do not wish to have a job, get an education, bring up children, live in reasonable housing or conform to any of the norms of the 'majority'. Although this definition has been challenged by others (Mann 1992), who maintain that there is no underclass as such, merely poor people who desire to conform but are restrained from doing so by lack of opportunity, ill health and disability, and lack of education and social support, the idea still persists that there is a stratum of British society which while it exists entirely on benefits is a 'class apart' and is excluded from citizenship (Morris 1994). We will return to this point later in this chapter.

The description of British society which has become much used recently is that of the 30/30/40 society described by Hutton (1995). He defines the groups as: the bottom 30 per cent who are living below the official poverty line and are reliant on state benefits for support, the next 30 per cent who are in low paid and part-time work with increasing insecurity and who are reliant on benefits to 'top up' income levels, and the top 40 per cent who are in relatively well-paid and secure employment.

The division between the highest paid and the lowest also increased during the 1980s. There has been a growth in total inequality and this has been divided on geographical as well as social lines. A recent survey conducted on the Rowntree Foundation (Goodman & Webb 1994) showed that the number of people living in households with below *half* the national average income rose from around 3 million in the mid-1970s to more than 11 million (1 in 5 of the population) by 1991. A regional analysis shows that the gap between the South of England and the rest of the country in living standards also increased in the 1980s. The 'quiet growth in poverty', as the Low Pay Unit has described it (1995), can be illustrated by Table 4.2.

As can be seen, it is the wage of the 'male breadwinner' which has fallen most dramatically. Women still, in 1996, earned less than three-quarters as much as

Table 4.2 Number and proportion of employees with gross earnings below the Council of Europe decency threshold 1995

	1979		1995	
	Million	%	Million	%
Full-time				
Women	3.00	57.6	2.69	49.0
Men	1.64	14.6	2.83	30.4
Part-time				
Women	2.99	79.0	3.63	75.9
Men	0.17	62.2	0.79	67.2

Source: Adapted from Low Pay Unit (1995).

men, especially as the majority of women workers are concentrated in the low-paid, no-security-or-benefits and part-time sector of employment. The much heralded 'genderquake' in male and female employment which has seen a growth in female and a decline in male employment has been constructed via the concentration of women workers into this sector. But low wages are not evenly spread throughout the country; London and the South-East have the highest rates of pay, with the North and Wales receiving the lowest. Indeed in Wales and the North of England over 44 per cent of all full-time employees earn less than the European decency threshold (Low Pay Unit 1995). Unemployment has a special significance for families in Britain; unlike other European countries it tends to be concentrated in households where all the members are unemployed. In 1993, households where no one had a job reached 20 per cent of the total and those where both adults were working was over 60 per cent (Gregg and Wadsworth 1994). Britain is therefore divided into 'work-rich and work-poor' households. But it must be remembered that even among the 'work-rich' it may require two adult wages to keep the family in the middle 30 per cent of the population.

This extent of poverty obviously has significance for the implementation of policies of community care (Mark Drakeford pursues this theme in depth in Chapter 16). In order to claim Family Credit as a 'top-up' for low wages, people must be in work, so that this mitigates against many giving up a job to care for a dependent relative. 'Community care' grants are available as an 'exceptional' payment to help individuals moving out of institutions and for families under pressure, although these are only available to those on Income Support. However, the single homeless, those with mental health problems, and the disabled often find this very difficult to claim (Bines 1994; Grant 1995). Homelessness has a direct connection to a history of institutionalisation: in 1995 half of single homeless people in hostels and seven out of ten of those sleeping rough had been in one type of institutional care (Kempson 1996). The decline in the amount of Local Authority on subsidised social housing built during the 1980s and the lack of repairs and maintenance to existing estates has rendered this type of housing, once of good-quality, as very much the 'last resort' for many.

Poverty, and its attendant disadvantages in terms of lack of housing, can be interpreted differently by people in inner-city and rural areas who objectively share many of the same conditions. A recent survey illustrates that people living in a small village in Scotland saw advantages in their lives compared with life in nearby Dundee even if they were just as poverty-stricken. The village where 'we never lock a door here' was compared with an inner-city estate twenty miles away; 'The area is not a good one to raise children. Kids start fires and race cars up and down...it's a rough estate' (Kempson 1996:62). The village, on the surface, appears to be an ideal setting for care in and by the community and to match up to the idealised conception which was discussed in Chapter 1; however, it had its problems: no public transport, no affordable housing, very few amenities including shops and presumably considerable remoteness for the delivery of care.

Figure 4.1 Percentage of weekly household income from salaries, benefits and pensions, 1965 and 1995

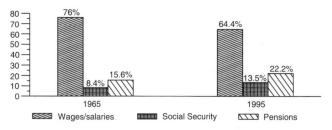

Source: Central Statistical Office

Britain, in the latter years of the 1990s, is a society in which dependency upon social security and other payments has increased and reliance on a wage or salary has decreased. This is both a reflection of an ageing society and also one in which employment, even if achieved, often carries a low wage, as Figure 4.1 shows. This growth in dependency upon state benefits runs counter to the belief, behind the reforms in the health service and other sectors, that market forces have produced a new relationship between the users and providers of services.

■ Consumerism and empowerment

There has been a wealth of discussion on the change in the *organisational* culture which the Health Service reforms have engendered (Strong and Robinson 1990; Walby and Greenwell 1994; Lewis and Glennerster 1996), and this is the subject of the following section. But have the reforms also initiated a changed relationship between the providers of services and the users? The aim of implementing an internal market into the Health Service was to change the nature of this relationship from one of 'passive client' to 'active consumer' (Saunders 1990). This has always been a focus of opposition from socialist writers (Plant 1990; Bartlett and LeGrand 1993), who have argued that the concept of 'choice' in welfare services is a flawed one given that the economic power which underlies true market choice is often missing. In the new rhetoric, the identification of a 'patient' as a 'consumer' is assumed to be unproblematic, but this is a change (if real) of enormous magnitude, because it alters the relationship between provider and user, as Table 4.3 illustrates.

Table 4.3 Dialectical relationships in care provision

Professional	Client or patient
Producer	Consumer
Seller	Buyer/purchaser
Provider	User
State	Citizen

The traditional relationship existing in the National Health Service between the professional and the patient, was, as the terminology suggests, one of the exercise of power in a downward flow. The role of the patient was to be compliant and obey orders and the role of the professional was to take responsibility for their decisions as they 'knew best'.

This alters radically with the creation of the title of 'consumer', however. A consumer holds the power; they can decide to take their custom elsewhere and it is the role of the producer to satisfy their demands. But is this a viable model in a welfare service, especially one which involves the delivery of health or social care? (Part II is concerned with this debate). As we have seen, those most likely to be in receipt of community-based care are the most socially and economically vulnerable and powerless. This point is thrown into even sharper relief by the rhetorical move in community care services from a *supply-led* service to a *user-led* service. In this construction, the users are both the person themselves and their primary carer, who according to the community care proposals must be consulted on the assessment of needs and provision of services (Department of Health 1989). The 'users' must not, in this instance, be confused with 'purchasers or consumers', who are the social services, GP fundholders, local health authorities or commissioners – those who actually purchase the services on the behalf of the users. This fragmentation of rights and responsibilities involved in the production and delivery of care has been defined by Fiona Williams (1994) as the introduction of post-Fordism into the social relations of care delivery and receipt.

The next point to take into consideration in this complex, almost Byzantine maze is that the demands of the users are controlled by a number of factors: knowledge of what services are available, the ability to articulate demands, the financial restrictions placed on the delivery of services. The 'empowerment' of such users would theoretically increase the level of demand for existing services and/or the demand for a range of alternative services and/or finance. For social care and community health care managers surely there must be an imperative *not* to empower, because this may place demands upon a system already under strain. The other change in the rhetoric which the move to a primary health and community-based care system evoked was that of a *needs-led* service. There are two problems to be addressed when implementing this shift in organisational direction: first, the question of how 'need' is determined, and by whom, and second, how to integrate an assessment of 'need' with a 'user-led' service, for in reality these two concepts are in opposition. The assessment of 'need' is undertaken by a professional (Lewis and Glennerster 1996), who has to make this assessment in the light of the services available: 'assessment must remain rooted in the appreciation of the realities of service provision' (Cheetham 1993). What happens if the individual user defines their needs differently? The question of the taxonomy of need is one which has been written on most clearly by Jonathan Bradshaw (1972), in which the differing levels of need identification can be clearly seen. But given a situation of financial restrictions, does a needs assessment take the form of targeting or setting up a 'hierarchy of needs'? The problem with this approach is that by targeting those in greatest need, those whose needs are just being met, thus enabling them to exist in a nominally 'independent' way, may find that that services are withdrawn so that they too 'fall' into the greatest need category (Kempson 1996).

■ Citizen consumers

There is one further point to be discussed; that of the match between citizenship and consumerism. The concept of citizenship is a relatively new one to the British political scene. Historically, it has always been connected with ideas of the 'rights of the free-born English*man*', and of a sense of a belonging to a nation state by virtue of birth or adoption. The address of 'man' is not an historical accident, for as Ruth Lister points out, women's economic dependency, which exists until the present day, fundamentally alters their claim to full citizenship rights (Lister, 1991). In the post-war welfare state, the idea gained a new currency with the extension of universal benefits and rights to health care, education and social security. The most famous articulation of the rights of citizenship and the relationship a nominal equality of citizens within an unequal class society was that of T. H. Marshall (1950). Marshall argued that the three dimensions of citizenship – civil, political and social – had been achieved in a chronological although uneven development. Citizenship therefore could coexist with social class inequality, in fact it could in a sense justify inequality. As long as a person retained their civil rights then any other aspect of their lives within which great inequalities existed could be negated as part of a democratic society.

In the 1990s in Britain we have witnessed the revival of ideas of citizenship. The Citizen's Charter and its corollary the Patient's Charter (note the terminology) have set out a list of standards which citizens are entitled to expect from public services. This in turn has led, so anecdotal and research evidence suggests, to an increase in people's expectations and demands of a service, an increase in complaints and a readiness to resort to litigation if citizens' demands and rights are not met. This 'Americanisation' of British social attitudes has affected the consciousness and behaviour of some user groups. In 1996, representatives of Elderly and disabled people challenged in the Appeal Court the cutbacks made by two cash-strapped local councils in the home help services previously provided; the rights of the citizen were placed above the ability of councils to provide services. The subsequent judgement however found against the plaintiffs, the so-called 'Gloucester judgement' in 1996 upheld the right of local Authorities to cease services if resources were not available.'

The complexities of a system in which some people get services free, while others have to pay towards them and others still have to pay the entire cost, and the extension of a culture of consumerism to users who pay for care services, have been extensively researched (Baldock and Ungerson 1994).

The relationship between citizenship and consumerism, between rights and duties, between protection and freedom is a complex and often contradictory one. An intellectual enthusiast of the right philosophy, sociologist Peter Saunders

(1993) admits however that they are contradictions; there is a problem in equating the principles of the economy (efficiency), the political sphere (equality) and the cultural (self-gratification) within an individualistic capitalist society. Theorists such as Marshall argued that the extension of welfare benefits and security to all prompted a sense of 'belonging' and an altruistic attitude to the collective (Titmuss 1970). 'I belong because I am looked after' sums up this attitude, but as Michael Ignatief has observed, 'Only someone who has not been on the receiving end of the welfare state would dare call it an instance of civil altruism at work' (Ignatieff 1991 : 34). It is undeniable that the old asylums, orphanages and workhouses offered a measure of protection for both the inmates and the outside society, but at the cost of the withdrawal of human rights and the exclusion of groups from full social citizenship. Protection, however, always comes at a price, often that of a restriction of freedom, and care too exacts a price, often that of independence.

■ Summary

In this chapter we have traced the growing state intervention into, first, the definition and then the protection and control of designated groups within the population. Policies which in the nineteenth century sought to define and give a measure of custodial care to children deemed 'in need', and to those with disabilities, have, in the twentieth century been replaced by 'protective' measures and more recently by an emphasis on 'rights'. Tables 4.4 and 4.5 may give an indication of this development in policy-making and implementation.

Like childhood, older age has been constructed as a specific chronological time in a person's life. Table 4.6 illustrates the changing direction of policies; state policies for older people were initially predicated upon the idea that a measure of economic protection was needed when a person's possible wage-earning capacity was diminished by age and infirmity. The payment of pensions was the first measure enacted by the state, but this developed during the twentieth century, first into a concern for the provision of residential care to an increasingly older population and now into the provision of formal and informal care in the community.

Table 4.4 State policies and children

1875	FORSTER EDUCATION ACT. Education made compulsory until the age of eight.
1878	FACTORIES AND WORKSHOPS ACT. Limits number of hours to be worked by women, young people and children to 56 hour week.
1880	School attendance legally compulsory. Truancy made an offence.
1889	PREVENTION OF CRUELTY TO CHILDREN ACT. Courts given power to intervene against parents to protect children.
1906	EDUCATION (PROVISION OF MEALS) ACT. Local authorities permitted to supply meals to non-pauper children.
1907	PROBATION OF OFFENDERS ACT. alternative to prison for first offence. Borstals set up for young recidivists.
1908	CHILDREN'S ACT. Set up special juvenile courts and gave child separate status in law. Abolished imprisonment for juveniles under 14, and established 'places of detention'. Parents prosecuted for neglect.
1918	FISHER EDUCATION ACT. School leaving age raised to 14.
1926	ADOPTING OF CHILDREN ACT. Child becomes legally and socially the child of adopting couple. No information to be given to child of identity of birth parents.
1944	BUTLER EDUCATION ACT. Tripartite system based on the 11+ exam. School leaving age raised to 15. Selective state grammar schools set up. Universal provision of school dinners and milk.
1948	CHILDREN ACT. Children unable to be with birth family yo receive high quality care. Foster or adoptive parents favoured and residential care provided. Children's departments set up.
1963	CHILDREN AND YOUNG PERSONS ACT. Move to preventive work with families. Family care as top priority.
1969	CHILDREN AND YOUNG PERSONS ACT. Children between 10 and 13 to be dealt with by care proceedings not in criminal courts. Approved schools to be amalgamated with local authority childrens homes and to be named 'community homes'. Probation orders replaced by supervision orders for 14–16 year olds.
1976	EDUCATION ACT. School leaving age set at 16.
1980	EDUCATION ACT. Free and universal provision of school meals and milk abolished.
1986	SOCIAL SECURITY ACT. No benefits paid to 16–18 year olds living at home.
1989	CHILDREN ACT. Child becomes the focus of concern. Children's evidence given parity in courts. Children consulted as to choice of residence after divorce. Emphasis on children's 'rights'.
1991	CRIMINAL JUSTICE ACT. Parents given responsibility to control under-16-year-olds. Financially responsible for their debts and fines, can be prosecuted if children not kept under control. Electronic tagging of 16-year-olds under curfew.

Table 4.5 State policies and disability

1834	POOR LAW AMENDMENT ACT. Distinction between 'able-bodied' and 'non-able-bodied' in order to restrict outdoor relief to the able-bodied and to separate and institutionalise the disabled poor as 'unfit' for work.
1845	LUNACY LEGISLATION. Madness could be certificated only by doctor. People thus defined could be institutionalised against their will.
1890	LUNATICS ACT. Local authorities to provide asylums in every locality.
1913	MENTAL DEFICIENCY ACT. Allowed statutory supervision of mentally handicapped people in their own homes. Created category of 'mental defective'.
1918–27	Special 'occupation centres' set up by voluntary organisations for mentally and physically handicapped (prompted by the increase during war).
1930	MENTAL TREATMENT ACT. Provision of out-patient treatment. Separation of 'mental illness' and 'mental handicap'.
1944	DISABLED PERSONS EMPLOYMENT ACT. Introduced vocational training courses and rehabilitation centres, set up sheltered workshops. Introduced quotas of disabled people to be employed and registered as disabled.
1948	NATIONAL ASSISTANCE ACT. Part III provision of residential accomodation as statutory duty of local authorities.
1954–7	Royal Commission on Mental Illness and Mental Deficiency – investigation into the viability of long-term institutional care.
1958	DISABLED PERSONS EMPLOYMENT AMENDMENT ACT. Increased quotas and set up Remploy.
1959	MENTAL HEALTH ACT. Emphasises voluntary admissions and community treatment.
1962	Hospital Plan – community-based provision proposed for 'mentally disordered and physically handicapped' and reduction in number of beds.
1967–72	Enquiries into numerous scandals concerning treatment in long-stay mental institutions – Ely, Farleigh and Whittingham.
1968	Seebohm Report – local authorities to accumulate data on size and nature of disability (mental and physical) and to develop service provision.
1970	LOCAL AUTHORITY SOCIAL SERVICES ACT. Based on Seebohm, establishes social services departments. Register of disabled people compiled.
1970	Chronically Sick and Disabled Persons Act. Social service departments to provide a range of services. People with disabilities given the 'right' to live in the community and to receive social support.
1971	White Paper *Better Services for the Mentally Handicapped* argues for ending of hospital-based care as primary system.
1972	Vernon Report recommends that visually impaired children be integrated into mainstream schools with 'special support'.
1974–78	National survey of day centres – included day centres for the elderly as well as sheltered workshops, adult training centres, family and community centres. Found that most users were of low educational achievement and low skills. Very little provision for young adults of 'mixed' nature.

1975   White Paper *Better Services for the Mentally Ill* recommends more out-patient and community-based services.

1981   EDUCATION ACT. Responsibility of local Education Authorities to provide services for children with special needs.

1983   MENTAL HEALTH ACT. places duty on district health authorities and social service departments to provide after-care for patients released from mental hospitals.

1986   DISABLED PERSONS (SERVICES CONSULTATION AND REPRESENTATION) ACT. Advocates to speak for people unable to make their own representation. Carers to be separately assessed (does not apply to carers of frail elderly people).

1995   DISABILITY DISCRIMINATION BILL ACT. Access to be provided on all new public buildings and transport. Illegal to deny disabled people provision of goods and services.

1995   MENTAL HEALTH (PATIENTS IN THE COMMUNITY) ACT. Appoints one key worker for every person released from long-stay care. Community psychiatric nurses have power to section.

1996   DIRECT PAYMENTS ACT. Payment for carers for mentally ill and physically and mentally handicapped people (not frail elderly).

Table 4.6 State policies and older people

1908 OLD AGE PENSIONS ACT. Provided non-contributory, non-pauperising pension but subject to behavioural acceptability. 5 shillings payable at age of 70.

1919 OLD AGE PENSIONS ACT. Repealed behavioural conditions and raised pension to 10 shillings.

1924 OLD AGE PENSION ACT. Removed earnings limit.

1925 OLD AGE WIDOWS AND ORPHANS PENSION ACT. Reduced pensionable age for women to 60.

1946 National Insurance Act. Entitlement to retirement pensions at 65 for men and 60 for women. 26 shillings for single people and 42 for married couple. Earnings restrictions.

1959 National Insurance Act. Introduced graduated pensions.

1960s Local housing authorities begin programme of sheltered housing for elderly.

1967 Report *Sans Everything* – documents elderly abuse in some residential homes.

1968 HEALTH SERVICES AND PUBLIC HEALTH ACT. Duty placed on local authorities to provide home help services and promotion of domiciliary services to elderly.

1969 Sheltered housing defined in government circular.

1972 Payment of Christmas Bonus to pensioners – £10.00

1973 SOCIAL SECURITY PENSIONS ACT. Introduction of earnings related sheme from 1978 (SERPS).

1981 White Paper *Growing Older* emphasises that care in the community must increasingly mean 'care by the community'.

1983 Discretionary payments of fees for voluntary and private residential homes by social services becomes statutory. Massive expansion of private nursing home sector.

1984 REGISTERED HOMES ACT. Regulatory body for private home sector.

1985 Audit Commission Report. '*Managing Services for the Elderly More Effectively*' – emphasises the need to include informal sources of care.

1986 Social Security Act. Reduced scale of SERPS. Income support replaces supplementary benefit. Half of earnings-related pension payable to widows. Incentives for people to opt out and buy private pensions.

1986 EC ruling allows married women to receive an Invalid Care Allowance but only until age of 60.

1988 Cold Weather Payments – first introduced in 1981, extended to apply to any period of cold weather – available to those on income support and disabled people.

1990 NHS AND COMMUNITY CARE ACT, those pensioners in receipt of Income Support have all costs of residential care met by local authority – after assessment. Those with assets of £3000 to £8000 have to pay a proportion of costs. Those with over £8000 must fund themselves.

1991 Cold Weather Payments – to be based on the weather forecast and so predictive rather than retrospective.

1991 Attendant's Allowance only payable to those carers under 65. Disability Living Allowance only payable to those under 65.

1993 SOCIAL SECURITY ACT. Following an EC ruling women can no longer be compulsorily retired at 60. Equalisation of pension ages to 65 for both men and women after 2010. Disability pension ceases at 60 for women until 2010.

Part I

Summary

We began by setting out the three main directions of community care:

- Care *in the community*.
- Care *by the community*.
- Care *for the community*.

We have seen how the responsibility for the delivery of health and social care has changed historically from being a 'private' matter, reliant upon charitable or voluntary effort and sited within the family and neighbourhood, to one where the prime responsibility was seen as that of the state and then finally, a reversal to a 'mixed economy' of welfare.

The changes that have been described and analysed can now be summarised as follows:

Changes in care in, by and for the community

Care *in* the community – change in sites of care

Institutions	Home
Long-stay hospitals	Hostels
Children's homes	Bed and breakfast
Nursing homes	Housing association

Care *by* the community – change in providers

Providers	Purchasers
Community nursing services	Social services
Social services	
Voluntary sector	Individuals
Market	
Informal care by family and friends	

Care *for* the community – the cared for

The frail dependent elderly
Mentally ill people
People with mental/physical handicap
Children 'in need'

The only really constant factor which remains throughout all the changes in both the siting and provision of care is the identity of the groups in receipt of care. But here too there has been a *cultural* change; these groups are now in the public rather than bounded by the walls of the asylum or the workhouse – they are visible and challenging. The development of ideas of citizenship and consumerism has transformed the relationship of rights and responsibilities between users and the state services. But the one factor which also has remained constant is the ever present reality of the threat of poverty. Poverty dominates the landscape of community and both restricts and at the same time creates the need for a real form of caring for the community.

In the Introduction to this Part we made a comparison to a new enlightened zoo to describe the policy of care in and for the community: a system of caring which allowed vulnerable people in need to live independently and roam free within their own habitat but which continued to control and 'protect' them. We are now placed in the position of having to think about a system which will enable people to be cared for and protected without imposing upon them a centralised and patriarchal power relationship, a system within which people as 'active citizens' have a say in their own lives but which also recognises the needs and demands of the majority (Part III takes up some of these themes).

There have also been great changes *within* the delivery and provision of care. The response of the professions, the deliverers of care, is looked at in Part II.

PART II

Professions and a changing world

Introduction

This part is the second of three on community care. The main theme is care by the community, which is seen as a developmental progression of the transfer of caring services from the private domestic environment to the public domain. In the following chapters the concept of 'care by the community' is interpreted as being care provided by professionals, and the voluntary sector, though in many instances the contribution of service users as co-producers of care is also acknowledged.

All of the contributors to this section discuss the challenges of providing care in community settings in the context of current policy for health and social care. Central to the debate are the constraints which public-sector management strategies and policy rhetoric are placing on professional carers, and the services for which they are responsible. Professional concerns are seen to be focused on the outcomes of service restraints for service users. As a result of this concern, it will be seen that professionals are involved in determining means to redress the current exigencies of policy for people to whom they have a duty to provide care.

In Chapter 5 social constructs of 'the professions' in contemporary society are unravelled, and the concept of professional power as a component of perceived professional responsibility for the provision of care is discussed. It is seen that although professional services appear to have been curtailed by the introduction of new policy, there is an increasing professional interest in structural causes of ill health and the prevention of social oppression. It is concluded that interest in factors which cause social oppression will motivate professional groups to work collaboratively for change, although it is recognised that collaborative care may alter the current distribution patterns of professional power.

Chapter 6 examines in more detail how public sector management reforms have curtailed traditional forms of professional service delivery. A collaborative model of care and service provision is suggested in order to overcome contemporary problems experienced by service users and those who provide care.

In Chapter 7 the social construction of management is unravelled, and it is shown that confidence in the infallibility of management and management strategies to rationalise the excesses of health and social care provided by professionals may be misplaced. It is concluded that the ideology of management is based on a theoretical model of management behaviour which is not evident in practice, and that the concept of management is socially constructed.

Chapter 8 discusses how professionals recognise that their clinical freedoms are threatened and restricted by changing policy. As a result of threats to their autonomy it is shown that community health professionals are developing an interest in a new form of social intervention known as community development. Community development is seen as an opportunity for professionals to play a full part in the management of new forms of social care. Integral to this chapter is an explanation of concepts such as empowerment, which exposes many of the myths surrounding community care policy.

Continuing the theme of contradiction found in the myth and rhetoric of community care policy. Chapter 9 deconstructs concepts of choice, rights and consumer power, which are central to community care policy and practice. The difficulty of having to work within the framework of such rhetoric is described as a problem for professional workers. However, it is concluded that a number of measures can be taken to alleviate constraints. Committed workers, it is suggested, can redress current problems through a true commitment to consumer rights.

In Chapter 10 the important role of the school nurse is identified as a means of improving the nation's health. It is pointed out that early intervention in adverse determinants of health have a potential to prevent ill health later in life. Currently medical orientations of primary health care (PHC) are shown to be limiting the potential of school nurses to expose structural causes of concern. It is concluded that expansion of the school nursing service would be a valuable contribution to achieving a healthy society.

Chapter 11 also identifies ways in which community nursing roles are limited by current interpretations of PHC strategy and a narrow view of community care interventions. It is concluded that, working in partnership with other professionals, community nurses have a potential to make the principles of PHC a practical reality.

Expanding on this theme, Chapter 12 describes how a grounded theory research study identified factors which interfered with the autonomy of community nurses. It is shown how working with GPs can increase the vulnerability of all nurses to subjugation by their medical colleagues. Although the researcher focuses attention on professional relationships between community psychiatric nurses CPNs and GPs, to prevent limitation of their roles, all nurses are urged to strive for their rightful status in the community team, and to insist on collaboration with their medical colleagues, rather than accept delegation of work tasks.

Finally this section of the book concludes with a discussion of the impact of market strategies on charitable agencies. Chapter 13 shows how these strategies affect relationships between voluntary agencies and health and social welfare organisations. It is concluded that professionals need to be aware of how changes in the voluntary arena, and fragmentation of voluntary services, are creating a divide between traditional charities and those establishen by disabled people. A 'shift' in the location of intervention from specialised services to the pursuit of rights and social and environmental change is seen as a desirable strategy for all agencies concerned with community care.

All the contributors to this part of the book show that professional workers have, to some extent been compromised by the policy and strategies of community care. However, the picture is not as black as it might first appear. The chapters show that innovative counter-strategies are being identified by professionals to overcome the worse exigencies of change. Armed with these strategies professionals are showing their capabilities to expand their interest in caring for the community.

Chapter 5

Concepts of professions and professionalism

Anne Kelly

■ Introduction

This chapter explores the concepts of professions and professionalism, and considers how these constructs may be changing as a result of new policy, which is perceived to be introducing different forms of organisational work patterns and changing traditional distributions of power between professional groups. It is concluded that although some change in the social construction of professional groups is inevitable, in the final analysis professionals are likely to maintain power because they are prepared to accept responsibility for client welfare.

The concepts of professions and professionalism are multifaceted; historical perspectives of these social constructs show they have a dynamism which allows them to change according to changing beliefs, ideologies and social patterns of society. For this reason, recent policy changes described in Part I, which support the idea that health and social care should be organised like any other commodity – rationally managed through a market – might be expected to bring about changes in the caring professions. In this new era, altruistic concerns of professionals for the well-being of service users may have to be subjugated to managerial concerns for the well-being of organisations controlled by the market (Kingdom 1992) Managerialism is seen as a transforming force opposed to old forms of power, characteristically held by professionals (Newman and Clarke 1994: 23).

Metcalfe (1992) suggests that the power of caring professionals is greater than that of managers because it is a byproduct of their responsibility for care, rather than an end in itself. This creates a distinction between the social construction of the caring professions and non-caring occupational groups, which might be a basis for suggesting that the new ideology of managed care could meet with resistance from professionals if it is judged to harm those who receive services. Fox (1993: 62) is of the opinion that in post-modern societies knowledge is central to the imposition of power, so that in the instance of patient care the professions which claim to possess expert knowledge may feel that they are in the strongest position and can expect to wield the most power. From this perspective the potential power clash between managerialists and professionals might be balanced on the perceived welfare of patients and clients.

Change does not of course occur in a vacuum, and we can expect to witness its effects on the organisation of the caring services. In community care services traditional power relationships between occupational groups appear to be gradually shifting. Powerful groups such as managers and administrators are claiming professional status and an 'expanded role' in service organisation and planning, sometimes overiding traditional boundaries between themselves and professional groups. The increasing dominance of a managerialist culture is evidenced by a diversity of new discourses designed to move the caring professions away from the ideological comfort of paternalistic welfarism to a less autonomous role in service provision. These discourses include new constructions such as 'community', the market, purchasers and providers, consumers, quality and outcome measures, all euphemisms for a new ideological hegemony of self-reliance and individual responsibility for health and social care. Those who support the 'traditional order' of caring services suggest that these euphemisms disguise the 'poverty' of a new social reality which is increasingly dominated by the concerns of global capitalism (Navarro 1984). Yet this social reality is imposed on professionals; it is a reality in which the values and concerns of caring people are viewed as anachronisms, and are placed on a scrapheap with other barriers to change, such as social housing, full employment, education grants, and numerous other-taken-for granted, soon-to-be-forgotten benefits of a bygone age. Supporters of the new ideology of community care proclaim the increased efficiency and effectiveness of change, yet, in many instances, the reality of change, as experienced by recipients of care and professional carers, discloses a pauperised vision of poorer care, poorer service, poorer health and poorer social status.

In this chapter we explore current constructions of the professions and professionalism, and examine how professional relationships may be changing as a result of organisational change. Finally, we focus on the likely outcomes of change, and how these might affect the future of professionals. The literature on professions who work in community settings, and the conflicts they experience as a result of paradigmatic change, has expanded considerably since the implementation of new policy. In this literature a consensus regarding professional instability caused by the abundant rhetoric of policy is evidenced (Calnan and Williams 1995). Table 5.1 illustrates examples of rhetorical constructs which have emerged from community care policy. A glance at the table shows that a divide exists between constructions and reality. It is in this divide, or vacuum, that all professionals concerned with community care services have to identify need, and to plan and deliver services. This chapter seeks to understand some of the problems involved with professional accommodation of ideological change.

■ Defining professionals

The question of what makes an occupation a profession has been frequently addressed. Social constructions of some occupations such as medicine have presumed that these workers possess specialist knowledge, attributes or traits

Table 5.1 Euphemistic community care discourses

Common discourse	Interpretation
Community care	Self-reliance
Primary health care	Responsibility to remain healthy
The market	Commodified rationalised care
Managerialism	Overseers of professional activity
Purchasers	Service/care rationers
Providers	Powerless professionals
Consumers	Empowered professionals (those deemed sufficiently loyal to hold budgets)
Outcome measures	Imposed activity targets
Quality	Minimum standards to prevent exposure/litiginous action.
Welfarism	Outdated altruistic activity

(Freidson 1970a) and a collective altruism which ensures that client or patient interests are paramount. For many 'the doctor' seemingly occupies a special place in the professions and may be as revered as was the priest in past times. Professionalisation processes of this group have sometimes been described as monopolisation of practice, self-regulation and autonomy. Glazer (1974) suggests that these qualities of professional expertise are found only in the 'major' professions of medicine and law, which sets them apart from 'minor' professions such as social work, professions allied to medicine, nursing and even professional management. Banished to the margins of 'professional' society, these 'service' class professionals have apparently been criticised for their non-rigour and dependence on academic disciplines superior to themselves. As a result of such social constructions the professionalisation of care is said to have been dominated by the medical profession, who have controlled the work of all other burgeoning occupational groups concerned with the public's health.

Traditional definitions of professionalism have, however, become outdated because they fail to reflect the social, economic, educational and political factors which currently precipitate new constructs of professional status, characteristic of changing divisions of labour in a post-modern society. Some theorists suggest that the change in professionalisation patterns may be part of a contemporary loss of confidence in professional knowledge. Schön (1992: 49) suggests that although society is dependent on professionals, doubts about professional ethics and expertise have recently led to scepticism about the adequacy of professional knowledge to 'cure the deeper causes of societal distress'. In particular, major professions like medicine have been criticised for being élitist servants of established interests, powerless to relieve the crises of poverty, environmental pollution and energy witnessed in today's society. These crises have been described as ill-suited to interventions that can be provided by traditional divisions of labour, dominated by powerful groups. As a consequence, a redistribution of interventional skills is suggested. Changes in community care policy, particularly the introduction of a 'mixed economy' of care, reflect opportunities for a redistribution of labour in health and caring services which may have the potential to alleviate the worst excesses of social crises. If, however, a redistribution of labour occurs, then traditional power sources may be undermined. As priests have been rejected in a secular society, so the more powerful professions may also be slowly rejected because they are unable to remedy all the ills of modern society.

■ Power as a source of professional superiority

According to Freidson (1970a, 1970b) medicine has secured its powerful status in the caring professions through social closure of the profession, that is by mono-polisation of practice, and restriction of access to its ranks. The power of the medical profession is such that it has also acquired the authority to define the tasks of other professions such as paramedicine and nursing. Why is this profession so powerful? Apart from being constructed as a 'major' profession because of its knowledge base and altruistic nature, the structural characteristics of the medical profession, namely class, gender, race and culture, match those of the policy-makers and leaders – that is, they are mostly drawn from the middle classes, and are male. Doctors are also seen as possessing high levels of 'indeterminate' knowledge, that is, a store of integrated knowledge, skill, attitudes and experience on which they can draw to meet any unexpected challenge (Schön 1992). As a consequence of this indeterminate knowledge, which Schön describes as profes-sional artistry, the medical profession has been able to maintain a social distance from other professions and maintain collegiate control of consumers (that is, to claim legitimacy for defining client need). This form of client control has been seen as superior to all others; it has allowed the doctor to determine client need, even defining clients' subjective requirements. In an era of new political ideology, the structural characteristics of the new managerial class also reflects that of policy-makers; therefore, it may only be 'professional artistry' which is the distin-guishing factor between this powerful class profession of medicine this powerful class profession and others. Yet this distinctive quality of care is increasingly emulated by some of the lesser professions, a point to which we return later.

Metcalfe (1992) adds another perspective to the argument regarding the superior status of medical power. In his view, medical hegemony is maintained because power has been earned through the acceptance of responsibility for clients. This form of power is, however, benign: it will only be used to discharge collegial responsibility, that is to defend patients and clients from the worse excesses of policy. The non-caring professions, such as managers or administra-tors, are prone to seek power as an end in itself. Non-caring professions are said by Metcalfe (1992) to be less keen to accept the responsibility that is integral to the provision of a caring human service. The power of the medical profession is, therefore, seen to be generated by responsibility which morally pressurises this occupational group to fight for the equal rights of all who require care. Yet there has been little evidence in recent times, that the medical profession is collectively organising itself against the social ills of society. In the view of Rifkin & Walt

(1986) this is because the profession has been socialised to work only within a paradigm of cure. Care, the essence of comprehensive primary health and well-being, has traditionally been conveniently delegated to lesser mortals, a service class, more suited to coping with intractable problems of society for which there are no 'magic bullet' cures. In many instances it is left to this 'service class' of occupations such as social workers and health visitors to defend society from social ills.

Elston (1991) believes that in past times the unique form of power possessed by the medical profession protected it from attack by all rival groups. Legitimate control over processes of care provided doctors with economic and political advantages, as well as clinical autonomy and a unique form of power which far outweighed that provided by traits of knowledge. More recently, critics of the unique power of the medical profession suggest that, contrary to common belief, their strength is not entirely motivated by altruism, but is facilitated by and contributes to capitalism (Navarro 1978). This is a view which coincides with that of Schön (1992: 49). These criticisms suggest that the powerful professions may be disabling client populations by conspiring to mask matters of social concern, and for this reason a redistribution of monopolised power would be an advantage. This is another significant recommendation and one to which we will return, as it is already being addressed by concerned professionals.

■ The stratification of professional power

For many the power of professionals who work in community settings has been unequally distributed. From a historical viewpoint, Witz (1992) equates institutio-nalisation of care from the domestic to the public arena as the death knell for women's participation in healing practices. In the public view, caring activities performed by women such as health visitors, district nurses and school nurses have come to be strictly controlled by men within the masculinist medical profession (Stacey 1988). Witz (1992) argues that the dominant male professions have protected their position by exercising intra-occupational control over their inter-nal affairs, and inter-occupational control of weaker professions, usually popu-lated by women. In this way the medical profession has been able to retain a solitary paternalistic form of autocratic leadership since the middle of the last century, when the professionalisation of care began. Struggles by other professions to undermine this form of leadership have continued since the Medical Registra-tion Act 1858 to the present day (HMSO 1992: known as the Winterton Report), but the hegemonic gender control of medical discourses has resisted challenge.

This hegemony is strengthened by other examples of discrimination between professional groups. Divisions of labour in health and caring are patterned by race and income. Iganski (1992) found that only 40 per cent of district health authorities who responded to a national survey of equal opportunities strategies monitored ethnicity, and of this number only 7 per cent had taken remedial action against discrimination of minority groups. Striking income differentials between professionals highlight status divisions throughout the caring services. The 1991 Pay Review Body on Remuneration (DoH 1991 a+b) determined that house officers (the lowest grade of doctor) should earn almost twice the salary of the lowest grade of nurse. Consultants were to receive twice the salary of the highest-paid nurse, excluding private practice income. Since the NHS and Community Care Act 1990, the caring services have been shaken by reorganisation strategies and stratified by 'market' paradigms. Employment contracts for staff have become short-term and insecure, but doctors supported by their professional organisations appear to be least affected by assaults on their status (Cox 1991: 106).

■ Current perspectives of divisions of labour and status in professional care

The ideological thrust of 'care in the community' has a potential to result in an increasing complexity of divisions in labour, as a result of a 'mixed economy' of care. Community care is, therefore, constructed as more than a mere altruistic form of health care; it can be interpreted as a culturally significant organisational move, emphasising prevention rather than cure and care rather than containment. This provides an opportunity for professions other than the medical profession to contribute to care. Strategies based on the Alma Ata declaration (WHO 1978) have been implemented to move health and caring services away from technological reliance and towards a recognition of the importance of prevention and social support as means of improving health and well-being (Smith and Morissey 1994). As a result, a new ideology or perspective has emerged known as the 'New Public Health'. Ashton & Seymour (1988) describe this new construct as an approach which combines the need for environmental change and personal preventive measures with appropriate therapeutic interventions. It recognises the importance of social aspects of ill health which affect lifestyles and thereby avoids the trap of 'blaming the victim' for frailty. The momentum for this new ideology has been a perceived need to tackle global health problems of the new millennium. Development of a new form of socialised care has been perceived as paramount to redressing the ills of modern society. This form of care will require both medical and social modes of intervention, while the mixture of skills required suggests that in future a 'team' approach to care will be essential. Such an approach would have the potential to redistribute monopolised power, currently said to be disabling client populations and masking social causes of concern.

In the view of Ashton (1991) the debate surrounding this renaissance of interest in public health and well-being is frequently polarised in adversarial terms between prevention and treatment, and between individual responsibility for health and structural factors beyond individual control. As a result of this polarisation, the broader integrative view of political, social, preventive and interventive strategies for health and well being are sidelined, and a modified, more pathologically orientated model of health care emerges. This model locates health and well-being in lifestyle factors of the individual, and it is criticised for being dysfunctional because it lends itself to professional intervention by medically orientated rather than socially orientated professional groups (McKeown, 1976). A team approach to care characterised by the concept of a 'mixed economy of care' could well redress this imbalance, but it would be likely to lead to a redistribution of power within the caring team (Turshen 1989).

Although the British government, in line with other governments throughout the world, accepted the need to take active steps to develop primary medical care, so that it became primary health care (an ideological shift away from preventive and treatment services provided by a team of health workers, to a social concept concerned with population health, involving a range of people other than health workers), the 'shift' controlled by the medical profession has been limited. Green and Baker (1988) argue that although the stage was set for increasing divisions of labour and responsibility in professional health and social care, change was occurring against a background of increasing cuts in the global economy. As a result of this crisis a comprehensive primary health care approach, which incorporated community development for health, was constrained to a narrower model of primary care based on rationalisation of resources, still dominated by medical orientations of care. Nevertheless, even this model represents a shift away from traditional medical orientations of individual intervention. It is also a model which creates opportunities for moderating health care expenditure through increasing divisions of labour in health and social care. In complying with this rationalised model of primary health care, Walby (1992) suggests, all professionals are being guided along a path from Fordist to post-Fordist patterns of work organisation. These post-Fordist principles represent a shift from the meeting of universalistic need by monolithic paternalistic professional bureaucracies, such as the medical profession, to a system of welfare pluralism, quasi-markets and consumer sovereignty (Williams 1994).

The phenomena described explain how the caring professions are being moulded into a pattern of work organisation which accommodates a move from welfarism to commodified care – that is, specific care provision for targeted care groups. This pattern of work organisation is not unique, but merely mirrors what is happening in the wider society. The restructuring of labour forces has become a common factor of industrial production where production lines have given way to 'specialist' products for 'niche' markets. Changes from Fordist to post-Fordist economic principles are significant in community care, as they provide the potential to cater for rationalised or targeted need such as that created by disadvantaged social groups. If this change, is insensitively managed, however, the 'seamless cloak' of care can potentially be torn into the 'rags and tatters' of makeshift provision by a mixed economy of care providers, organised according to post-Fordist principles. On the other hand, if the potential contribution of all professionals is recognised then seamless care could become a means of unifying holistic care provision and addressing intractable social problems.

■ Post-Fordism in professional care

In professional service organisations post-Fordist patterns of work organisation mean the introduction of 'skill mix' patterns which substitute cheaper labour, or less-qualified assistants, for more highly qualified staff (NHSME 1992a). It is a strategy which seeks to develop a core of highly trained staff with a periphery of less-qualified assistants, the rationale being that this type of organisation provides a more flexible workforce which can quickly respond to rapidly changing needs, characteristic of service users in community settings. However, the strategy is a potential threat to all professional groups, because they run the risk of being diluted by the addition of technical assistants. For example, nurse practitioners are undertaking some medical roles and care assistants are undertaking tasks which were the responsibility of nurses. A system similar to 'outworking' is being developed whereby care processes formerly undertaken by 'experts' are broken down into components which can be carried out routinely according to protocols and procedures. The resource advantages of this type of organisation are obvious. But the dangers involved with this system are that the quality of care provided may be undermined (Carr-Hill 1992). It is apparent that in many instances assistants do not have the necessary levels of integrated knowledge, and skills to cope with 'indeterminate' problems, to make sound judgements or to 'manage' risk. For these reasons professional staff may be more difficult to replace than reformist managers believe. Hunter (1991) argues that mediation in professional affairs through the process of post-Fordism, may be more difficult than was first envisaged, because not only will higher grades of professional staff be difficult to replace, but consumers of services may not take kindly to change. Attempts to interfere in 'collegial' relationships between professionals and clients may be resisted, because it is perceived that professionals possess superior knowledge. Possibly, for these reasons, bureaucratic efforts to control professionals are currently limited (1) to strategies of 'charterism', that is, to attempting to make client populations more aware of their rights, so that they can control the excesses of the professionals, and (2) to surveillance techniques, characteristic of Foucault's idea of disciplinary power (Foucault 1980a: 155). In most instances this 'disciplinary power' is taking the form of audit and information technology control, to monitor professional behaviour. However, these sophisticated devices appear to be failing to capture and decipher the complicated patterns of professional judgement and decision-making. Professionals may, therefore, challenge these new forms of bureaucratic control as antithetical to the goals of the NHS and professional responsibilities.

As a result of the more undesirable aspects of post-Fordist change, professionals may be more than prepared to mobilise political and public support to highlight resource restrictions which curtail client need. A notable example of such action is evidenced by consultant psychiatrists' demands for an increase in resources to deal with the mentally ill who are severely disadvantaged by community care arrangements (*Independent* 16 July, 1996). Examples such as this show that although processes of social change are restructuring the organisation and work practices of caring professionals, there is little evidence to show that professionals are completely subjugated to new regimes. Neither is there evidence to show that 'consumers' of care are blaming professionals for perceived shortfalls in services. On the other hand, there are criticisms of the cost of an 'internal market', and of excessive bureaucratic management, from consumers perceiving that care services have been 'pared to the bare minimum' (Coulter 1996). Thus a post-Fordist, mixed economy of care organised on a primary health care model may have the potential to dilute professional hegemony, but it also has a potential to improve interprofessional and collegiate relationships between clients and professionals to the extent that they will be able to resist the excesses of ideological change and of managerialism.

■ The 'new managerialism'

A new style of macho, interventionist, private-sector management, characteristic of late-modern post-Fordist organisations has been introduced into the caring services to facilitate change (Millar, 1995; DHSS 1983). It has replaced a diplomacy model of administrative management which was permissive, reactive, problem-solving, introverted and aimed to facilitate professional practice. Porter (1992) suggests that 'new managerialism' has endeavoured to make professional services more businesslike by attempting to shift the values and culture of professional staff from altruistic care to rationalised care management. This has been achieved by imposing a plethora of management techniques to increase professional productivity and efficiency, in order to benefit the organisation rather than patients. Strategies such as 'market mechanisms', 'purchaser – provider' splits and 'consumerism' are being used to curtail professional autonomy. Consequently, professionals have to conform to targets, comply with purchaser requirements, submit to audit, suffer consumerism and in many cases be accountable to line management rather than senior professional colleagues. For these reasons professional responsibility criteria are sometimes threatened, and gendered divisions of labour are exacerbated (or emulated, in the case of the female professions) by hierarchical bureaucratic management patterns. According to Porter (1992), these developments are a bitter irony when at a micro-level there were already signs that more egalitarian inter-professional relationships were developing as the shift towards primary and community care became more apparent. The drive for cost containment may, therefore, be having a serious impact on professional work. In Porter's view purchasers of services, that is those who purchase the services of care providers, are prostitutionalising professional workers by selling their expertise – in the form of 'care packages' – to the highest bidder. All workers, even the medical profession, appear to be affected by managerial efforts to reduce unit costs, and in some instances even their jobs are at stake (*Western Mail*, 6 August 1996). In the professional hierarchy, however, it appears that the paramedical professions and nurses may be more disadvantaged by this phenomena than the powerful medical profession in particular, nurses in primary health care teams are finding that their work patterns are increasingly dominated by funded GP purchasers (Symonds 1997), who have adopted managerial roles. Yet, worse of all, consumers of services are doubly disadvantaged by reduction in services and interference in fiduciary relationships (trust relationships) between themselves and professional carers.

■ Outcomes of change

There is plenty of evidence from both professional journals and the press to show that there is concern over the fact that the devolved power of the new managerialist class may be outflanking the power of professional groups. For this reason, it is suggested that the claims made by Navarro (1978) and Schön (1992) regarding the powerful professions' facilitation of and contribution to capitalism may not be as damning as first supposed. An alternative proposition might be that a deliberate capitalist process of proletarianisation of professionals, through managerialism, is the perpetrator of increasing contributions to capitalist development of the caring services. According to this argument, it is managerialism which is reducing the status of all professional groups to that of workers in a production team, so as to create care packages to suit 'niche markets' (Walby 1994). Certainly it appears that there may be some evidence to support this hypothesis.

Increased bureaucracy in the form of managerialism seemingly, then, has the potential to interfere in inter-professional and collegial roles of professionals, and to undermine professional judgement, decision-making and responsibility. Current evidence shows that non-caring professionals, such as managers are challenging the supremacy of the caring professions to direct and control all action (Tudor Hart 1994). In particularly services have developed a top-heavy management structure. During the 1970s administrative staff increased by 50 per cent; in the 1980s this increase rose to 100 per cent. Overall administrative staff increases have risen by 19.5 per cent of the total number of hospital doctors. Professional and technical staff have risen by 29 per cent, while the number of doctors has risen by only 13 per cent, the number of qualified nurses has dropped by 5.2 per cent and there has been a 17 per cent increase in unqualified staff (OPCS 1992).

These changes obviously reflect policy change (see Figures 5.1 and 5.2) and how it has impinged on professional status, stratification patterns and potential labour divisions in care. There are many reports of professionals criticising 'new reforms' for the way in which they have diminished professional power and are geared towards cost savings (Browse, 1996). Other criticisms are that changes have 'turned off' NHS altruism (Lee-Potter 1996), have forced doctors to become clerks (Hughes 1996), have undermined the principles of the NHS (Hajioff, 1996) and have turned the service 'into a sweatshop', where, according to Johnson (1996:37), professional morale and goodwill have been damaged beyond repair,

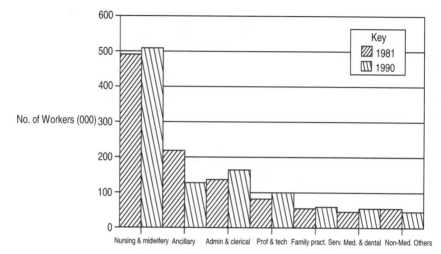

Figure 5.1 Composition of NHS workforce, 1981–90
Source: OPCS Adapted from (1992).

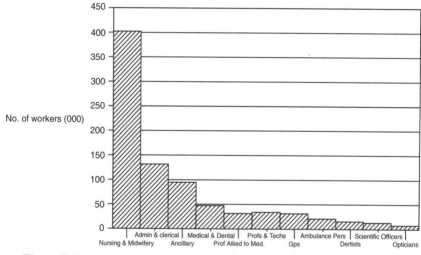

Figure 5.2 Numbers of different occupations in the NHS in England in 1990
Source OPCS (1992).

and quality care has been curtailed by efficiency savings. At face value, it would seem that a process of proletarianisation may be affecting all professionals and that professional autonomy has been curtailed. A more favourable scenario is that mediative processes will emerge in which managerial excesses may be moderated by consumer demand for professional services and by professional concerns for the welfare of consumers. Harrison and Pollitt (1994) also suggest that although change has been traumatic it may utimately benefit both professionals and consumers. Professionals may benefit because change has the potential to bring about a more democratic distribution of power within care teams.

Whereas previous stratification patterns of professional teams permitted medical dominance, in post-Fordist organisations 'lower-status' professions may be allowed more autonomy. This will mediate power excesses, and will have the potential to improve patient care through the provision of more holistic services. A shared power base would increase the power of all professionals and also provide a mechanism whereby many of the social problems currently affecting health and well-being could be addressed.

■ The proletarianisation/autonomy debate

Throughout the 1980s a recurrent theme of literature on the American medical profession noted increasing state and corporate involvement in medical care. According to Elston (1991), in Britain also patterns of work organisation and decreasing public confidence in the medical profession combined to change the market position of doctors and bring about a reduction in their autonomy. Writers such as McKinley and Arches (1985) believe that the factors described by Elston (1991) are bringing about deprofessionalisation and proletarianisation processes internationally. It is suggested that medicine in particular is a victim of social trends affecting all occupations of privileged status. Sociological analysis of the process of change argues from a Marxist perspective that in accordance with capitalist development medicine is undergoing a transformation of its labour process comparable to that which affected independent artisans in the Industrial Revolution, that is, it is being incorporated into a factory-like production system, with progressive loss of autonomy and skills. Evidence of change is based on de-skilling alleged to occur because of increasing specialisation, technology, ceding of control over decision-making to managers, and increasing challenges to doctors' social and cultural authority from the lay public, all of which are supported by recent government reports (NHSE 1996). Running alongside the proletarianisation thesis is the deprofessionalisation thesis; McKinley and Arches (1985). This argument suggests that increased lay knowledge of health undermines the cultural authority of medicine. The limitation of this thesis, however, is its lack of specificity, which makes it hard to test. According to Elston (1991), neither the proletarianisation nor the deprofessionalisation theory is amenable to testing; the value of either is merely to stimulate debate, but the debate has important consequences for the future organisation of services. In Britain there is certainly some current evidence for proletarianisation and deprofessionalisation; professionals' relationships with the state are definitely changing. The efficient and effective use of professional resources has been questioned, and there have been increased demands for professional accountability; interference in general and clinical freedom is evidenced by the issue of a limited list for prescribing; and demands for greater value for money have introduced evaluation techniques such as QAs (quality assurances), PIs (performance indicators), DRGs (diagnosis-related groups) and QALYs (quality-adjusted life years measures), all of which signify intention to circumscribe clinical freedom through bureaucracy. Many other examples of professional curtailment are available. Assessment of these factors led Trevor Clay, General Secretary of the Royal College of Nursing, to comment that the Griffiths Inquiry in 1983 signalled the demise of professional power in the NHS. In Clay's view, 'Doctors are deemed important only, so far as they can be nudged into management.' Nurses were deemed monumentally unimportant – from the time of this report. The situation may not be as bleak as it appears, but there may be cause for concern.

In a study of GPs' perceptions of changes since the introduction of the new GP contract and Patient's Charter, Calnan and Williams (1995) found that themes of loss of control and autonomy, perceived constraints on freedom to organise work, dissatisfaction with the administrative workload and an emphasis on pecuniary gain were all factors perceived by doctors to be affecting their practice. However, it was the view of these researchers that so far overall economic and clinical freedoms of general practitioners were still intact, though the style of doctors practice had changed, which was a matter of concern and dissatisfaction.

■ Contemporary and future developments in professional community care

In this chapter we have seen how social constructs of the professions can be moulded by social, economic, educational and political factors, which collectively shape policy relating to health and caring. Although society is still dependant on professionals it may become increasingly sceptical of their ability to alleviate societal distress and environmental problems. Scepticism stems from two sources: first, the major professions like medicine have been seen as servants of capitalism who are powerless to relieve crises of poverty and disadvantage, and second, the scope of contemporary problems is seen as too broad to be dealt with by traditional divisions of labour. As a consequence the 'lesser' professions are claiming an expanded role in primary and community care, and there is some evidence that changing organisational structures, such as post-Fordism, are facilitating more democratic patterns of professional role distribution in a mixed economy of care. These developments suggest that the balance of power between various professional groups may be changing. Although the medical profession is seen by some to hold superior status by virtue of its 'professional artistry', collegiality and acceptance of responsibility, other 'developing' professions, such as nursing and social work, may also exhibit increasing 'artistry' or expertness, by virtue of improved education, and may therefore be granted more autonomy and responsibility (Kelly 1996). Metcalfe (1992) suggests that it is the acceptance of responsibility for patient and client care which is the unique quality distinguishing professionals from non-professional groups. In particular, acceptance of responsibility is equated with superior status and power. It is pointed out that the non-caring professions such as managers are less keen to accept responsibility for decision-making in caring human services. Thus, it is reasoned, the power of professions is arrogated, that is, it is earned for the expert services it provides. Despite these assertions there are still critics who believe that the power of professionals is facilitated by capitalism, rather than motivated by altruism (Schon 1992). The argument for this accusation is supposedly based on assumptions of conspiracy to mask social concerns, thereby disabling specific client populations. However, exploration of the implementation of new strategies reveals that in many instances professional expertise is controlled by managers, the implementors of policy change.

Ideological thrusts of new policy, such as community care and primary health care, are seen as culturally significant organisational moves emphasising prevention rather than cure and care rather than containment. As a result the concerns of all caring professional groups are seen to be 'shifting' from the pathology of the individual to the social pathology, recognised to be seriously threatening health and well-being. The consequences of this shift are that social as well as medical causes of ill health are recognised, and multi-disciplinary development schemes are emerging to meet community needs (Labour Party Document 1996). Professionals who recognise their responsibilities to exert their power in defence of client impoverishment are keen to expose gaps between the 'rhetoric' and 'reality' of new strategies. Many examples of exposure of defects in policy are available: to take two, critics of policy suggest that ghettoisation of those with mental health is a serious threat (Nettleton 1995:245), while exploitation of the elderly has also been made apparent – research shows that between 40 000 and 50 000 houses are currently being sold by elderly people to fund residential care bills (Health Visitor 1996). Arguments based on the shortfalls of policy demonstrate how the foci of the argument (people) are valued, and how the reality of care in the community is exposed by professionals as a potentially mythical vision (see Figure 5.2). In such an environment the provision of services becomes a travesty of social justice.

Table 5.2 Myths of community care characterisations

Rhetorical myth	Contemporary meaning
Warmth	Not being snubbed/avoided by neighbours who no longer have a moment to pass the time of day.
Support	Buying in of social care at prohibitive cost.
Safe	Being fortunate enough to have avoided incidents of 'street terror'.
Secure	Being fortunate to be able to afford installation of burglar alarms and security devices.
Care	Affordable at a cost of sacrificing all other possessions such as the family home and contents.

Armstrong (1995) believes that recent evolution of professional constructs of ill health and social well-being are removing the cause of pathology from the individual to the communities in which individuals must live their daily lives. Professionals have accepted standards for the attainment of health and well-being (WHO 1978) which suggest that 'care should be based on scientifically sound and socially acceptable methods made universally accessible to individuals and families in the community by means acceptable to them through their full participation' (Basch 1990: 20).

Armstrong (1995) also suggests that to address contemporary constructs of illness which are identified as structural in nature a 'new' medicine based on the surveillance of normal populations is emerging. This new 'surveillance' medicine will involve redrawing the relationships between symptoms, signs and illness, and the localisation of illness outside the corporeal space of the body. As a result diseases such as poverty, unemployment, breakdowns in social cohesion and discrimination which breed in the extra-corporeal spaces of the community can be dealt with. Thus, according to Armstrong (1995), a new model of pathology has been constructed, which shifts the 'professional gaze' from the interior of bodies to the social body. Use of this model will ensure that professional client contacts, relationships, home visits and support will become as important as treatment (Oakley *et al.* 1994; Whelan 1993). This model of professional intervention supersedes that of the British government's *Health of the Nation* strategy, which Williamson (1996) describes as flawed, because of its failure to recognise structural problems of the environment and poverty. According to Williamson, the future goals for all professionals concerned with community care policy are equity and subsidiarity. Working together, professionals have the potential to become a powerful source for change. Increased collaboration between medical and social sciences professionals, agencies and populations will mean holistic care which will require better integration between organisations and between professionals and lay carers. This kind of collaboration has the potential to increase collective professional and lay intervention in community care, and to supersede strategies which are flawed because of their failure to recognise structural problems. To remedy this situation, Williamson (1996) recommends that all professionals learn the techniques of community development. Working together, professionals and the community are a powerful force for change and for reducing the excesses of managerialism. The government has challenged the professions (WHPF 1993) to make decisions in strategic issues, specifically:

- The context in which they will work.
- The contribution they will make to meeting community needs.
- The effect of substitution on their role.
- The reaction of the public to the proposed changes.
- The extent to which teamwork with other carers in health and social fields will be developed.
- The degree to which professional accountability and authority will be altered.
- The impact regulation will have on quality of care.

Professional responses to these challenges have recently been published (Welsh Office 1996; Scottish Office and NHSE, 1996). The desire of professionals is:

- To promote high-quality services organised by a mix of primary care professionals.
- To provide opportunities for professionals to use their skills to the full.
- To provide more flexible employment opportunities in primary care.

■ Conclusion

From this overview of professionals and professionalism in community care, it is apparent that the nature of professional care is changing in accordance with the demands of society. Although economic controls and market strategies are identified as curtailing professional autonomy, there are plenty of examples to show that where clients are seriously disadvantaged professionals are not hesitating to exercise their powers of responsibility. This suggests that professionals still possess a rational power which may be difficult to undermine.

Post-Fordism has brought about a restructuring of the labour force in community care. Improvements in the education of the nursing profession and an extended scope of professional practice (UKCC 1992) are removing some of the traditional exclusion and demarcation strategies used by the medical profession to maintain power. This may mean that the potential for unification of professionals may improve social collaboration.

Finally, lay groups are encouraged to become more articulate consumers of community.services, and overall consumer perceptions of professionals remain high. This is an advantage which professionals should be pleased to foster, as it may be their strongest defence against the worst excesses of change and excessive managerialist strategies.

Chapter 6

Professionals and the changed environment

Anne Kelly

■ Introduction

In this chapter the new 'private sector management strategies' intoduced into the health and caring services to bring about rationalisation are criticised for their adverse effect on professionals and service users. In order to restore equilibrium it is suggested that excessive managerialist strategies should be mediated, professional collegiality with clients should be increased, and service users should be encouraged to become more participative service patrons. In this way collaborative care can be enhanced and community participation in the planning of service provision increased.

■ Background

Social reform in the guise of rationalisation has caused upheaval in health and social service organisations since the late 1970s. A particular source of stress is that private sector management strategies introduced to create rationalisation of the caring services are seen as unsuitable for improved state administration of public services. (Harrison *et al.* 1990:60). New strategies, intended to create a revolutionary attitudinal change from 'welfarism' to a belief in the effectiveness of a 'market' in health and social care, are criticised because the public domain of care provision is constructed as being different from the private sector, which market strategies are designed to serve. The necessity for change has been presented as concern to halt escalating costs; changing demography, which is creating unbalanced demands for services; and a professional demand for increased technology (Turshen, 1989). There is, however, an opposing view that the real 'change driver' is the political ideology of individualism, based on the teachings of Bentham (Kingdom 1994). According to Kingdom ideology has generated the economic theory underpinning change, and is criticised for being more concerned with maximising profit, than with the moral demands of society. Public administration, in contrast to private sector strategy, is characterised by its 'particular sense of mission' (Waldo 1971), which means that it is concerned with:

- Identifying and balancing conflicting demands in decision-making.
- Informing the public without bias.
- Voicing the demands of latent groups.
- Facilitating and encouraging participation.
- Constructing compromise solutions to maximise consent.
- Safeguarding citizens' rights.
- Promoting social justice in the allocation of goods and services.
- Promoting social intergration.
- Preserving ethical standards in administration.

While private sector management strategies are criticised for their focus on financial economy, reduction of public spending, and a desire to 'roll back the state' (Harrison *et al.* 1990 : 62), public sector management is seen as enhancing individual rights, promoting citizenship, a sense of community spirit and facilitating social democracy. Yet, since change has been introduced, constructs of public sector management responsibilities have been viewed as anathemas despite the fact that individualist policy appears to have brought about the demise of social democracy which characterised the National Health Service (NHS) and the welfare state (Kingdom 1992). Evidence to support the view that social democracy has declined is substantiated by cuts in social provision and the privatisation of national assets.

For example, social institutions such as hospitals and social care provisions have been affected by 'cuts' in funding which are described as a covert form of privatisation. Baratt Brown (1991) suggests that these 'cuts' have opened the way for a market in welfare provision, but this form of market is seen as having the potential to create a social divide between those who can afford private care and those who have few resources. As a result, it is forecast that a new 'underclass' may emerge comprised of the elderly, the mentally ill and the disabled who cannot afford to pay for care, and have 'no voice' to remonstrate against reductions in welfare provision.

Kingdom (1992 : 115) suggests that institutions such as the caring professions have been demoralised by the social changes described, because they are aware that social divides disadvantage service users and compromise professional responsibility. In this chapter we consider whether public sector management reforms should be mediated in order to 'inject' some substance into what may currently be described as an ethereal spectre of community care. For 'normal' service to be resumed, it is Kingdom's opinion that three essential changes should occur:

- Those that manage services should have empathy and first-hand experience of social provision.
- Those that receive services should have opportunities to contribute to service provision, and have real opportunities to be involved in democratic local government and decision-making.
- Faith in the professions needs to be restored.

The feasibility of these changes will be explored and strategies for change identified.

■ Management in the caring services

According to Harrison and Pollitt (1994), managers of caring services who are involved in the mediative control of professional workers should be mindful of the fact that their security is integral to that of professional care providers and the welfare of service users. Mediative control of professional activities is said to have the capacity to undermine relationships between professionals and service users, which have been built on trust. Poor mediation may interfere with professional judgement or with the use of services and may, therefore, create professional dilemmas and client dissatisfaction. It is the view of Harrison *et al.* (1990:83) that the 'Griffiths' prescriptions for change (DHSS 1983) were meant to change the culture of the caring services. Following the implementation of new management policy, professionals became responsible only for the provision of advice, while they were accountable to general managers for the day-to-day performance of their work. The perceived outcomes of change are that professional carers have lost much of their autonomy; they are now no more than members of a team, and, beyond that, of an organisation. It is presumed that professionals will be subject to the rules, plans and priorities of the organisation. It is the opinion of Tudor Hart (1994) that the new managerialist strategies have moulded professional practice into a model of industrial commodity production. New developments are observed to have the potential to bring about deprofessionalisation and reduce the status of professionals to that of workers. (McKinley and Arches 1985). However, these changes, which are controlled by management, do not appear to be benefiting service users (Jordan 1995). Change has been characterised by a rise in the cost of services, which is blamed on 'internal markets' controlled by teams of accountants, managers, and 'contract' experts, needed by 'purchasers and providers' of services. Another example of the cause of escalating costs is the 'means testing' of clients for their eligibility for services. Jordan suggests that although there has been little organised mobilisation of professionals and service users against the new system, aquiescence cannot be presumed, because a number of sporadic protests have been reported. (*Western Mail*, 11 February 1997). This is a view which predicts that current policy systems may fail, not because they are hurting those affected by them, but because those affected will ultimately reject the policies

Tudor Hart (1994:82) warns that a serious price might be paid for impaired professional and user morale, motivation and independence. If caring professionals and those they serve continue to be controlled and disrupted by the soul-destroying efficiencies of 'commodified care' then it is predicted that the effects of managerial strategies could be minimised by uneconomic measures, designed to reunite fragmented relationships and restore a sense of shared human activity in community services. These somewhat extreme sentiments raise the question of how unecessary conflict might be avoided.

It is the view of Shapiro (1996) that a new model of care management is essential, one in which healthy partnerships are developed between managers, professionals and service users. Concurring with this view, Harrison and Pollitt (1994 : 137) predict that management control of professionals will be self-limiting. It is their view that 'management' itself will change because it is 'not monolithic, and managers are not a single interest group or even ideologically homogeneous'. Seven reasons are given for the likely restraint of the management era in the caring services:

- Professionals still possess considerable powers to resist managerial control.
- NHS managers are likely to become increasingly dependent for finance on private patients.
- New contractual arrangements provide an opportunity for professionals to set up independently of managagement hierarchies.
- It may not be in management's interest to extend their control to all areas.
- The interests of managers themselves are likely to become fragmented.
- Government may find that extension of management power will not offer relief from political pressure over the NHS.
- Empowerment of consumers may create an important new source of legitimacy. NHS politics to challenge management dominance

Many of these points will be returned to later in the discussion, but for the moment the last four will be addressed briefly. Managers may be reluctant to extend their control to all areas of patient care, because they may be understandably reluctant to take responsibility for unpopular choices such as 'care rationing' (Harrison and Pollitt 1994 : 142). Neither do managers have the expertise to make decisions over individuals' treatment; at most they appear only to be willing to set broad priorities, thus avoiding the stress of taking responsibility for implementing uncomfortable decisions. Taking on responsibility of this nature would expose managers to criticism from many quarters. It is the opinion of Harrison and Pollitt that for the above reasons managers will be very cautious about drawing up general guidlines, pursuing this activity only when they have a reasonable consensus of opinion with professional and service user interests.

Acceleration of decentralisation of the caring services may lead to fragmentation of management interest, as is already apparent, between purchaser and provider units, between the management of competing provider units, and between top and middle management. Middle management is seen to be particularly threatened, because it is under pressure from rationally self-interested top management, from professionals turned managers, and from empowered service users. Finally, it is very noticeable that recently there has been much criticsm of bureacratic public management by government. It is suggested that this might be due to evidence of higher administrative costs since the introduction of new strategies, and it may be a signal of withdrawal of previous support for managers, together with a rekindling of interest in better service user management by professionals. If there is a crisis of public confidence in the NHS, Harrison and Pollitt suggest that government may not support managers.

Although it is not possible to be certain that any of these possibilities will come about, they may support a case for mediation of current excesses in management strategies. Mediation of 'new management' interventions would have advantages for all concerned with caring services, because as we have seen current strategies impoverish many client groups. An analysis of what is happening in the health and social services is too complicated to be explained by a simple bipolar analysis of management and professional conflict. As we have seen, the conflict embraces many client groups. professionals, service users and various groups of managers themselves. Outcomes of this conflict could well result in the formation of different alliances. What is certain is that bureaucratisation is currently stratifying many relationships and causing incipient damage. If good quality care is desired then there is a case for mediating management excesses. Managers may benefit from taking account of processes employed to achieve better services and care outcomes. It could be the case that facilitation rather than subjugation of professionals is a better choice of strategy. A return to a public sector management style of administrative management is one possibility, whereas an alternative consideration might be the encouragement of more professionals into management. The latter would comply with Kingdom' s suggestions for essential change, particularly that good management of caring services requires empathy and experience of sevice provision.

■ Service users

To improve caring services, in Kingdom's view, service users should have an opportunity to contribute to service provision, and have real opportunities to be involved in democratic local government and decision-making. This is a position shared by Tudor Hart (1994) and by Harrison and Pollitt (1994). The involvement of service users in the planning and management of care is one of the 'pillars' of community care and primary health strategies (Macdonald 1995) Baggot (1994:201) suggests that there should be 'a greater emphasis on care and support in the home and the mobilisation of the community itself, both individually and collectively, to care for those in need'.

Harrison and Pollitt recognise that if user participation is to become a reality then service users may have to be encouraged to use their power as consumers of services to participate in the planning of care. Professionals should work with 'consumers' to define their needs and to provide them with equitous services, that is service provision to meet individual need. This model of care is based on a belief in citizenship and equality rather than an ability of the 'consumer' to pay. It demands a commitment from all to working together. Tudor Hart (1994) agrees with this model, but considers that at best 'consumers' can be 'co-producers' of care as they often do not have enough knowledge to make informed choices. Under the present system it is recognised that the socially deprived, the elderly, the chronic sick and the disabled may be barred from the care 'market' by lack of means. Increased prescription rates, charges for dental treatment, home care and residential placements are limiting consumer choice, and individual rights. It appears that in reality the current concept of consumerism is no more than a myth, for many comparable to that of the emperor's new clothes. The question of why consumer empowerment is such a prevalent issue of community care strategy is thought by Harrison and Pollit (1994 : 125) to have an obvious answer: originating under a populist government for which control of the professions was a natural extension and cover for attempts to totally control the unions it is seen as the best way of controlling professional power and autonomy. However, the whole concept of 'consumerism' appears to be misconceived; whereas true consumerism might control any excesses of professionalism, the model we have does not appear to transfer any positional power. So far consumers have only been given power over issues that are not important to professionals, such as waiting room facilities, or food preferences. These issues do not infringe on the autonomy of professionals in the way that allowing users to make choices which interfere with clinical judgement would. Increased consumer power could, however, also impact on managerial discretion if, for example, consumers had a greater influence over administrative issues like staff appointments or resource allocation. These are activities that would allow service users to become involved in democratic decision-making, and control managerial excesses. However, notions that consumerism could ever become a means of controlling professionals are dismissed by Harrison and Pollitt, because they recognise that consumers are dependent on professionals. It is their view that consumer allegiance will, always be likely to be directed to those who are seen as 'experts' in relation to care provision. For this reason attempts by managers to interfere in client–professional relationships could 'backfire' on managers, leaving them in an uncomfortable position. In the long term it is suggested that service users may use the 'key' of consumerism to reverse the effects of deprofessionalisation strategies. In spite of all the rhetoric surrounding the concept of consumerism, it appears that service users are being given few opportunities to contribute to their care or to take part in democratic decision-making. How could this deficit be remedied?

Williams *et al.* (1993) identified the benefits of consumerism as increased choice, quality services and sovereignty for the service user, while the organisation may also benefit from increased efficiency, effectiveness and value for money, which are byproducts of providing a service which meets the need of its users. This is a model of consumerism which allows users to have sufficient authority to assess the process of care and to judge it's outcomes. Using such a model, it is suggested that users might be expected to become knowledgeable patrons of professionals and organisations. Patronage allows the service user more power, because it is recognised that without patrons a service is worthless. Johnson (1972) believed that patronage was essential to any organisation, as it is a means of creating equality in service relationships. Opportunities for patronage in caring services should provide users with a greater chance to become co-producers of their care as well as consumers of care. Tudor Hart (1994) saw the 'co-producer' role as a legitimate one for users as it allows them to play a responsible 'partner' role in the planning, implementation and evaluation of care. As co-producers of care, consumers have increased responsibility for the informed use of professional services. Using their authority as co-producers, consumers can also control and minimise the technical bias of professional carers and the excesses of public sector management strategies. Patronage, therefore, has the potential to be a leveller of both professional and public norms. It provides opportunities to recognise the essential role that users play in care production, and illustrates how professionals and managers can become 'clients' of the service user to facilitate their needs. Studies show that most people want to be involved with the planning of services. (Bowling 1996). Above all, service users wish to see managers working with, not against, professionals, specifically when decisions related to prioritisation of services are an issue. In Kingdom's opinion, informed consumers should be given real opportunities to be involved in making a contribution to their own care, as well as having an opportunity to be involved in democratic local government decision-making about care provision. Consumerism is a fairly new concept in community care, the extent to which it may be adopted is likely to depend on the degree to which a patronage model of consumer involvement is appreciated. Harrison and Pollit (1994) have predicted that: 'Empowerment of consumers may create an important new source of legitimacy in NHS politics to challenge management dominance' and private sector management ideals. If professionals recognise the importance of making people partners in decision-making about care then a patronage role for service users is likely to emerge. This will strengthen both professionals' and service users' power.

■ Professional service providers

As we have already seen, Kingdom (1992), has recognised the importance of restoring faith in professional service providers, who have been severely criticised for inefficiency, ineffectiveness and self-interested behaviour. In his opinion, this is the only way to restore principles of public sector administration, and thereby equitable service provision for all service users. To what extent, then, has faith in the professions been undermined? This question is to some extent rhetorical, because there are few empirical studies which provide proof of the phenomena. Literature, however, provides many examples of observed outcomes of change. Monks (1996) believes that a campaign to weaken the power of professional groups was mounted because it was perceived that professional 'power' limited the current economic policy. The nature of the new policy has been described by a number of observers as one which was aimed at creating professional subservience and had the potential to downgrade the status of all caring professional groups. Agreeing with this view, Macara (1996) comments that 'General manage-

ment has been seen as the ideal force to eliminate restrictive professional practices, and to ensure that professionals submit to organisational objectives. '

Outcomes of change, as has already been mentioned, are widely documented.
Tudor Hart (1994) notes how the first wave of New Right policies from 1979 to
the mid-1980s imposed on public services a drive for 'cost improvement'
programmes and emphasised short-term strategies, which were tightly costed
and made professional interventions more difficult. Large investments were also
made in computerised management systems to provide information on
professional activity. Lee-Potter (1996) comments that these strategies had limited
appeal for both professionals and the public. Professionals resented restriction
of their autonomy, while the public were quick to realise that increased
public administration had the potential to direct funding from care. Widespread
demoralisation of professionals was said to have resulted from perceptions that
serialised cuts in the name of efficiency and economy were attacks on professional
status.

■ Other strategies to limit professional strength

Another source of attack on professionalism identified by Tudor Hart (1994) is
the discourse on quality. This discourse has been utilised to encourage professionals to deconstruct care processes and question their effectiveness. Underlying
this strategy is said to be an inference that 'management' adopts a more responsible position than professionals, and will protect the public from exploitation. In
Tudor Hart's opinion, although the 'rational' public may have been prepared to
consider the need for improved efficiency, they have not been easily taken in with
the 'quality' discourse. Monks (1996), agreeing with this view, provides examples
of episodes which have undermined public faith in management strategies. In his
opinion, 'Reports of patients dying whilst being shunted around the country in
search of suitable care', have done little to instil confidence in the public mind.
On the contrary, such reports are seen as exposing the poverty of a discourse
which shakes the roots of an ideology opposed to welfarism. As most people have
a social reality based on 'fair play', morality and a sense of responsibility, it is
concluded that the hegemony of a 'market ideal' is a poor comparison to the
ideals of professional care.

It would appear that current interpretations of quality discourses are far
removed from those of the management gurus Deming (1982) and Juran
(1986), who interpret 'quality' services as based on the 'expert' contribution of
professionals to service production. According to this view professionals are seen
as essential to 'problem-solving' in any service; only they can improve 'products'
and services, and ensure that customers will return to the 'market'. Thus it is
argued that the livelihood of caring organisations depends on 'empowering'
rather than 'proletarianising' professionals. In relation to the quality discourse,
currently perceived to be disadvantaging professionals, Harrison and Pollitt
(1994:11), suggest that quality in public services should mean satisfying users

throughout the process of care. Users are said to be not easily 'taken in' by ideological devices such as quality discourses, designed to create an avuncular image of policy and its strategists. It is concluded that both users and professionals are likely to be disillusioned with quality standards that do not measure up to those intergral to professional responsibility. As a result, professionals may decide that they have a responsibility to protect users from lesser standards imposed through new management strategies (Metcalfe 1992).

The purchaser–provider culture has also been identified as a strategy which undermines professional carers. Specifically, this strategy introduced to create a 'pseudo-market' environment in the caring services means that equitable professionals employed in different camps as purchasers or providers have different levels of status and authority. For example, following the general practitioner (GP) contract (NHSME 1992b), some G. P's were given purchaser status, which provided them with a great deal of power in relation to hospital consultants, now providers, and their 'unfunded' colleagues. This means that the tables of professional hierarchies and culture have been overturned by monetarist means. Also, as a result of market strategies, the health service has been divided by a two-tier culture. Mohan and Woods (1995) describe how 'fund-holding and 'trust' status strategies provide some professionals with opportunities to secure better services for their clients. In some instances, these writers suggest, service users have been covertly coerced into acceptance of these divides by the introduction of a market in health insurance schemes. If this evidence is correct then it would appear that service users are being moulded into a different form of creature, namely 'consumers' who provided that they have the means also have a degree of 'choice' in relation to services. In many instances, however, Tudor Hart (1994) observes pseudo-consumers are unable to recognise their own need, or the services they require to meet their needs; confronted with social catastrophe, it is likely to be the case, that service users are in an 'alien' land where their experiences are outside their own frames of reference.

It is concluded that although the strategy of 'consumerism' may have a potential to undermine professionalism, it is likely to be less damaging than the 'purchaser–provider' split, which has upset the natural order of events. Introduction of multi-divisions in professional care labour is not only a means of power redistribution; it is also a means of introducing post-Fordist work organisation principles into the caring services. As described in the previous chapter, these principles represent a shift from paternalistic and bureaucratic professional services to a system of plural provision, often by lesser qualified or non-professional staff (Williams *et al.* 1994). As a result of this change the hegemonic power of 'old' orders may be diluted, and professional carers and their clients may be confused as to the natural scheme of things. For example, local government has been stripped of its' duty to provide care, and is now constrained to comply with an 'enabling authority' model of brokerage, which purchases services for clients on a competitive basis from a variety of competing public, voluntary and commercial agencies. Thus it appears that there is a consensus of viewpoints which perceive that professionals have been undermined by changing policy in health and social care. Kingdom (1994 : 51) comments that the 'market', which is a construct of 'individualist' policy, is alien to those who have communitarian ideals; it is

> a denial of any form of communal planning, its produce [or outcomes] result from myriad small decisions made by individuals with no thought of wellbeing for one another – individuals are expected to do each other harm through a process of unrelenting competition.

Unsuprisingly, the 'market' has been criticised for the way in which it has a potential to limit professional decision-making, to undermine professional solidarity and relationships with clients (Coulter 1996). The British Medical Association (BMA 1996) expresses the opinion that the hardest burden for professionals to bear is the curtailment of freedom to deal with social injustice caused by structural reform.

Harrison and Pollitt (1994) add that new policy implemented through the medium of managerialism is intent on driving professionals from their moral 'high ground'. For the first time in their history primary care medical practitioners have become managerially accountable to Family Health Service authorities. Although the BMA. originally welcomed this development for its potential to redistribute resources from hospitals to community services, the system has been criticised subsequently for the way in which practitioners are now responsibe for rationing services (*Guardian*, 30 Sept p. 12 1994). Smith and Morrisey (1994) suggest that GPs have become no more than 'interest' advocates with a brief to practice distributive justice. Management objectives such as 'limited list' prescribing and 'health gain target' bandings are criticised for changing the ethical frameworks which previously guided decisions about care. Thus it is not difficult to see how changes have a potential to undermine faith in professional practice. In retrospect it can be seen that since the 1970s policy changes have been slowly moulding a different model of professional services. Table 6.1 shows clearly how change has been brought about. Most recently service cuts, and managerial strategies such as the quality discourse, purchaser–provider and consumerist cultures, have all appeared to contribute to undermining faith in professional care. For professional carers this is a serious situation, as the service they provide is dependent on the quality of their fiduciary relationships with clients. That is, the essence of professional care stems from trust.

Table 6.1 Policies of the last two decades which have shaped professional services for community care

1969	Mayston Report – introduction of management structures into community nursing.
1970–84	Setting up of health centres; development of primary health care teamwork; health visitors attached to GP practices; first school nurse training courses established by CETHV.
1970	Peel Report – review of domiciliary, midwifery and maternity beds needs.
1970	EDUCATION (HANDICAPPED CHILDREN) ACT. Transfer of responsibility for education of mentally handicapped children from health to education services.
1970	CHRONICALLY SICK AND DISABLED PERSONS ACT. Provision for this group in the community.
1971	*Better Services for the Mentally Handicapped* – discussion of plans for services in community settings.
1974	NATIONAL HEALTH SERVICE REORGANISATION ACT. Integration of local authority health services with hospital services and transfer of school health services to area health authorities.
1975	*Better Services for the Mentally* III – exploration of care alternatives.
1976	ADOPTION ACT. a review of adoptions procedures.
1976	*Sharing Resources for Health in England* – investigation of resource allocation.
1976	Court Report – recommendations for improvements in child health services.
1976	*Prevention and Health Everybody's Business* – advantages of preventive care.
1976	*Priorities for Health and Personal Social Services* – identification of strategic objectives in health and social care.
1978	*Declaration of Alma Ata* – report of the International conference on primary health care.
1979	NURSING, MIDWIFERY AND HEALTH VISITING ACT. UKCC established with national boards responsible for training, further-training, professional discipline and maintenance of a single professional register.
1980	*Organisational and Management Problems of Mental Illness* – investigation of care strategies.
1976–81	Development Teams for the Mentally Handicapped. Development of care strategies for mental health.
1980	Black Report – working group report on inequalities in health status.
1981	EDUCATION ACT. Provision for meeting the educational needs of all children.
1981	*Care in the Community* – consultative document on moving resources for care in England from institutions to the community.
1981	*Care in Action* – policies and priorities for the health and personal social services
1981	*Report of Study on Community Care* – feasibility of care in community settings.
1981	*Growing Older* – an innovative report on alternative forms of care from the ageing.
1983	MENTAL HEALTH ACT. Emphasis on care outside of institutional settings.

1983	Griffiths Report – An enquiry into management of the NHS.
1983	*Health Care and its Costs.* An investigation of factors underlying increasing health care cost.
1985	Government response to the Second Report from Social Services Committee on Community Care.
1985	WHO targets for 'Health for All'.
1986	DISABLED PERSONS SERVICE, CONSULTATION AND REPRESENTATION ACT. Increased right for disabled persons.
1986	WHO health promotion targets identified in Ottawa Charter.
1986	SOCIAL SECURITY ACT. Review of benefit provision.
1986	Audit Commission – *Making a Reality of Community Care.*
1987	*Promoting Better Health* – discussion on the benefits of preventive health.
1987	FAMILY LAW REFORM ACT. Review of family law.
1988	*Public Health in England* – report of inquiry in the future development of public health function.
1989	CHILDREN ACT. Unification of all previous law relating to children with emphasis on meeting the individual needs of all children.
1989	*Caring for People* – discussion of community care for the next decade.
1989	*Working for Patients* – improving health with emphasis on prevention and improved primary health care.
1989	Medical Audit Working Paper – introduction of audit procedures.
1990	*NHS Workforce in England* – review of resources.
1990	*Strategic Intent and Direction for the NHS in Wales* – identification of strategy for health gain.
1991a	The Patient's Charter – identification of patients' rights in terms of service expectations.
1991	*Equal Opportunities for Women in the NHS* – discussion on the equal opportunities of female employees.
1991	*Return of Written Complaints By or on Behalf of patients* – procedures for managing complaints by patients.
1991	*Women Doctors and their Careers* – investigation of career patterns of women doctors.
1991	Review body on doctors' and dentists' Remuneration.
1991	Review Body on Nursing Staff, Midwives and Health Visitors renumeration.
1991	*Research for Health* – identification of a research and development strategy for the NHS.
1991	*A Regional Strategy for Northern Ireland* – preventive health care strategy.
1991	*Working Together under the Children Act* – collaborative strategies for health and social care agencies.
1991	*The Health of the Nation* – An investigation of causes of ill-health and a strategy for targeting preventive care in England.
1992	*Child Protection* – guidance for senior nurses, health visitors and midwives regarding detection and management of intervention.
1992	Extension of the hospital and community health services elements of the GP fundholding scheme.
1992	*Households Below Average Income* – statistical analysis of householders near or on the poverty line.
1992	*Scotland's Health: A Challenge for All of Us – preventive health care strategy.*
1993	*Making London Better* – report on the need for rationalisation of institutional health care provision in London.
1993	EDUCATION ACT.

1993	*Ethnic Minority Staff in the NHS* – a programme of action for redressing ethnic inequalities in health care services resources.
1993	*The Patient's Charter and Primary Health Care* – extension of charterism to primary health care provisions.
1995	MENTAL HEALTH (PATIENTS IN THE COMMUNITY) ACT – improving community services for the mentally ill.
1996	*Primary Care in the Future* – discussion on extension of primary health care services and contribution of the nursing services to primary care.

Yet all may not be lost; as we have seen from the above review of strategies to curtail professional power, service users are often aware of the fact that it is the implementation of new policy that is causing disadvantage, not the action of professionals. Harrison and Pollitt (1994) therefore believe that professionals still possess considerable powers to resist managerial control. Tudor Hart (1994) also is of the opinion that the futility of current rationalisation strategies in the NHS. must soon be recognised. Evidence is provided to show that between 1946 and 1974 administrative costs in the NHS. were only 2 per cent, while following reorganisation in 1974 costs rose to 6 per cent, but were still moderately low as clinicians managed their own work. Since management reform, however, NHS costs have risen to 11 per cent in 1994 and are still rising. Between 1987 and 1993 administrative costs rose by £1.44 billion to over £3 billion, and senior management costs rose from £25.7 million to £494 million. Although public service staff may have conceded that the NHS was undermanaged, remodelling the service on business lines has no doubt depleted resources for care. Harrison and Pollitt (1994) therefore suggest that to a large extent the future of professionals in the NHS lies in their own hands; if service users still have faith in their services then there are still many opportunities for professionals to strengthen collegial relationships with clients.

In particular, it will not be in managers' interests to extend their control into all areas of patient care because there is little profit to be made from long-term care of many specific groups. In addition, new contractual arrangements provide all professionals with opportunities to set up practices independently of management hierarchies. For these reasons it is apparent that managers may increasingly be dependent for finance on private patients, who may not materialise if it is perceived that expert professional care is unavailable. Professionals appear to have much to gain from improving collegial relationships with their service users.

■ Current professional reactions to change

Although for GPs preventive services are said to have become lucrative options since the introduction of 'banding payments' (DoH, 1989), while services for the chronically sick are overlooked because they are less productive and a drain on resources (*Guardian*, 30 Sept 1993, p. 12), there are those who perceive that fundholding can provide service users with more scope to receive services. This article makes the point that it should not be assumed that all fundholders are intent on profit-making. Yet, to guard against funding excesses a counter-policy of corporisation has been adopted by government. By amalgamating district health authorities and Family Health Service authorities, activities of GP's have been realigned with policy. This may be a disadvantage for professionals, as corporisation increases the bureacratic establishment and increases the threat of proletarianisation of doctors, through management imperatives such as documentation, productivity, cost efficiency measures and increased specialisation. Under these conditions many GPs may run the risk of becoming salaried and losing more autonomy. Already non-funded GPs are said to percieve that both their patients and themselves may be disadvantaged by change. (Monks 1996). On the other hand there is evidence to show that although GPs are irritated by increasing bureacracy they are confident that relationships with patients are not yet undermined (Calnan and Williams 1995). More encouragingly, Armstrong (1995) describes how doctors are becoming increasingly interested in social problems which cause ill health. Despite attempts at subjugation by managerial strategies, it appears that doctors are rallying.

■ The position of nurses

Nurses appear to have experienced mixed benefits from policy changes. On the negative side, professional advantages which had been conferred by management opportunities presented in the Salmon Report (MoH 1996), the Mayston Report (DHSS 1970) and the NHS reorganisation were negated following the Griffiths Report (DHSS 1983) which discounted the role of nursing in management (Webster 1993). An added setback for the nursing profession was that neither the Cumberlege Report (DoH 1986) or later reports prescribed a definitive role for community nurses. In fact, recent reports have been GP-centric, and as such are contrary to WHO directives (WHO ICN 1989), which emphasise the crucial role of nurses in primary care. The General Secretary of the Royal College of Nursing complains that reforms have produced major negatives for nurses. There have been: a damaging loss of skilled nurse posts; fragmentation of a national service into competing trusts; abandonment of the public service ethos; explosion in management costs; staff insecurity fuelled by chronic change; short-term contracts; local pay bargaining and the 'gagging and victimisation of 'whistle-blowers'. (Hancock 1996 : 35). As a result many nurses are said to be demoralised.

Yet for the last three decades there has been a proliferation of documents relating to the professional development of nursing (see Table 6.2.). From an analytical viewpoint it is interesting to speculate why a specific role for community nurses has not been identified, despite the fact that improved educational opportunities (UKCC 1986, 1992, 1994) have created professional opportunities for nurses (Walby 1992). All of the changes in professional nursing represent a move away from a rule-focused approach to one of critical clinical judgement, which should enable nurses to provide holistic, autonomous care, as participative members of a primary health care team. Specifically, it is suggested that the contribution of nurses to community care provision may be appealing to managerial classes because the developed nursing role has a potential to provide community care at a lower cost. In some instances nurses could substitute for medical provision, and there are a number of people who believe that nurses can make an invaluable contribution to the public health challenges of the next decades. More importantly Fry (1993) suggests that nursing interventions will be essential adjuncts to the limitations of medical models of care which currently underpin *Health of the Nation* strategies (DoH 1992). This observation is based on the specialist model of nursing emerging from educational change (UKCC 1994), which responds to the challenges of the Heathrow Debate (NHPF 1993), for nurses to make decisions on a number of strategic issues related to their future role. Yet *Choice and Opportunity* (DoH 1996), the most recent report on primary health care, makes no mention of an expanded nursing role; it is completely GP-centric. However, all is not completely lost, because a corresponding report from the Welsh Office (DoH 1996) identifies a need for all professionals in the primary health care team to use their skills to the full. For the moment, then, the 'way ahead' for nursing is not clearly delineated, but many opportunities are apparent. The Report, *Choice and Opportunity: Primary Care–the Future* (DoH 1996 : 1) recognises that 'employment arrangements have not kept pace with the changing needs and aspirations of GPs and other professionals who work in primary care.

Table 6.2 Landmarks for professional practice development

1956	Jameson inquiry into health visiting – investigation of function and recommendations of staffing ratios.
1959	*Report of the Working Party on Social Workers in Local Authority Health and Welfare Service* – recommendations for social work roles.
1962	HEALTH VISITING AND SOCIAL WORK (TRAINING) ACT – new regulations, retraining and setting up of the Council for the Training and Education of Health Visitors.
1968a	*Report of the Royal Commission on Medical Education* – recommended changes for future education.
1968b	*Psychiatric Nursing Today and Tomorrow* – a way forward for the psychiatric nursing profession.
1970	Mayston Report – recommended changes in management structures for nursing services.
1972	*Guide to Syllabus of Training for Health Visitors* – recommendations for social science as well as health science framework for health visitor education.
1972	Briggs Report – recommendation for future education of nurses.
1975	Morrison Report – an inquiry in the regulation of the medical profession.
1978	The Warnock Report – inquiry in the educational needs of handicapped children.
1979	JAY Report – inquiry into mental handicap nursing care provision.
1979	NURSING MIDWIFERY AND HEALTH VISITING ACT – unification of governing bodies of all branches of nursing. UKCC established with national boards responsible for training, professional discipline and a single professional register.

1981 *Health and Prevention in Primary Care* – indication of change in the focus of general medical practice.

1981 *Prevention of arterial disease in general practice* – introduction of preventive care strategies for general practitioners.

1981 *Prevention of psychiatric disorders in general practice* – preventive care in the community for psychological problems.

1981 *Family Planning* – an exercise in preventive medicine expanding the role of GPs into family planning provision.

1982 *Healthier Children: Thinking Prevention* – transfer of child health care to GPs from local authority provision.

1983 *Promoting prevention* – extension of preventive services.

1985 *Health For All* – identification of targets for health gain.

1986 Ottawa Charter – a strategy for health promotion.

1986 *A New Preparation for Practice* – recommendations for changes in nurse education (Project 2000).

1986 The Cumberlege Report – review of community nursing.

1986 *A Midwives Code of Practice* – a code of professional practice for midwives.

1987 *Nursing in the Community: A Team Approach for Wales* – Recommendations for changes in community nursing in Wales.

1989 *Paper 30: Requirements and Regulations for the Diploma in Social Work.*

1990 Post Registration Education and Practice Project – recommendations for the post registration educational requirements of nurses.

1990 *Paper 42: Ensuring legally competent practice in social work.*

1991 Project Health: the role of the school nurse in the community.

1992 *The Principles of Health Visiting. A re-evaluation.* An investigation of the continuing relevance of theoretical principles of health visiting practice.

1992 Tomlinson Report – an inquiry into London's health Service, medical education and research.

1992 *UKCC Code of Professional Conduct* – a review of the code of conduct for professional nurses.

1992 *UKCC: The Scope of Professional Practice* – confirmation of an extended role for nurses.

1993 *New World, New Opportunities* – a discussion of practice opportunities for nurses.

1993 *A Vision for the Future* – the future contribution of nursing and midwifery to health and health care studies.

1994 *The Future of Professional Practice* – identification of standards for the education and practice of nurses following registration – all community nurses to be educated to degree level.

■ The position of social workers

New policy developments also appear to have curtailed the authority of social workers. Emphasis on a 'mixed economy of care' indicates that the role is increasingly administrative. Mohan and Woods (1985) suggested that curtailment of social work services would be an ideal way of deregulating the private sector, and placing a stranglehold on statutory welfare services. Henwood (1995 : 23) suggests that the 'mixed economy of care' is already disadvantaging some groups who expect to receive community care services:

many older people feel insulted about the fact that they now have to pay for services to which they have contributed all of their lives and are now cheated out of by changing rules. The result is a great deal of anger because people are afraid of the financial implications of asking for help.

As a result of situations like that described, social workers are perceiving that collegial relationships with clients are threatened, and that there is too much mediation in their professional affairs.

Although all professionals may appear to be disadvantaged by the outcomes of community care policy, and are particularly threatened by new styles of private sector management, which have been introduced to the caring services, even critics of professionals such as Illich (1977 : 27–38) argue that the primary motivation of professionals is to matters of social concern. It is apparently also recognised, that professionals have internalised codes of ethics which allow them to work without protocols and procedures required by other groups of workers. These are reasons to suggest that the role of professionals cannot be lightly dismissed. On the other hand, some weaknesses in professional groups are noted, particularly continued conflicts between professional groups, and stratification in divisions of care labour are criticised, because these are said to be unhelpful in terms of a public image. Another weakness is that some professionals are said to define pathology as individually rather than socially constructed. This is potentially a serious weakness, as pathology framed in biological or individual contingencies can only be blamed on individuals, and thus the state is exonerated. If professionals begin to locate pathology in socio-structural concerns they may become a considerable force to pressurise for communal concerns (Harrison and Pollitt, 1994).

It is suggested, therefore, that to increase their strength professionals should improve inter-professional and collegial relationships. Occupational homogeneity or skill mix should be redefined in relation to user requirements and collaborative patterns of care, rather than as a response to demand for increased 'commodity' production. Developments of this kind have a potential to create mutual respect between professionals, and provide an understanding of the roles and professional aspirations of colleagues. Harrison and Pollitt (1994) suggest that outcomes of these endeavours would be the development of common objectives, goals and strategies, all of which have a potential to infuse a reality into community care. In the opinion of Kingdom (1992 : 116),

Without professionalism ... care ... must return to the dark ages. Much of the 'New Right' espousal of managerialism was really a mission to undermine professionalism. ... The derision of professionalism was, of course, part of this grand strategy. Yet when we are sick, ... it is not the managers who will treat us, or give us comfort.

■ Conclusion

In this chapter we have seen that social reform, in the guise of rationalisation of the caring services, has caused upheaval in these organisations since the 1970s. In particular, private sector management strategies introduced to bring about change, have been seen as unsuitable for public sector services concerned with the provision of care, because the public domain of care provision is constructed as being profoundly different from the private sector which they are designed to serve. The necessity for change has been presented as concern to halt escalating costs, to cater for a changing demography and to curb increasing professional demand for expensive technology. It was shown, however, that there is an opposing view; the real 'driver' of change is a political ideology based on a belief in individualism, or a minimalist state. This ideology is criticised for being more concerned with profit than the moral demands of society. What is important is the ability to address social need through a model of administration that has a particular sense of mission, so that individual rights are enhanced, and a sense of community spirit and social democracy are generated.

To re-establish equilibrium in the caring services, three essential reforms were advocated:

- Mediation of an overenthusiastic style of public management.
- The opportunity for service users to develop the skills of patronage (a democratic form of decision-making).
- The restoration of faith in professionals.

In discussing these factors it was found that a model for change should, therefore, consist of mediation, patronage and collegiality. Each of these factors, respectively, characterises a role for managers, service users and professional carers.

■ Mediation

It was found that poor mediation on the part of managers interfered with professional judgement and collegial relationships with the public. This had a potential to create user dissatisfaction with services, which ultimately might rebound onto service managers, rather than professionals. Current strategies were seen to be excessive, and were likely to mould professional services into a model of industrial production, at the expense of failing to benefit service users and of raising costs. It was concluded that if mediation does not occur then professionals may react adversely. Several reasons were also presented for the fact that managers themselves may also suffer. Thus mediation of 'new managerialist' strategies was seen as a desirable option, and it is suggested that managers should be socially reconstructed as mediators.

■ Patronage

To improve caring services it was recommended that service users should be given increased opportunities to be involved in democratic local government and decision-making. Involvement of users in care planning was described as a 'pillar' of community care strategy. Users should be encouraged to use their power as 'consumers' to define their own need, though it was perceived that this action needs to be facilitated by professionals who will allow users to become co-producers of care. In this way, both professional and managerial excesses can be controlled. Service users were seen as being more likely to give their allegiance to professionals rather than managers. This is a 'key' which professionals might use to turn back the clock, and reverse the effects of deprofessionalisation strategies. It was concluded that patronage not only improves the lot of the consumer; it also has has the potential to benefit professionals and to improve the efficiency and effectiveness of the organisation. The social reconstruction of service users as patrons is recomended.

■ Collegiality

The importance of restoring faith in professionals was seen to be integral to the quality of professional–client relationships. Despite many of the strategies employed by the 'new managers' to weaken collegial relationships with service users, it was seen that the public are not easily 'taken in'. In the last resort service users still have faith in professional service providers. Current professional reactions to change appear to show that although in many instances professionals are irritated by increased bureaucracy, they are not entirely subjugated to managerialism. Professionals may even be able to identify some positive indicators for change and development. In particular, a new social construction of the collegial professional provides an opportunity for professionals to become advocates for matters of public concern.

The model of mediation, patronage and collegiality has the potential, if used mindfully, to underpin professional principles and to establish better partnerships in care. If a goal of communitarianism in care can be accepted as legitimate then it is predicted that working together for mutual benefit will follow. Kingdom (1994) suggests that before communitarian ideals 'the market' and 'public choice' models of care collapse like a house of cards. Communitarianism achieved through adherence to a model of mediation, patronage and collegiality has a potential to bring all the players in community care closer together , so that a moral reintegration of society becomes possible and welfare is once again the right and responsibility of all.

Chapter 7

The social construction of management

Nancy Harding

■ Introduction

The intention of this chapter is to explore the model of management which has developed over the course of the twentieth century, reaching its zenith in the last two decades of the century, when management has been deemed throughout the world to be essential to those health and social services organisations which had previously managed without 'managers'. The second part of the discussion will analyse how this model has affected managers themselves. Finally the impact of a new style of management upon health and social care services will be considered.

■ The twentieth-century model of management: management as technical rationality

The political philosophy of the New Right maintains that private sector organisations operate within the model of competitive markets and are thus efficient, wealth-generating and rationally managed. Public sector organisations such as health and social care agencies are deemed inefficient because (1) they are not subject to the discipline engendered by the 'market', (2) they are dominated by powerful groups, notably the professions, politicians and trade unions, and (3) they are administered rather than managed and so emphasise altruism, concern for humanistic objectives and safety rather than efficiency (Flynn 1994). Table 7.1 summarises the presumed differences between private sector management and public sector administration. It follows that for maximum efficiency at minimum expenditure those public sector organisations which cannot be removed to the private sector must be subjected to the tutelage of those economistic, rationalist and generic managers assumed to exist in the private sector (Farnham and Horton 1993; Flynn 1993). In this New Right philosophy the manager is seen as a 'transformational force counterposed to each of the old modes of power' (Newman and Clarke 1994 : 23). Managers 'do the right things: that is, they are able to make judgements, decide priorities and use resources flexibly and wisely to achieve an end result' (ibid.). They are the 'necessary corollary' in the restructuring of the welfare state to dismantle the previously dominant interests of bureaucracy, professions and politicians. The introduction of managers with a 'right to manage' is not the only factor in opening up the state sector to rationalising forces – those people, especially members of professions, who have been barriers to change are now expected, themselves, to learn the tenets of management and thus start to think and act as managers (Hunter 1994). Altruistic concerns of professionals for the well-being of patients must be set at nought against managerial concerns for the well-being of organisations.

Table 7. 1   Presumed differences between public and private sector management

	Private sector (management)	Public sector (administration)
Driven by	Market	Government
Environment	Market – dynamic and ever-changing	Political
Criteria for success	Economic success	Relative to the goals set by politicians, and sometimes unobtainable
Requirements for success	Customer satisfaction, surplus of revenues over costs, capital investment programme	Often left vague, so as to allow for the reconciliation of various interests
Management function	Management driven by economic dictates	Carrying out policy decided upon at political level
Statement of goals	Easily defined	Complex, vaguely defined and often conflicting
Strategy	Planned and rational strategy	Defined by politicians but implemented by managers whose skills must often be more political than rational
Structure	Coherent	Complex, multifunctional, interrelated with other public sector organisations
Accountable to	Through law to their shareholders, and in part to employees, suppliers and customers	The public, over whom they may have great power, through legal, political, consumer and professional powers
Management function	Rational, technical	Technical, political
Legal position	Can do anything not prevented by law from doing	Can do only what law permits and prescribes for them
Ideology	Economistic	Political and social: Social welfare

This belief in the efficacy of incorporating private sector management systems and managerial techniques into the public services assumes that major changes in strategy, structure, measurement of outcomes, cultural change from collectivist to individualistic, and changes from supply-led to demand-led services will follow their introduction (Farnham and Horton 1993). This ideology *about* management, that is the belief in the validity of the truth – claims made by and for managers and managerialists – is the apolitical and technical basis upon and through which the structure and culture of public services are being recast (Clarke *et al.* 1994).

■ The evolution of managerialism

The roots of this managerialist hegemony lie in classical management theory, and indeed in Weber's analysis of bureaucracy (Anthony 1977). Classic management theory, developed and expanded throughout the twentieth century by managerial and social scientists, analyses the functions of managers and focuses on ways of increasing efficiency; it allows managers to assert that they possess precise knowledge and highly specialized and technical skills based within a science of management, which are generic and therefore generalisable to all organisations. This theory, labelled by Reed (1989) 'the technical perspective of management', is *the* dominant school of managerial thought – most books about management and most management training courses are based within its perspective (Anthony 1986).

The history of management thought has its beginnings in the work of F. W. Taylor and the introduction of assistance from the social sciences is repeated, *ad infinitum*, in texts on management and need be rehearsed in no more than its essentials here. It relates that, as organisations grew, they became too large for one person to own or control. This led to the appearance of

- Shareholders, to share the burdens of ownership.
- Managers, to share the burden of control.

On what can managerial authority be based, however, in the absence of the legitimacy of ownership – as is the situation in health and social care organisations? How can management's position be legitimised? The answer to both these questions is simple. Managers' authority is legitimate, Weber argued, because managers use the resources of the organisation wisely, ensuring that all members of society benefit. Further, because organisations become bureaucracies it is the case that only the most capable workers are promoted to managers. By being in charge, managers demonstrate, because of their ability and experience, that they are the best people for the job.

This is a model based on a 'science of management'; it is underpinned by knowledge from the social sciences and the applied physical sciences, which serves to legitimate management's standing (Child 1969). The model is particularly important in the present context, at a time when people working in health and social services are questioning the legitimacy of the authority of the newly imposed management dicta (Laughlin 1994).

■ The ideology of managerialism

According to this philosophy the centrality of the role of management has been labelled 'managerialism'. It comprises 'a set of beliefs and practices, at the core of which is the seldom-tested assumption that better management will prove an effective antidote for a wide range of economic and social ills' (Pollitt 1990:1). This antidote 'encompasses a set of ideas and values justifying a central role for managers and management within organisations and society'. The belief in managerialism, and its elevation to the status of *ideology*, is not confined to the New Right; managerialism draws its adherents from several points of the political spectrum (Clarke *et al.* 1994). For example, international support has been provided by the World Health Organisation (WHO) which advocates efficient management as a way of achieving world-wide improvements in health (McMahon *et al.* 1980; Chase and Carr-Hill 1994). Consequently, the introduction of markets and management into the health sectors of developing countries is currently being explored (Broomberg 1994). In Britain the practices and language of management are becoming common, if not dominant, in the National Health Service (Harrison and Pollitt 1994) in general and in community care services in particular.

■ The hidden assumptions of the ideology of managerialism

The functionalist school of thought within which the claim to a science of management is based is inextricably intertwined with analyses of organisations. According to this view, management and organisations are seen as synonymous. The emphasis is upon *structure* and how that structure should work, not upon the people within it and how the world of work, including managerial work, is a social world. The model has evolved out of the attempts to understand organisations and how they can become more efficient. The earlier management theorists attempted to find one general theory of management (that is, management as a task) which would be universally applicable. They assumed, that there was no such thing as an *informal* organisation, only a formal one. They took it for granted that the structure of the organisation would determine how people within the organisation would behave.

Thus according to this type of analytical approach managers as people are invisible. It is only by digging within the interstices of the model that the model of management implicit within the theory can be perceived. What emerges from this exercise is a construction of the person as the manager who:

- is rational.
- requires a formal organisational machinery.
- aims at large-scale coordination of people in order to achieve long-term stability in society; therefore management is a control system.

- is concerned about means (achieving technical effectiveness) rather than ends – how tasks are done rather than why they are done.
- focuses on constituting a neutral social technology for achieving goals which could not be achieved without management.

There is little within this model that reflects the real world of managerial work, which, self-evidently, is occupied by human beings. Management ideology, therefore, portrays organisations as 'a neutral social technology' in which managers are implicitly seen not as human beings but as machines – they have no feelings of their own; their only wish is to serve the organisation. They have no values other than those of the organisation, and the organisation's values are always assumed to be right. Managers are seen as almost God-like – they are all-seeing, omnipotent. The manager is, in this model, a highly rational automaton possessing precise knowledge and highly specialised skills. It is this model of management which underpins managerialism; it makes an interesting contrast with views of the professions, politicians and bureaucrats whose partisan powers are seen by the New Right as preventing rational and effective organisation of community care services. In order for New Right strategy to be adopted in relation to health care the irrationality bred by the power play of these groups had to be overcome, and who better to intervene and to introduce logic and objectivity than those disinterested persons envisaged in the dominant model of management?

■ Socialisation process of management

The model of management portrayed here is one which is taught to managers and it pervades everything they read about themselves as managers (Anthony 1977, 1986). It is a model which is not based on research, but on armchair theorising (in the case of Henri Fayol and Urwick and Brech) or on subjective observations of very limited samples (as in F. W. Taylor's famous observation of one Belgian immigrant labourer). It is, however, peculiar to only part of the world. It is a concept 'invented in the USA at the turn of the century' which is 'neither timeless nor endemic to all parts of the world' (Hofstede 1994:12). It does not exist in Germany, Japan, in France nor perhaps in other countries either. It is an American model, which sees the manager as 'a culture hero of mythical proportions' whose presence 'is supposed to be a precondition for other people to do their work' so that 'the concepts of 'manager' and 'management' are products of one particular culture' and the 'only universal component is the employed person' (ibid.).

We now have one half of the socially constructed picture of the manager. We are given to believe in the manager as a rational-technical automaton, selflessly applying a science of management, and without whom organisations cannot function, because workers will not work unless they are managed. This is the model of management which dominates social policy in late twentieth-century Britain. It is a model which when examined closely, as I will now show, is seen to be of dubious authenticity: because its claims to status rest upon a science which is not a science; upon a presumed universality which does not exist; and upon a model of the human which strips away all the realities of human nature. What happens when this model meets the real world of work?

■ The social construction of management and the manager

□ The claim to scientific knowledge

Let us begin by examining the basis upon which management's claim to rationality rests: possession of a scientific body of knowledge claimed by managers. The debate within the sociology of science concerning the social construction of science (Mulkay 1991) alerts us to the need to examine how and why 'scientific facts' emerge, and when examining 'management science' we must go one step further and examine also how the 'science' is applied. So, we must ask:

- How do theories of and for management emerge and become incorporated in management science?
- Why do such theories emerge?
- How is 'management science' applied?

The answers to these questions must be tentative. However:

1. Management theories emerge through the application of methods and theories from the other sciences, both the physical and the social, to organisations.
2. They are developed not so much for purposes of understanding, but for their utility in application – the emphasis is upon improving organisational performance.
3. The improvement of organisational performance through the application of 'science' could enhance management's claim to possess a body of knowledge and the necessary skills to apply that knowledge – their rational-legal status is thus enhanced.

There are problems in application, however. First, theories adapted from the physical sciences and used to structure the flows of inputs, throughputs and outputs are designed for mass-production industries where the human input is minimal and control is maximal (Eldin and Beheshti 1981). They are not designed for the diffuse organisation structure necessary in health and community care services.

Second, many of the theories and practices of the social sciences drawn upon did not emerge as, and were never intended to be, applied sciences; they developed as part of that search to increase knowledge about how societies work. Thus, there is a huge conceptual gap between trying to understand how people interact and using that understanding (which can probably be no more than approximate, given the complexity of the human animal both as an individual and in groups) to change people's behaviour at work. This may explain why these theories do not appear to 'work'.

Finally, the people responsible for applying the theories are middle-level managers. Studies show how managers conform not to expected behaviour patterns but to what could be construed as irrational behaviour patterns, built upon talk-and-task-orientated work patterns which are subject to constant inter-ruption (Stewart 1982). Within this pattern of work there is little prospect of applying the theories of management science in the form in which they were designed. Short cuts have to be made, corners cut and the edges shorn off, so that what remains is a shadow of the scientific method which is supposedly being applied. In other words the superficiality of the applied theory of management questions its credibility.

Indeed, many of the theories of currently fashionable management gurus fall by the wayside when they meet the world of middle management. One after another management theories become fashionable, are implemented, fail and are replaced by other theories. As a result, one commentator reviewing the history of failure suggests management theory is little but 'fad and fashion' (Ramsay 1996). Tom Peter's *Thriving on Chaos* (1998) has proved impossible to implement even by managers keenly committed to its implementation (Harrison, *et al.* 1994). Michael Hammer, whose *Re-engineering the Corporation* (1995) led to massive redundancies around the world as organisations adopted his recommendations for 'downsiz-ing', has recanted. The evidence is now overwhelming that application of his theory led to business stagnation or even failure – the most successful organisa-tions in the decade of downsizing had in fact maintained and even increased their numbers of employees (Keegan, *et al.* 1995). If all these criticisms are taken together it can be concluded, albeit tentatively, that 'management science' is a mixture of models, designed to help mass-production organisations, and half-understood theories borrowed from other sciences, some of which were never meant to have practical application. They are used, perhaps with some degree of effectiveness by senior managers responsible for strategy, to enhance the status of managers in the Anglo-American world. When they are applied by middle managers responsible for the day-to-day operation of the enterprise the already tentative nature of the theories is further decayed, so that what is applied bears in many instances little relation to science. What remains is a claim to scientific status, a claim which serves to buttress the legitimacy of management. An analogy to this situation would be the game of Chinese whispers, where what starts out as a rational statement becomes distorted into garbled nonsense when it is repeatedly whispered down the line.

☐ The real world of the manager

Let us now explore the real world of the manager. At a behavioural level of analysis, relatively few empirical studies of managers exist, but those which do have shown that far from applying a rational science managers are involved in work characterised by fragmentation, talk and reaction to events. They also show the human side of managerial nature, and reveal it to be aggressive and ambitious (Mintzberg 1973, Stewart 1982;). The political model of management which attempts to explain these characteristics suggests that managers are not selfless automatons. Instead, they are seen to be highly ambitious and competitive people who organise themselves into groups or coalitions the better to achieve their ends. These groups or coalitions are often in conflict, so that a continually shifting balance of power and interests within management is observed (Reed 1989).

Implicit in this model is one of the most consistent empirical findings about managers, that is, they are male. The labour market is segmented both horizontally, into 'men's jobs' and 'women's jobs', and vertically, so that more highly graded jobs are typically held by men. Very, very few women are represented in senior management positions, and although women are in some countries becoming better represented in middle management positions, they are still very much under-represented in terms of numbers. Women, inevitably, seem to hit a 'glass ceiling' which prevents their promotion to higher level jobs. The vast majority of part-time jobs, jobs which are characterised by lack of security and inferior benefits, are held by women. Women consistently earn less than men, despite the existence of legislation requiring equal pay for work of equal value. In sum, the real world of the manager is one where work is fragmented and differs markedly from that cool functionality of planning, organising, staffing, co-ordinating and controlling seen in management texts. It is a world where men predominate, and where jockeying for position and promotion takes place constantly. To understand management and whether it can achieve the objective of bringing rationality into non-rational organisations we therefore need to understand the world of men, and how they work together and with other (often male-dominated) professional groups. Yet the issue of gender in organisations is so ignored in the 'classics' on organisation and management theory, that its avoidance appears 'bizarre' (Hearn and Parkin, 1986). Therefore, it is to feminist writers that we must turn for explanation.

☐ Analysing the real world of management

Feminist writers attempt to understand a world which has until recently been analysed and understood in some instances through a Western 'phallocentric' image. The term 'androcentric', can therefore be applied to a concept of management understanding which merges the two sexes, male and female, into one model which is congruent only with the masculine (Grosz 1988a). This model is then generalised across many if not most of our fields of knowledge so that seemingly all life forms are understood only in terms of the masculine. In management theory this 'androcentric' (male as norm) bias, which rarely describes the female experience of management, also prevails. Indeed, management theory cannot be described as any thing other than androcentric, in that it assumes that the experience of all managers will be similar, so female managers are elided with the male.

This bias can be seen if we look at how research into management has been undertaken. Research samples are drawn mainly from the corporate world or the military. Mintzberg's highly influential research into what managers do consisted of a study of five male managers. Maslow's famous 'hierarchy of needs' is essentially a reflection of male norms, with the needs ranked in such a way as to place those typically seen as 'female' at the lower end, with 'higher-order' needs being biased more towards the male than the female perspective. F. W. Taylor in his role as founding father of management theory wrote exclusively about men, about the 'management of men' by 'scientific methods'. 'Managers should fully plan out each work*man*'s work at least one day in advance, after 'giving' 'a model of men and [a] model of masculinity [which was] precise, behavioural, controlled and instrumental'. In Taylorism, 'women vanish, or very nearly so. The prescriptions made are for men and for male society. This is especially significant when such models are applied to community health and social services, which as we have seen are essentially female, both in provision and use. Women are both the majority providers and receivers of community care services. Taylorist models of management may therefore serve to subjugate and control women.

It is only in the 'caring' departments of organisations that women have any status, notably in personnel management, which continued to be a female preserve until a profession of well-paid personnel, or human resource, managers developed, at which time men took over the personnel function (Anthony and Crichton 1978). So the ethos of organisations has traditionally been male, but a specific type of male – the élite, small in number, who 'put their rules, their stamp, and their model of behaviour on organizational "expectations"'. This ethos of management then has been one of 'masculinity, strength', [and] 'aggression' [which] 'themselves' have become linked to dominance and its micro forms – management and leadership' (Mills and Murgatroyd 1991 : 135).

Of the papers and books which do focus on women in management, two dominant perspectives can be seen: those which have a strong feminist perspective, and those which view being female as a problem which necessitates certain adaptive techniques if women are to succeed in a male world (Adler *et al.* 1993). In this latter perspective, because femaleness is problematised, it has to be controlled. Maleness is not seen as problematic, as it is taken for granted. There is an assumption in this literature that only women are gendered, giving an 'implicit formula' of gender equals sex equals women equals problem (Calas and Smircich 1992).

☐ **Management as a gendered practice**

Management is a gendered practice which determines how its members act. This is shown in studies emerging from the discipline of 'men and masculinities', which have shown how the world of the male manager is created (Hearn and

Morgan 1990 : 7) These studies have revealed a paradox: that although social studies have been primarily male-dominated, men have been as invisible as women. This is because studies which are routinely about men, in that men constitute the acknowledged or unacknowledged subjects, are not necessarily about men in a more complex, more problematised, sociological sense. That is, they do not provide a great deal of information about the real experiences of men. Writers in this field have started to fill in some of the gaps in our knowledge about men, a crucial task if we are to understand the world of management.

Mills and Murgatroyd (1991) suggests that as adults at work, organisations require us to act in 'appropriately gendered ways' (Mills and Murgatroyd 1991). Males dominate in management, displaying one of a possible range of dominant 'hegemonic masculinities', that is historically and culturally the way men have been conditioned into forms and practices of masculinity (Hearn and Morgan 1990). Today's dominant hegemonic masculinity is 'white, heterosexist, middle-class, Anglophone, and so on' (p. 11), which describes the archetypal manager. The gendered behaviour of such a manager is a masculinity 'shaped around notions of rationality', i. e. 'detached, logical, unemotional and absorbed in the work process'. If we turn this around, we have a managerial self-identity based on a rationality defined as being masculine and therefore beyond being attained by women. It is a rationality which serves a double purpose, as it provides a manager with an air of superiority over manual workers who are supposedly less rational, and it excludes supposedly irrational females' (Mills and Murgatroyd 1991). It is a rationality embedded deep within Taylorism, where the 'ideal workman would appear to almost lose physical presence, or would be a mere disembodied bearer of role, in effect part of a machine system' where a very explicit model of masculinity is given, one of stable, taken-for-granted power and authority, as in the patriarchal family (Hearn and Parkin 1986 : 18–19). In this world, males 'are expected to exhibit male-associated characteristics of toughness, competitiveness, aggressiveness and control. These concepts make up part of our understandings of management – a concept that is riddled with notions of masculinity' (pp. 78–9). It involves a dedication to work – being in the office up to eighteen hours a day. Most men in late-industrial societies rely on work as a 'prop' for their masculine identities, as work is one way of 'securing self in gender identity', but it appears to be a very fragile self, with its masculine identity being precarious, artificial and fragile (Collinson *et al.* 1990 : 202). It is a type of masculinity modelled upon that of the leader, with whom subordinates must identify and whose behaviour they must mirror in order to stress their potential for success and their masculinity (Mills and 1991).

In these men-only domains, Hearn (1992) argues somewhat contentiously, managers can be involved in 'gathering together, as managers and/or work-mates, standing up, strutting, performing in public, orating, arguing, saying your piece, [which] in the competitive world of men involves a symbolic waving around of the penis ... as a display of power to others, women and men, but most importantly men.... The whole sordid little show is a "phallusy" – a desperate complex of moves by men to take the public stage by storm, to dominate the material world of reproduction' (Hearn 1992:207). (Here we have a metaphor, the organisation as a herd, with the males strutting and displaying themselves in order to prove their supremacy.)

The thrust of the above argument is that:

- Organisations are dominated by members of one sex, the male.
- Men have to conform to certain learned behaviours which determine 'masculinity' and how men should behave. Organisations dictate a certain model of masculinity, based upon that of those most senior in the organisation, to which all other managers must conform if they are to be successful.
- Those who have reached the top have done so because they are the most aggressive, the most competitive, the most rational, the most able to separate out their needs for warmth, companionship, and so on and who are most comfortable in the world of men. This is the model which other men in the organisation must adopt.
- This is a model which excludes women. Women, however, can be seen as a challenge to it, but only those women who pose an alternative model of management. As Cynthia Cockburn has shown, many women in management adopt identical male strategies or female strategies which emphasise their femininity. Such women are visible as community care managers (Cockburn 1991).

☐ The battle for managerial power, or the search for legitimation

When management was introduced into industrial organisations its status and authority had to be legitimated and managers similarly have to seek such legitimation in community care services. Where legitimation cannot be achieved then power may suffice. Managerial power is a 'complex and multi-faceted power' (Cockburn 1990), which includes the power of class, power of colour, power over the managed, and the power of the male which allows women to be dominated. When analysing community care services, we are analysing a situation where management, a largely male-dominated institution, has been introduced into, indeed imposed on, organisations which in terms of numbers are largely female-dominated, and in terms of power are dominated by professions, some of which may conform to a different model of maleness. Early evidence regarding the introduction of managers into hospitals suggests that they are gaining power over nurses but the power of medical consultants remains undiminished (Pollitt 1993). Does this allow a tentative conclusion, that the introduction of management into professionally dominated organisations results, not in the greater rationality of service provision, but in the introduction of yet another group vying for status and authority? The result appears to be that female professions can be overpowered, whilst male-dominated professions maintain their status and position. The result can only be an intensification of the problems which have bedevilled health and social care services in the past, and which managers were, naïvely, presumed capable of solving.

■ Conclusion: the social construction of management in community care services

The introduction of managers into community care services should, in theory, result in a new rationality which will supersede the supposed anarchy created by the competition between bureaucrats, politicians and professions fighting for territorial dominance. However, we have seen that the model upon which this assumption is based is fundamentally flawed, for management is a socially constructed phenomenon having two aspects. The first is its position as an ideology within a society, and the second is that which has been constructed in practice.

At the ideological level, management is a belief system which preaches that management is an absolutely necessary and vital function peopled by rational – technical functionaries – managers – who possess a body of knowledge and skills without which organisations cannot function. The doubtful nature of these claims suggests that they may be ideological. Management emerged in the United States and is thus culturally variable and time-specific; it is also applicable to only a few countries. For these reasons, it may not be the absolutely necessary and vital function that is a taken for granted assumption in those countries in which it is dominant. Its body of knowledge and skills is not of the claimed scientific type. The ideology of management is based upon a theoretical model of managerial behaviour which is not evident in practice.

At the level of the organisation, the world of management is socially constructed by managers who conform to the social construction of the role. This is a role which is synonomous with the dominant model of masculinity within the culture in which managers are located. To be a manager is to act the part of a man, doing masculine things.

Chapter 8

Community development and health professionals

Stephen Clarke

◾ Introduction

In this chapter professionals are urged to adopt innovative strategies to overcome problems created by a new form of management and control by restricted resources. A recommended strategy is that of community development, which is described as a means of overcoming the oppression of current policy and of creating a reality of concepts such as 'empowerment', health promotion and professional risk-taking. It is concluded that community development presents an opportunity for professionals to play a full part in the management of new forms of social care.

◾ Background

The community health professionals are discovering that their freedom to assess need and set general health targets is being restricted (see Chapter 6) both by the resource levels at their disposal and by a new form of management and control. If they are limited to providing predefined services for a priority group of 'those with the greatest need' then they may have to drop others to whom they now offer care and support. What will happen to those left out? Despite the pressure to limit their practice, professionals can and should seek new methods to bridge the gulf. Community development is one such approach, and it has the benefit of building new relationships between professionals and citizens, which is to their mutual advantage.

Community health professionals are beginning to realise that a raft of new questions have recently emerged concerning the way in which they practise. These arise from the changes of policy regarding the provision of health care within the framework of the NHS and Community Care Act 1990. None of these questions have easy solutions, and many practitioners may feel that they are being pulled in a number of contradictory directions all at once. This chapter does not seek to solve these dilemmas at a stroke, but health practitioners may consider that, if they seek a broader answer, they may begin to find a way through. This chapter addresses the nature of a number of concepts which are current today: empowerment, health promotion and professional risk-taking, among others. A fresh approach to the meaning of these terms, and how they relate to the new realities of practice, might call for some profound changes in the way the work is done. There is growing interest in the health professions in a form of social intervention known as *community development*. A number of writers have singled it out for special attention, and it has been referred to, obliquely, in a number of closely associated publications on promoting healthy communities. And yet it does not feature on the pre-registration training curriculum of any strand of nursing, nor is it developed much further in the post-registration syllabuses for community nurses (MacDonald 1993; McMurray 1990; Open University 1991). Interestingly enough, community development is a method of intervention not much favoured by the social work profession, either. This is despite the fact that much of the literature on the subject has been produced by people working directly in the social welfare field. Many of these are, in fact, social workers. So what is the mystery? What do health professionals need to know about community development, and can it work for them? We attempt here to describe what community development is, and what it is not. We also describe the circumstances under which it might be appropriate for health professionals to adopt it as their primary intervention mechanism.

■ Community development

Community development combines a number of elements which set it apart from other health or 'caring' professions:

- First, it constructs people primarily as citizens, and not as the objects of a health or curative strategy. Each individual involved is free to take part, or walk away, as is felt preferable.
- Second, it targets aggregates of people, or groups, known as 'communities'. These may be defined by their geographical location, but they may comprise or include those from any area who share common interests, or who experience common circumstances. A segment of any of these aggregates may constitute a 'community' for development purposes.
- Third, community development is about change, and not about defending the status quo. Many health and welfare interventions are limited in their intentions; to restore a form of stability, rather than advocating and ensuring that real change takes place.
- Fourth, the *development* strategy in the community is directed at empowering the citizens to engage in their own analysis, planning and delivery (or control over) of services/activities. The targets may involve structural changes in the relations between interest groups in society, in order that change objectives can be reached. It *will* involve the creation of citizen-based organisations which will be the vehicle for instituting these changes, either on their own, or in concert with other groupings.

- The professional is not in *control* of the process of social change (development). The role of the professional is to enable the change to happen through applying skilled intervention and supportive techniques such that the 'community', so defined, can bring about their own, preferred arrangement of the resources that are available to them (Clarke 1996; Jones and Tilson 1991; Midgley 1995). Building the community from scratch may be the first requirement of the intervention process (Henderson and Thomas 1987).

For many professionals, the suggestion that such a dramatic departure from established practice be introduced into their repertoire may appear to be a baffling, extraordinarily radical and unnecessary step. Many professionals are presently comfortable with their roles. The methods are clear, and their objectives are manageable. Training is geared to the attainment of these objectives, and the established pattern of activity is in keeping with the need for a profession's own stability and self-image. In any case, many of these suggestions for a new approach to practice have been advocated for settings outside the UK. They can, therefore, be of little relevance here. There are profound reasons why this outlook is deeply flawed, but if this opportunity for reappraisal is ignored then lasting damage to professional life in the health and welfare constituencies may occur. Here we attempt an analysis of the context as it presents itself today, and then show that the adoption of the community development approach might be the only feasible way forward.

■ Why should professions change?

The implementation of the NHS and Community Care Act 1990 has transformed the relationship between the health and caring professions and their client constituency. This is most apparent at the level of community nursing and health visiting, where the introduction of an arbitrary financial element into the planning and allocation of health services is setting limitations on their scope for intervention. The ability of professionals to manage, for themselves, the nature and extent of their relationships with those in need of their services, is now under pressure. The descriptive language which heralded these changes carried a two-edged message. Much of it sounded friendly enough. There can be little to argue with over such phrases as 'health gain', 'resource effectiveness', or 'people-centred' (West Wales Health Commission 1993). In the same vein, the notion of services which concentrate on those with the 'greatest need' appeared to be a humanistic and rational proposal when it appeared in 1989 in the White Paper, *Caring for People* (Department of Health 1989). In the event, this 'reform' proved to be a mixed blessing when it was discovered that it was to be combined with 'market mechanisms' for the delivery of care. This shift of approach recast the world of health care from a unitary approach into separated 'purchasers' and 'providers', not to mention trusts, charters, and work process recording (Mayo 1994; Wistow *et al.* 1991).

If health professionals in community nursing contexts are considered to be health care providers, and if their services are to be purchased by those that plan the health care of others, then their precise contribution to the care process will have to be measured and costed. The measurement of health care practice in terms of process, and the agreement, in advance, of its monetary value as part of a financial contract (Department of Health 1994:6), will surely restrict the amount of authority which health professionals can retain over the role for which they are trained. And yet, the retention of professional authority is a recommendation of the Department of Health, which also asks for innovation in the workplace (Department of Health 1993:7 and 14). The market logic of this situation is that supply will not exceed demand for very long. Health care professionals will be recruited according to their cost to the 'purchaser', and then restricted in their practice to only those classes of 'need' to which they are then referred. There will be limited scope for work outside this remit. It seems that there is a glaring contradiction somewhere between the expectations of the vocation of nursing, the scope of human suffering, and these growing restraints on professional freedom.

There is a need to create a balance between these competing forces. If professionals are to play a part in establishing that balance to fit with their own professional needs, then they themselves will have to play a much more assertive role. To be effective, they have to know what the options are, and be prepared to use those which are most appropriate. The framework offered by the *Health of the Nation* strategy (DOH 1992) identifies key areas for priority targeting under the reorganised Health Service. This includes certain high-vulnerability groups in the community, such as women, 'certain socioeconomic groups', and ethnic minorities. The follow-up publication, *Targeting Practice*, identified a regime of good practice to be promoted by the employers of health professionals working in the community (Department of Health 1993). This included building *healthy alliances* within, across and beyond the health sector. This gives professionals something on which to build.

■ Assessing need

In community care, the nature of need is now being determined centrally by the planning mechanisms of the (de)centralised local social service and health authority management. Financial boundaries are set, costing guidelines agreed and the allocation of community health resources made between the competing interests. The actual level of professional health care depends largely on the deployment of sufficient resources to meet the demands of 'assessed need' in any particular area. It is likely that this definition of 'need' will not coincide with that discovered by health professionals in their daily visits to the homes of their clients and patients. In addition, as community care becomes established and various bridging mechanisms expire, they are likely to find that the extent of their resources may vary from year to year. This will also arise if, and when, priorities change between national and local intervention targets. In this way, the degree of freedom to attend to the known needs of the community will rise and fall.

This may entail being able to respond to a particular assessed need in year one, being deprived of the resources to do so in year two, and then, perhaps, being able to resume support in year three. Some will get no care at all, if their 'assessment' finds them below a certain needs rating. This is a baffling and distressing prospect for the patient who, as a citizen, must wonder how the definition of a personal state of health, or need for social support, can be varied through the manipulation of completely arbitrary and disassociated factors. In addition, at the present time, there is little that the individual can do to respond, save to exercise an individual right through the Patient's Charter. In a recent ruling, the courts have decreed that public authorities have no obligation to provide a 'statutory' service if they lack the resources so to do (*The Times* Law Report March 1994). Health professionals are placed in a double-bind situation.

Their problem stems from the conflicting pressures that arise from their training, their status and their contractual position within the newly restyled services. Primarily, they have the right and duty to protect their role in the assessment and treatment of health conditions in the community. The parameters of the 'medical model', and the progress of medical science, have provided professionals with a great deal of justifiable faith in their methods, values and integrity. They have the expectation that if only they could get the space and the resources to function properly then they could alleviate most of the situations which so tax their scarce resources today. To some large extent, this right, and responsibility, is being eroded, or being made impossible.

■ Professional blindness?

There is another dimension to this discussion. This is the notion that the nature of 'cure', or health support, is a culturally determined one. In a recent visit to the UK, community workers from India remarked that they were confused by the apparent toleration, or even collusion, of our professionals with the conditions of poverty that prevailed in cities like Glasgow. They claimed that the questions surrounding poverty could not be solved by 'experts'. Rather, they had to be addressed by the people, themselves. But they were unable to do so, as they had been dispossessed by the social forces which consigned them to their poverty – dispossessed of the awareness and the power to act. All around the poor, it was claimed, danced the professionals, offering only palliative support. The complex health problems attached to poverty remain uncured, just alleviated temporarily. In 'professional' terms, however, the intervention was 'successful'.

These visitors were not preaching revolution, merely the need for a change of approach. It was the community as a whole that had to grapple with these deep-seated structural issues. Professional intervention brought no changes, just stability to the status quo. It was the duty of the professionals to induce a state of awareness in the community. This awareness was the necessary first step if they were ever to overcome the legacy of oppressive conditions which stood in the way of change (Freire 1972; Miller 1995; Smithies and Adams 1993). Ivan Illich described the 'disabling' professionals who, in conjunction with other élites, had usurped the role of the community in the articulation of social concern. This, in turn, inhibited the people from confronting their situation (Illich 1977). People are turned into mere consumers of the latest, and most perfect, products or cures. Despite claims that the 'medical model' has been left behind, and that 'processes' of alliance and dialogue have been brought in to replace it, professionals have failed to break free from their traditional approach to practice, even to a limited extent. The consolidation of power has led, instead, to the glorification of professional expertise, and the inhibition of social innovation (Illich 1977 : 27–38).

In his recent study of research on the subject, Watters emphasises the need for much closer attention to details in applying professional skills and judgement (Watters 1996). He describes the experimental interventions in the mental health field (the government's Mental Health Task Force projects), where members of ethnic minorities were first involved in innovative, short-life projects in order that the specific needs of these groups could be addressed. It had become apparent that large numbers of compulsory admissions to hospital, and evidence of dubious diagnoses, were creating victims of whole communities because of cultural differences and pre-judgements by health professionals at every level. Targeted assessments were made of communities and groups, and developmental methods used to create fresh and responsive structures to provide community support and appropriate service mobilisation. Once the approach had been developed and consolidated by the end of the project period, the whole experiment was dropped. Mainstream services were unable to accomodate flexible methods, and, anyway, the demands of the'mixed economy of care' were absorbing everybody's effort. The emergence of a health intervention model which showed signs of actually working was nipped in the bud. This a stereotypical example of the 'residual need' gap being recognised and ignored.

■ WHO sets the standards

The UK is a member of the World Health Organisation. The Alma Ata *Declaration on Primary Health Care*, the Ottawa Charter *Health for All by the year 2000 and Beyond* and the WHO European Regional Office for Environment and Healths *Healthy Cities Project* all are initiatives which fall under its auspices. The WHO sets the international standards for health attainment of its subscribing members and it has consistently pursued a line which values citizens' participation in, and shared responsibility for, their own health. Thus: 'The people have a right and a duty to participate individually and collectively in the planning and implementation of their health care' (Alma Ata *Declaration*, 1978, I. IV, in Bryant 1988). Or: 'Health promotion is the process of enabling people to increase control over, and improve, their health' (WHO 1986).

It depends on how an individual's rights are defined, but in the UK the new policies of community care seem to have driven a wedge between the abilities of the people to realise their 'duty' to play an active part in the health process, and their 'right' to health care that meets their true needs. The limitations of parliamentary democracy consign their role to being the passive recipients of a system of care rationing, overseen by an echelon of health professionals who are hired by the hour.

There is scant evidence that at least one of the action recommendations of the Forty-first Assembly of the WHO (Riga) is being realised in Britain (art. V):

> Empower people by providing information, technical support and decision-making possibilities, so as to enable them to share in opportunities and responsibilities for action in the interest of their own health. Give special attention to the role of women in health and development. (Text quoted in full in Bryant 1988 : 137)

Thus, the professionals find themselves facing more than two ways at once. They have power and skills which give them the best possible insight into the needs of the people for whom they are trained to serve. They subscribe to a value system which transcends the boundaries of their own national service. They are searching for a way in which to attain their vocational objectives. But they remain tied to the health and community care delivery system which denies them the freedom to act according to their talents. Which set of interests is of the greatest importance? Is there any way in which a balance can be restored? Is there some way in which they can modify their approach to health issues which will enable them to comply with the new agenda of the employers, allow them to maintain their vocational desire to protect the health interests of all those with need? One way of seeking a way forward is to consider the implications for practice of the term 'empowerment', which is used to define good practice.

> Health services should fully involve communities: in defining problems, about which communities often have intimate knowledge; in decision-making, in which communities have both a right and a responsibility.... Health personnel must learn how to organise and support community involvement... People should participate in determining what kind of information and education they need for their individual community development. (Bryant 1988 : 79)

The statement above is from the affirmation of the Alma Ata *Declaration*, at the WHO Conference in Riga, in 1988. In community care the term empowerment has been described as '(participation)... to the maximum degree possible in the choice to be made about how his/her needs will be met' (Smale et al 1993 : v). The Health Education Authority commissioned another definition:

> At the heart of health promotion is the empowerment of communities, their ownership and control of their own endeavours and destinies, and their direct involvement in the process of change. (Adams 1991 : 142)

The significance of these statements, and the ensuing absence of any policy follow-up, reflects the reluctance of those in power to admit the community into the policy debate, especially over the setting of criteria for need and the level of care to be provided. The fact that there has been no professional clamour for the adoption of intervention methods which actually bring lasting alleviation to social problems reflects the relative weakness of the professions. It also reflects the inappropriateness of training for, and professional ignorance (which may, in part, be deliberate) of, a successful practice method which can be used to address the structural causes of bad health (poverty, isolation, bad housing, illiteracy, lack of social cohesion). These are 'social illnesses', which the 'needs-based' community care strategies are supposed to somehow get around (Thomas 1995). The apparent clarity of vision that comes with the 'needs-based' model is only displacing lesser needs which will return to put pressure on health professionals in the future. They need to be addressed now, and not left to fester. Professionals are using a model of resource allocation which fixes the social relations of care firmly within a financial framework and which precludes flexibility. But no impact can be made on these issues without strategies that bring *actual* social change. To achieve this, the professional model needs to be modified. The power and skill of the professional must be applied at another pressure point in the health system. If there are not sufficient public resources to meet the needs of those who fall below the assessment threshold, then the community itself must be brought into the equation. If community resources are to be utilised, they have to first be organised and mobilised, and, when they are, then they are free to give or withhold their consent to be so engaged. Achieving both these objectives requires some of the skills of community development.

Health professionals might draw on the outlook of a related group which also has a close interest in community care. When the Joseph Rowntree Foundation commissioned two eminent social work professors to consider the place of 'empowerment' in the range of social work practice, the following emerged. First, they described the nature and function of empowerment as lying within a very narrow perspective, amenable to a restricted role for social workers as compliant participants in a needs-based community care, as described above. Second, they expressly ruled out a social change dimension, and deliberately avoided a single mention of community development as a means of achieving their form of 'empowerment' (Stevenson and Parsloé 1993). If the structure of social welfare professionalism presented in this report is accepted by the social work profession, then the dispossessed, the critically disabled, the poor and the mentally distressed have nothing to fear. They can look forward to a continued, social-work-assisted life with palliative support, which will fluctuate not according to professional guidelines, but on the whim of governmental priorities. If professionals are to tackle this challenge then they will need to reappraise their model of professional intervention

■ The power to define need

Empowerment is a word which links both the exponents of radical politics, and those who expound total quality management (Howkins 1995; Morgan and Murgatroyd 1994; Wallerstein 1993). It maximises the resources available and it enlists the energies of citizens in the achievement of wider, social goals. We admit that it does throw up some awkward questions of its own. For example: does empowerment mean the power to act against the prevailing structure of health and community care services? Does it mean that citizens (health care professionals are citizens, too) might seek a definition of need which does not conform to a politically determined scale of resources? Might 'they' seek to require that services be planned and delivered with their own stamp upon them? Are these questions, in themselves, good for the future of community care?

■ Community development for a professional future

What is at stake in this? It could be that each question above might produce an ambiguous answer. If 'enabling' a self-help support group to emerge is good practice and valued health promotion (Ewles and Simnet 1985), then who draws the line to cut off sponsorship if the group turns into a political pressure group? What if the response of such a group is to demand responses from the system which are beyond its remit? Is the nature of professional assistance for such mechanisms limited only to those of the 'coping' variety? It is at this point that the professionals will have to consider taking risks, or, rather, putting more faith in their capacity to develop the trust of the community. They need to spend some time in dialogue with its members about the real nature of the care which they strive to provide. The demand for excellence is ranged against the sheer impossibility of achieving it (Wilson 1995). A sense of realism needs to be injected. In a world of diminishing resources, 'work measurement and evaluation', *value for money*, and the contract culture, what place can there be for professional 'success'? If the pressure for achieving ever-narrower goals within an ever-narrowing resource base is to be sustained then it is time for health professionals in the community to seek out, actively, the only source of support that they have not, as yet, exploited – the community itself. There will be professional risks involved in this. It may be, that to be between the rock of a limited role, within boundaries of contracts and creeping de-professionalisation, and the hard place of 'consumer' dissatisfaction, potential scandals resulting from enforced neglect of certain categories of need, professionals may be required to take some risks. Otherwise, the situation may get out of (professional) control. A good example of this has been highlighted by Bryar and Fisk, which was a 'low-tech' response to the more general needs of community health. A 'community health house'was established to act as a focus for community health services and for the members of the community to apply local knowledge, neighbourhood cultural interpretation and indigenous effort in managing the social and individual tensions which arise in the management of health care (Bryar and Fisk 1994) By seeking to exploit the real needs and the power of citizens, health care professionals may play an 'important role in enhancing and mobilising their clients' for their own survival. There might be substantial health benefits in this process as well (Stewart 1993).

Community development presents an opportunity for professionals to play a full part in the management of new forms of social care in the community, in partnership and as experts, rather than as dispensers of elixirs of wonder. They will have to develop new methods and negotiate fresh relationships with the people who rely on them for very different forms of service today. They are unlikely to be given the time or the space by their employers to do this, unless they make the necessary moves within the care system to force change upon it. It will also take time for health professionals to digest and react to these thoughts. Every day that goes by will find the prevailing approach more and more entrenched, and the room for manoeuvre restricted. The politics within health care professions are complicated enough, and will delay many changes (Howkins 1995). It is down to those on the patch, who know the true nature of need, and who see it on a daily basis, to take the initiative.

Chapter 9

Rights and rhetoric of practice: contradictions for practitioners

Tim Stainton

■ Introduction

This chapter highlights contradictions in the rhetoric of community care policy, and is concerned that practitioners should understand their own limitations in relation to redressing the ambiguity of social constructions such as 'choice', 'rights' and consumer power, and its negative effect on service users.

■ Background

It is difficult today to find an article or policy document on community care without encountering florid rhetoric on consumer choice, empowerment and rights. The stated objective of the 1989 White Paper *Caring For People: Community Care In the Next Decade and Beyond* (Department of Health, 1989), the precursor of the NHS and Community Care Act 1990, is to help 'people lead, as far as possible, full and independent lives...to stimulate public agencies to tailor services to individuals' needs...[and to]...promote choice as well as independence.' In countless articles and guidance on assessment social workers are exhorted to 'work in partnership with service users' and to 'empower the citizens to be fully involved as an equal partner' (Smale *et al.* 1993:7). Admirable and desirable as these goals may be, there is little in the way of structural safeguards or guarantees. Social workers in local authority social service departments, who have the primary responsibility for community care assessment and case management, will often find themselves embroiled in a host of contradictions and conflicts which prevent them from forming any real partnership with service users or from giving them any significant choice in how their needs are defined or met. As one commentator notes, there are 'Tensions between the objectives of self-determination, independence and the need to ration services' and 'the problem of maximising choice for individuals and their carers at the same time as taking into account ... "the local availability and pattern of services"' (Beardshaw 1990:1).

In this chapter we consider some of the contradictions between the goals of choice, rights and consumer power and current community care policy and practice. While some suggestions on how these contradictions may be remedied will be given, the main purpose here is to highlight the contradictions so that practitioners can both understand their own limitations within the current system and begin to take steps to counter the negative effects these have on service users. Before we begin, though, a brief look at what consumer rights and power actually mean will help to frame our examination of policy and practice.

■ Autonomy, rights and citizenship

The subject of rights is complex and fraught with arguments over their nature, application and basis. A comprehensive review of these arguments is beyond the scope of this chapter; however, a general position on what constitutes a right will be useful in framing our consideration of the structural contradictions faced by social workers working in community care. Most of us are familiar with the idea of 'human rights' as basic entitlements we share with other human beings by virtue of our status as 'persons'. Similarly, most of us share a basic understanding of the idea of civil and social rights. One of the key distinctions between the two (although they will often overlap) is that civil rights are encoded in and enforced by specific political entities such as a nation or the EU and are set down in specific legal instruments such as the American Bill of Rights or the recent Disability Discrimination Act 1995 in the UK. Rights of these latter types have been much more influential in social policy in the US and Canada than in the UK. However, citizens in general and consumers of social services in particular are increasingly characterising and demanding service as a matter of right rather than as a charitable or paternalistic handout from a benevolent state. This distinction between what is often called the 'best interest' or the 'welfare principle' and the liberty principle, that is the principle that a person's liberty or individual freedom is the paramount consideration, is central to the debate on the role of social welfare and indeed all areas of state action. It is, however, a mistake to view the two as exclusive poles. A balance of the two is achieved through a concept which should be familiar to all social workers and social work students, that is, the notion of personal autonomy, which is gaining a central place in the debate on the proper role of the state and social policy.

Autonomy can be understood as the capacity to formulate *and* pursue plans and purposes which are self-determined. In other words, this goes beyond what is often called 'negative freedom', that is merely the absence of restraint, and encompasses the notion of 'positive freedom', that is, having the means to act. Another significant aspect of this definition is that it is concerned with capacity rather than outcomes. Certain outcomes will become important if they preclude further autonomous action, but they become important because of their impact on capacity, not because a particular outcome is disliked.

Autonomy is a familiar concept to social workers. What is often ignored, however, is that it is central not just to social work but also both to the function of the state and – therefore social policy – and to the derivation of rights. Simply put, rights can be conceived of as those basic goods which provide the basis for autonomous citizenship. Some of these will be explicitly codified, however the vast majority will be implicit in the structures, including social policy structures, which regulate relations between citizens and between citizens and the state. The idea of equality is also important here. In democratic societies this infers a basic equality of opportunity, or more specifically, of basic capacity, for autonomous citizenship. This implies the idea that equal treatment will not result in equal capacity. Hence, differing levels of state-supported health care to different individuals can be justified on the basis of what is required to provide a basic level health necessary for autonomous action. In other words, 'equal treatment' does not satisfy the claims for equal citizenship, because different people require different types of treatment to achieve the same basic capacity. A person who requires a wheelchair for basic mobility can claim the 'right' to that wheelchair on the basis that it is a basic need in terms of equal capacity for autonomous action.

This perspective requires that as we shift from a welfare-based to a rights-based approach, social policy must be concerned primarily not with protecting the welfare of the individual, but with enhancing their autonomy. While social work has long held self-determination as a central value, little regard has been given to how the structures themselves impede or restrict the autonomy of the individual or groups, or, conversely, how social welfare systems and structures can be designed to enhance and safeguard the autonomy of the person. Social policy has traditionally focused on outcomes or ends. The concern has been with number of residential beds, of day centre spaces, and so on. While the ends themselves have changed, the focus on defining the ends have not. When services have changed, they have changed in relation to changing perceptions of a collective rather than individual definitions of need. For example, institutional provision for people with learning difficulties was seen as the 'best' means of meeting 'their' needs throughout the 1950s and much of the 1960s. When this began to change to group homes provision it changed on the basis of 'what was best for this group'. In other words, services and structures to support people were defined on the basis of a collective welfare principle, that is of what was 'best for them'.

This focus on ends, or 'supply', is also reflected in funding structures and mechanisms. Traditionally the services have been funded directly by the state and it has been up to the individual, their family and perhaps a social worker to access that service. In practice this has often meant waiting lists, stigma and, in the end, that the user is forced to accept what is on offer. If their needs are not met and there is no alternative service then the person has few options. This process leaves the service provider as the *de facto* definer of needs and how best to meet them. If the person does not fit then they are either shown the door or choose to take their chances elsewhere, or else are left to make do with an inappropriate service. There are few structural means for the person to influence the nature of the services. We can call this 'structural paternalism' in that no specific person is dictating what is in one's best interest but rather it is the structure which inherently makes this determination.

The issue for community care then is not simply a question of more resources or services or of 'allowing consumers to participate'. What is required is a restructuring of the system to a 'demand-based' model in which the individual has control over both the means and the ends of determining legitimate needs and the nature of the 'ends' provided to meet those needs. The challenge for community care practice and policy is to create a structure in which individuals can articulate their demands directly *and* which allows the state to adjudicate and meet legitimate claims in a manner which does not in itself infringe the autonomy of the person. In essence, what is required is a structure within which an ongoing dialogue on legitimate claims can occur between the individual and the state, as the representative of the collective. Further, once claims are established, there must be means to satisfy those claims in ways which the individual chooses, which are to a degree self-regulating, and which allow both the individual and the state to monitor and adjust as needs change.

In practice, then, what this position implies is that the consumer should be able to define not only their needs but also how those needs are to be met. The role of the local authority as represented by the social worker is not to define what a person's needs are or how they are to be met, but to negotiate with the individual on what needs are legitimate claims against the state and to support the person in meeting those needs deemed legitimate in ways which are acceptable to them. What defines a need as legitimate is (1) whether it is required to protect or promote the person's autonomy and (2) whether the need is consistent with ensuring that the individual has an equal capacity for autonomy as any other citizen. In other words, the issue is not whether the state can afford a particular service requested, but whether it is consistent with what any other citizen can reasonably expect in terms of autonomy. So I may wish to have an unlimited access to funds, and that would surely enhance my capacity for autonomous action, but the claim is not valid because it would give me more than what most other citizens can reasonable expect. On the other hand, if my claim is for services which only ensure my equal participation in the community, for example a wheelchair for basic mobility, or a personal care assistant to help with daily living tasks which I am unable to do directly for myself, then the state can only deny that claim if it denies that it is a reasonable expectation for any citizen in our community to have, given the relative economic position of our society.

■ Rights and structure

As noted in the introduction, current community policy and practice seeks to enhance consumer choice and empower the client to live as independently as possible. Although no explicit right to community care exists, rights to services, assessment of need and specific forms of support such as benefits exist in various health, social security and community care legislation. The question is whether within the current structure individuals rights can be sufficiently promoted and protected. The social worker involved in community care as a service planner, assessor, or care manager has an ethical obligation to respect the client's individuality and self-determination. However, they also have a legal obligation to their employer, the local authority and personal interest in maintaining their work and career prospects. So long as the individual's interest and the interest of the local authority coincide then there is no difficulty; however, only the most naïve among us would suggest that this is always or even normally the case. The social worker, from a purely structural perspective, is in a clear conflict-of-interest position. In this section we consider some of the key areas of conflict.

☐ Care management

Care management is now the system within which most local authorty (LA) social workers function. Although there are wide variations in forms and structure, most share the same basic characteristics. (see Beardshaw and Towell 1990; Rose 1982). Case management generally refers to a mediating structure which provides a variety of planning, assessment and service coordination functions. As the name suggests, it is essentially a model for more efficient management and coordination of existing resources and has more to do with the drive for efficiency of the 1980s than the current demands of consumers for a more rights based approach. Although there is no statutory requirement that the case management function be carried out directly by the LA, this is generally the case. Located within the 'system', it is structurally – and frequently ideologically – connected to the funders or providers of services, as opposed to a neutral position, or allied to the consumers of service (Rose and Black 1985:74–7; Salisbury, *et al.* 1987 : 19–20).

While there is much value in many of the techniques and general approach of case management – such as better coordination of services, a more individualised approach to planning and assessment and improved efficiency – the basic approach remains structurally, and in practice, a more efficient form of welfare paternalism. Challis and Davies (1986), in their research study on a much-replicated 'enhanced case management model' where the case manager had considerable control and flexibility in the determination of need, allocation of funds and selection of resources, demonstrate, although inadvertently, the basic conflict between this model and an autonomy-based system. After detailed analysis of a range of indicators of quality of life and well-being, they note that 'there were significant positive changes in favour of the community care scheme'; there were however, three exceptions: diet, anxiety and *felt degree of control over own life*. (1986 : 157).

This result should not be surprising given the extraordinary degree of power and control invested in the case manager. A clear example of this can be seen in the following quotation. The same authors note that 'A particularly difficult task was trying to balance the client's ambivalent feelings of need for care and drive for autonomy'; addressing this 'problem' they state with approval that:

Goldfarb (1968) has described as 'pseudo-independent' behaviour that which renders the person unmanageable because of their failure to accept help, advice or relief. He suggests that in such cases help can only be given by establishing 'even in a disguised form . . . some dependence in a protective relationship'. (Challis and Davies 1986 : 47).

This is consistent with Abramson's (1989) findings on the work of Adult Protective Service workers in the US, where paternalism was generally favoured over autonomy.

This is not to suggest that the 'welfare outcomes' of this model are insignificant, or that there is not much of value which could be retained; the problem stems from a lack of structural safeguards which protect the potential autonomy of the person against conflicts of interest and abuse of power through a lack of balance. As Dowson notes, there is a conflict of roles and a high degree of professional control inherent in the case management model (Dowson 1990 : 20–1; see also Peck and Smith, 1989).

■ Funding

There is also a serious conflict of interest where the case manager and/or the assessor is also a representative of the funder of services. Traditionally we have funded the services directly and the consumer has had little power to determine the nature of the service provided or if and when they can access it. This has resulted in a failure to serve many people, in ways appropriate to their needs or even at all. It has also precluded any real accountability to the person or influence the individual can have on the service or the system. Finally it has led to a very fixed system, with little flexibility or portability of funds between services. This type of funding also increases dependency and stagnation within the service system (Salisbury *et al.* 1991: 11–12; GARI 1991 : 50–2; Bosanquet 1984 : 9–13).

One means of increasing choice and flexibility currently advocated in is the notion of 'devolved budgets'. A variety of models have been discussed, such as the 'budget holding case manager' in the Kent model, and the splitting of purchaser, commissioner and provider roles (DoH 1991c). The devolution stops at the case manager, however rather than devolving down to the individual. The Independent Living Fund has been one of the rare examples of consumers having direct control over their own service funds. This may change with new Direct Payments Bill which came into force in April 1997, though the scope and effectiveness of this is as yet undetermined. Most authorities now have some form of purchaser–provider split; in some cases this means the case manager as purchaser of contracts with a specific provider, while in others the purchase is made *en bloc* by the LA and the case manager simply negotiates for a 'space'. While this certainly lessens the conflict from when the LA was assessor, funder and provider, in many cases the split is merely an internal device where the case manager negotiates with other LA departments or cost centres. Where budgets are devolved to the case manager or the team, a further conflict arises between clients, because the case manager must decide which of their clients get scarce resources, so that in essence they have to 'rob Peter to pay Paul'. The block purchase arrangements are also limiting, because they are purchased not directly to meet the needs of a specific individual but rather for a predetermined general need. In other words, for the consumer such arrangements here do not differ significantly from when the LA developed large services for a general population without any attempt to ascertain specific individual needs.

A further problem with these arrangements is their limiting effect on choice. By and large it is the LA which determines who will be contracted to provide services, and the consumer is left to choose between them. This is further limited by availability and charges. Even if a consumer identifies a service which they feel will meet their needs the new system does not preclude a waiting list. The introduction of user charges will also limit many people's choice, with most authorities unwilling to pay beyond social security rates or to contract with services which are perceived as more expensive. A final problem with these systems is the lack of portability. As it is the LA who contracts with the provider and not the individual, the service user has little power to change the nature of that service or to change providers once they begin receiving service. While this is not precluded there is no incentive for either the LA, the case manager or the provider to encourage change, and for the consumer change can often mean lapses in service, time-consuming reassessment and delays in implementation.

While these approaches recognise the need for a separation of powers and seek to facilitate consumer choice, the user remains a marginalised actor with no real power to control their allocation of funds. As noted by Peck and Smith (1989 : 1502), the conflict of roles where assessor and budget gatekeeper are mixed creates a serious disincentive to meeting individual needs. This problem becomes even more acute if the devolution is merely within a single entity such as a health authority or local authority.

If people are now to assert a 'right' to service, then for that right to be at all meaningful they must also have the ability to actually get service, and to strongly influence its nature, which means control of needs determination and funding approved for the meeting of those needs. As Salisbury *et al.* note: 'The most compelling way to ensure system flexibility, responsiveness and accountability is for government to allocate funding to the person served rather than to programmes, services or agencies (1987 : 13).

■ Assessment

The LA has a statutory duty under the NHS and Community Care Act 1990 to provide an assessment to anyone in need of community care services. They also must, under the recent Carers (Recognition and Services) Act 1995, assess the ability of the carer to continue to provide care if requested to do so. Assessment is the key gate-keeping activity of the LA. While the LA is responsible for ensuring an assessment is carried out, it does not have to do the assessment itself (HMSO 1989 : 21), though in practice most retain this function.

The conflict here is an obvious one. The LA is going to be largely responsible for arranging and paying for any needs which are identified and are provided for under current community care legislation. They have then a serious material interest in minimising assessed need regardless of the degree of goodwill or professional commitment on the part of the assessor. This is not to suggest that willful underassessment of need is a common practice, but simply to point out the structural conflict inherent in this arrangement.

In its report, *Community Care: Choice for Service Users*, the House of Commons Social Services Committee (1990a) describes the potential problems with assessment and case management. The contingency of consumer involvement is noted with disapproval, as is the potential for conflict of interest if the case manager is both responsible to the person and the authorities budget. A local authority social services director is quoted referring to the need for rights of representation which, he notes, 'are necessary because at present too much power rests in the hands of the bureaucrats... The balance of power needs to be adjusted towards disabled people' (p. xiii).

There is much talk of involvement and partnership with consumers in the assessment process, but this is, technically, purely rhetorical. While LAs are encouraged to involve users and carers and to take their wishes into account during assessment (DoH, 1989 : 19) there is no duty to comply with their wishes. Under current legislation the LA has only a statutory duty to invite health and housing authority representatives to participate if these services are deemed relevant to the specific individual. In their study of assessment and community care the Social Services Inspectorate found serious gaps between the rhetoric and reality of user and carer involvement (SSIa 1991). Again the fear of creating a very powerful class of manager/professionals is a very real one with little in the way of structural safeguards. While we may strive for equality in the assessment relationship, the reality is that the power is virtually exclusively the preserve of the LA assessor.

As the quote above suggests, representation in the form of an independent advocate or assessor would serve to redress some of the power imbalance. However, in practice, the use of independent representatives or advocates is rare (SSI b1991 : 25) There are no rights to representation in the current legislation. The Disabled Persons (Services, Consultation and Representation) Act 1986 provided for the appointment of an 'authorised representative' by the disabled person, or in the case of children, their parents. These representatives were to be included, at the disabled person's discretion, in meetings and discussions regarding service provision, and were to have access to all information that the disabled person themselves would have access to. However, the government decided not to implement the sections of this Act on representation, or those on the right to ask for service, despite repeated calls to do so from the House of Commons Social Services Committee (1990a:xii–xiii; 1990b::xxvi–xxvii).

A final point on assessment concerns the use of standardised forms for different types and levels of assessment. These, it is argued, ensure fairness and even-handedness. Unfortunately, they also mitigate against highly individualised assessment which takes into account particular needs and wishes. While in an ideal situation the form will be an outcome of the assessment, too often the form drives the process itself. While the current rhetoric is about needs-led assessment, the factors discussed above strongly weight it towards a resource-based assessment, albeit with an extended range of choices in most cases. What is the point of a needs-led assessment if service outcomes will not be related to particular needs so much as to resources available?

■ Participation

One means of trying to bridge this gap between the rhetoric and the reality of consumer rights and power is through what has become known as 'consumer participation'. The immediate problem with this approach is that 'consumer participation' rarely means consumer power. Indeed, as McGrath (1989 : 72–3) points out, many who participate in the process feel their views are disregarded. Numerous problems with this approach have been noted, such as the lack of knowledge about the system and difficulties in attending meetings (McGrath 1989), 'tokenism, economic constraints, poor communication and the diversity of views of 'consumers' (Valentine and Capponi; 1989). This raises the broader critique that such a strategy often essentially requires consumers to become 'pseudo-professionals', and to deal with general needs rather than their own or their family member's needs. Croft and Beresford make a similar point, noting that 'User groups are increasingly conscious of the problem of being sucked into the operational and organisational detail of agencies, when what they actually want is more control over their own lives and their dealings with them' (Croft and Beresford 1989 : 15–16).

One obvious problem with this approach is that the inherent assumption that any given group of consumers speaks for all consumers within the defined category. In this regard, this approach goes little beyond the older system of local authorities or health authorities determining what services a defined group of people may require. A further problem is that consumers groups are often dependent on the local authority for grants to function, giving the authority a large degree of influence over who is the 'voice ' of the consumer. While this does not imply that consumer organisations should not be involved in service planning, it is important to recognise the limits of this approach and not confuse it with consumers' rights or power.

■ Conclusion

This chapter has tried to point out some of the contradiction between the rhetoric and the reality of consumer rights and choice with which workers in community care will have to contend. While it paints a rather bleak picture of the current scene, there are hopeful signs on the horizon. Laying out an alternative structure is beyond the scope of this work, but a few suggestions can be made (Stainton 1994). A key issue is to increase the separation of powers between the various elements in community care such as removing the assessment and case management function from direct local authority control. Systems such as the service brokerage model, or the independent living model, offer hopeful directions. As noted, the advent of direct funding is a welcome development, although it remains to be seen how far this will be extended. It is interesting to note that few of these types of changes are precluded in current legislation; rather, the LAs have chosen to retain the power invested in these functions directly.

For the worker in the field this may represent a depressing picture. While it is important not to minimise the constraints, the committed worker can seek to redress the imbalance of power through a true commitment to consumer rights. Practically, they can actively seek to involve advocates and personal representatives and ensure that consumers and their supporters are fully informed as to the process and its limitations. Creativity in using funding and finding support outside normal pathways will foster a more individualised approach to both assessment and meeting needs. More importantly, they can advocate within their own system on behalf of individuals, and for overall structural changes. Finally they must be honest with themselves and their users regarding their abilities, their limitations and their conflicts.

Chapter 10

Professions and school nursing

Irene Webber

■ Introduction

This chapter discusses the role of the school nurse in relation to community health care for children of school age. A historical perspective illustrates how school nursing, like all of the health care professions, began its development in the second half of the nineteenth century. Initially the service grew out of philanthropic and voluntary efforts to improve the health of children. Legislative policy to formalise these philanthropic efforts followed, as the advantages of a healthier child population were acknowledged by society. Thus the care of well children in the community began. It will be argued that throughout its history school nursing has contributed a valuable service to the community. Additionally, the service provided has been of a dynamic nature, changing its focus and interventions to match the changing needs of society. The philosophical principles which are currently adopted by the service to direct its goals are examined and said to be robust (HVA/UKSC 1992). Yet, despite the soundness of principles which facilitate a community development approach to school health, the effectiveness of school nursing interventions is being marginalised by selective primary health care strategies and the 'market'-orientated policies of the New Right. It is suggested that a comprehensive service for schoolchildren should be firmly located in preventive care strategies, but for this to take place attitudes and strategies need to change.

■ From private to public responsibility

Historically, the responsibility for the health and social care of children lay in the private sphere of home and family, or when this was inadequate with charitable and philanthropic organisations. Throughout the latter decades of the ninteenth century, increasing state intervention occurred which placed parental responsibility into the more public sphere of surveillance and accountability. By the early twentieth century growing public and political concern over the health and education of children (and mothers) culminated in policies and legislation which sought to provide a measure of state-sponsored health and social care to working-class families. Collective child care or care for children in the community soon increased public awareness of the poor health of children.

Social policies which covered the training of mothers, the institution in schools of compulsory physical training and team games, and the provision of meals to poor (but not pauper) children, were enacted before the outbreak of war in 1914. In the post-war period concerns over the general state of education and health of the working class once again re-emerged, following the medical evidence of the state of recruits. As a consequence, the Education Act 1918 (the Fisher Act) was passed; it provided medical treatment and inspection for primary school children and medical examination for those at secondary school. In addition treatment for visual problems, dental defects, minor ailments and enlarged tonsils and adenoids was provided. Throughout the inter-war period various policies aimed at improving child health were passed, but the advent of mass unemployment, economic crisis, and increasing social division in Britain meant that some children remained grossly disadvantaged. In the 1939–1945 war children from deprived industrial areas who were exposed to the public sphere as wartime evacuees were still found to be suffering from ill health, to be verminous and to have severe behaviour problems stemming from years of political neglect and educational deprivation (see Table 4.4 for details of state policies and children).

Over a period of seventy-five years, although children's health was brought into the public sphere, and care in the community was made a reality, care 'by the community' was targeted only at those who were obviously living in poverty. Consequently, a situation arose which could be likened to an iceberg. In other words, those children who appeared to be in the direst need (previously defined as paupers) may have recieved a residuum of health and social care, but the vast extent of need remained unidentified. A public and political disinclination to directly link social factors to health and educational achievment has meant that the prime responsibility for childcare continues to be placed firmly in the private sector for the majority of children. This dichotomy of responsibility still appears to pervade service provision. Care in the private sphere is always subject to social rationalities of what supposedly responsible parents should provide. Care in the public arena is rationalised to be merely that which is essential to prevent 'significant harm'. While the failure in provision by parents is deemed to denote individual moral ineptitude, on the other hand, failure in provision by the state simply denotes a duty to ensure that parents uphold their responsibility. It would appear, therefore, that the rules for public and private spheres differ according to the source of provision.

■ Developments in school nursing

Section 48 of the Education Act 1944 required all local education authorities to provide regular medical inspection at appropriate intervals for all children, and to make arrangements for free medical treatment when necessary. Specific duties of the school nurse were to include identification of children suffering from disability, blindness, partial sightedness, deafness, subnormality, epilepsy, physical handicap, speech deficits and delicateness. However, in the case of school children, despite the evidence of the past the comprehensive health care provided by the 'rolling in' of the state was short-lived. By 1959 regular health checks for all children were stopped and a system of selective inspections was instituted because of rising costs. In 1976, at the time of the Court Report, HMSO (1976) school medical inspections had fallen by 25 per cent (Nash et al, ·1985); this gives the impression that there had been a constant retreat in provision from the public sphere. Since the National Health Service Reorganisation Act 1974 the school health service has been integrated into the NHS and controlled by the DHSS. Local area health authorities became responsible for the coordination of all health services for children. Following the 'Patient First' reorganisation of 1982 the responsibility for school health services was transferred to district health authorities. There are, however, apparent disadvantages with current systems, as it is often the case that district areas are not coterminus with the boundaries of local education authorities. Local education authorities retain responsibility for assessment of children in need of special education, but despite some positive developments services may not be forthcoming because of a lack of resources.

■ Current perspectives

The whole history of child health therefore appears to be one of rather motley progress. Despite the 'enlightenment' of the nineteenth-century which, on the basis of the philosophies of Locke and Rousseau, revolutionised child education, child health appears to have remained on the boundaries of public care. It would appear that the ultimate responsibility for the health of children lies with parents; only when they fail to meet their children's needs does the state intervene (DOH, 1989). At the end of the twentieth century children still appear to have many health needs which are not successfully met. According to Nash et al, (1985) children are often brought up in box-like homes or high-rise flats which exacerbate family stress; they have few safe play areas, there are many families who have difficulties in 'making ends meet', and 37 per cent of families with children have half the average income (Kempson 1996 : 2). All of these factors play an important part in the determination of the state of children's health (Kempson : 40). In relation to health problems there are also a number of other concerns. For example, although there is evidence that the rate of pregnancies among under-sixteen's in England and Wales is falling (see Table 10. 1), in comparison with other European countries , such as the Netherlands where sex education is part of the early school curriculum, rates of teenage pregnancy in the UK remain high.

Other problems which challenge the health of teenagers are alcohol consumption, drugs and smoking. In all instances health education directed at individuals is proving to be lacking in effectiveness. Many problems are underpinned by

Table 10.1   Rate of pregnancies

Year	Rate of pregnancies
1990	10. 1/1000
1991	9. 3[a]
1993	8. 1/1000[a]

[a] Latest year for which figures are available.

Source: Office for National Statistics 1996.

structural and social deficits evident in today's society. These deficits are to some extent increased by expectations of material benefits which have been confounded by a reversal of economic trends, and many adolescents may have nothing to look forward to other than unemployment

■ Challenges for school nurses

School nurses are therefore faced with many challenges. Current interest in promoting healthy lifestyles and preventing ill health and disease in children is stimulated by an appreciation of the cost to society both financial and in skills lost – of premature ill health and death. Knowledge of morbidity and mortality rates in other countries of the European Union and the developed world leave no room to doubt that there is considerable scope for improvement in health care in the United Kingdom. School nurses in the United Kingdom may appreciate the need to make increased collective efforts to ensure that children remain in good health.

It is believed that a child in good health has more chance of gaining the full benefit from their education and of reaching their employment potential if health status is maximised. The Court Report 1976 (Nash 1995 : 17) suggested that: 'The connection between health and education is one of the most important aspects of paediatrics.'

■ School nursing and social contexts of health

The significance of the social context of health has been accepted by a series of community nursing reviews over the last two decades. The Cumberlege Report (DOH 1986), for example, recommended using the neighbourhood or community as a focus for assessing and addressing the health needs of populations. In particular, school nurses believe that children are an integral part of any functioning community, and that responding to their health needs by targeting the school population will both reach a large number of individual children and also reach into their families, which are the 'heart' of the community. It is reasoned that success in health matters is more likely when the community is tuned into health concerns and where supportive services exist to reinforce health messages. School nurses are convinced that their practice has the potential to make a substantial impact on the health of the nation. They believe that they have the skills to help school children develop a positive sense of health and that they can stimulate participation in health gain activities to teach children how to use available health resources appropriately and effectively. Further, school nurses perceive that by involving adults (parents and teachers) in their health care interventions for children these groups may also be stimulated to make improvements in their lifestyles.

Given the nature of their role, school nurses are convinced that they adopt a public health or proactive perspective to health care. In many ways the role of the schoolnurse complements that of the health visitor; although the target populations are different, both concentrate on health promotion and the prevention of illhealth. Because of this phenomenon the principles of school nursing within a community setting have been claimed to be the same as the principles of health visiting, namely

- Searching for health need.
- Stimulating an awareness of health need.
- Influencing policies affecting health.
- Facilitating health-enhancing activities

(In the case of school nurses the community is defined both by the school population and by its catchment area.)

The legitimacy of this claim has been endorsed by both the United Kingdom Central Council for Nurses, Midwives and Health Visitors (UKCC) and the NHS Management Executive (Health Visitors' Association 1992). However, in applying these principles to practice school nurses may encounter resistance from a number of sources because the principles expose structural factors affecting health status both within the school community and its wider environment. Nevertheless, school nurses are determined to show that previous reliance on medical models of health is limiting. The use of a broader concept of health, one which includes educational social and environmental issues, is seen as ultimately more productive because, as Seedhouse (1986) states, 'People are part of their whole surroundings, like cells in a single body.'

The culture and expectations of the population determine how they respond to health issues. Social context must therefore be seen as an integral part of health and health needs assessment. Failure to recognise these aspects will result in the provision of services which fail to meet the real needs of people. It is therefore important, that school nurses should be identified as a profession 'which sees clients in their social context' (Standing Nursing and Midwifery Advisory Committee HMSO 1995 : 6).

Many believe that their aims can be achieved through application of those principles identified by the health visiting profession in 1967. Thus structural deficits in state provision as well as individual behaviour will be made explicit, but how to take a more proactive stance towards the identification of health needs is a challenge for school nurses.

■ Searching for health needs

When searching for health needs, school nurses like other community nurses need to use some form of assessment. The compilation of school profiles has become increasingly widespread; these are a collection of epidemiological and social data which characterise health status within a school population and the wider environment.

> Profiles of schools and the surrounding communities can be used as an informed basis for the purchase of relevant services especially as they conform to local, current information about the needs of specified care groups. These should then supplement the long term epidemiological data usually asked for by health authorities and others to assess priorities and determine services. (Association and United Kingdom Standing Committee for Health Visitor Tutors HVA/UKSC 1992)

A properly researched and analysed profile would obviously be an invaluable tool in the setting of health priorities, the planning of objectives and the implementation and evaluation of nursing input. However, its value is dependent on whether it is accurate in its identification of local health need and whether resources can be directed to addressing the needs found. If, regardless of the profile findings, 'others' perceive the work of the school nurse to consist of traditional health screening, and surveillance activities which do not relate to the priority health needs of the specified population, then school nursing practice is devalued and it will fail to realise its potential to make a substantial impact on the health of the future nation. The improvement of health cannot take place in a medical vacuum, yet it is often the case that 'new contracts' for nursing services provide purchasers with what they require, in this case the targeting of health gain areas identified in the *Health of the Nation* White Paper (DoH 1992) rather than providing for the specific needs of individuals and families and communities. If contracts are not questioned then the likelihood of long-term health gain will be marginalised by structural deficits.

According to Hall (1996) a properly constructed health profile, that is one which records social as well as health deficits within a defined community, will identify objectives for the service over a period of time and include markers of achievement and of non-achievement along the way. Nursing staff will know where those activities are leading and so will the pupils and staff and families served. This clear understanding of the purpose of intervention is of great importance, especially since the NHS reforms have emphasised the need for professionals to measure the outcomes of their service interventions. The profile, then, as well as recording health and Social deficits within a community also incorporates an assessment of health and social needs and a plan of action. Therefore the profile can be recognised as an invaluable tool which overtly displays nursing skills and activity. As well as describing pretty accurately the health status and needs of school attenders, the profile may include information classified as sensitive, for example the teenage pregnancy rate and/or some indication of risk-taking behaviour such as drug and alcohol abuse, smoking and social and structural deficits. Which have an adverse affect on health. Thus the profile has the potential to be viewed as a double-edged sword, on the one hand it can be seen as a valuable tool which has the potential to expose factors detrimental to health, and to make explicit the worth of nursing activity Whilst on the other hand it may be a threat to head-teachers and school governors who may not be best pleased if such rates are higher than average in their school especially if parents have access to this information. However, the school nurse who values the principles of preventive practice has a responsibility to make unmet needs apparent to those who have the power to influence intervention in social and structural factors, which adversely influence the lives and health of children. A comprehensive profile, which clearly details the health status of pupils and the health-promoting nature of the school setting, may therefore be a 'hot potato' which challenges the school nurse to place professional responsibility and accountability above considerations of organisational demand and loyalty.

■ Stimulate the awareness of health needs

School nurses have the expertise to inform parents, teachers and others of the normative needs of schoolchildren as they pass through various developmental stages. They also have the skills to determine possible 'extra needs' for vulnerable pupils; for example an increased number of children are entering school having been diagnosed as having asthma or diabetes or other chronic illnesses and disabilities such as cystic fibrosis. More children with enhanced or special needs are now attending so-called 'normal' school, and the school nurse will have access to knowledge about their conditions and can contribute to decisions which facilitate their potential in the education setting. Specifically, resources or adaptations to the environment to enhance quality of life for these children may be advised. The school nurse allied to the special school must also highlight the normative needs of children so placed; for example an adolescent with spina bifida or deafness needs to be aware of sexual health issues or substance abuse issues no less than any other adolescent.

To be effective school nurses must have knowledge of societal issues which directly affect their target populations if they are truly to offer a needs-related service. Often recognition of societal issues may challenge the '*status quo*'; for example, the number of children living in poverty in the UK is about 37 per cent at the present time, and, as was shown in a recent Rowntree Foundation study, childhood poverty is often accompanied by poor health, poor diet and poor housing (Kempson 1996 : 40). The school nurse must be able to identify vulnerable children and trends in risk-taking and/or health-damaging behaviours and she needs to adapt her working practices to accommodate the needs of these clients.

Unfortunately, 'new management' dictates characteristic of community care organisation strategy determine that resources may be allocated only on the basis of activities or tasks that can be counted. For example, check lists of screenings and so forth may be the only evidence of school nurse activity. Such a limited indicator of inputs can not reflect the work that school nurses do or should do. To address many of the social issues outlined above, school nurses should develop indicators of their real activities, that is the whole process and emphasis of their work, which is individual- and community-focused. In addition they must be able to demonstrate that their practice is evidence-based so that it achieves measurable outcomes of relevant health gain in the target groups. These outcomes should also acknowledge links between health, education, needs, fulfilment and resource input. To be effective, then, school nurses must participate in the construction of indices of deprivation relevant to their schools, and in decisions made about how to address the resulting health issues. This type of intervention often challenges the bureaucracy of organisations, whose limited methods of information gathering conceal the true nature of the roles of many professional workers. Therefore there is a potential for the *status quo* to be disrupted and for the role of the school nurse to be controversial.

■ Facilitating health-enhancing activities

Whether the school nurse works in an inner city comprehensive of two thousand or more pupils, or in a more rural setting – perhaps visiting thirty or forty small rural schools – the principles of school nursing can be utilised to deliver an appropriate and cost-effective service. Whether she is helping teachers to interpret and deliver national curriculum topics or offering a screening and health surveillance service, these principles provide a range of strategies from which to choose appropriate interventions. It might be argued, however, that this is an aspect of school nurse potential which needs to be further exploited in education and training, so that the school nurse can offer a less directive service and encourage more participation by consumers in order to address structural inequality. The school nurse may need to increase her confidence and skills, to develop group or community approaches to health maintenance and lifestyle changes if current health and social care strategies are to be combatted. A knowledge of varied health promotion strategies, especially using a multidisciplinary community approach in health initiatives, could improve the confidence and service delivery of the school nurse. This means that as well as the traditional health promotion activities, school nurses should involve themselves in activities such as lobbying the local authority to provide facilities which enhance health and social well-being. Above all, school nurses should remain active in identifying structural inequalities if they are to prove that their services are effective in the long term. It is important that children should not be given mixed messages by encouraging them to attend clinics only to be met by negative staff attitudes, questionable confidentiality, and services which their parents cannot afford. The objectives of this type of school nursing will be unlikely to be achieved unless they work in collaboration with other community practitioners. Fragmentation of service provision, such as that typified by changes in health care policy provision, may seriously hamper school nurses' attempts to improve care for children in community settings. For example, many fundholding GP practices are now undertaking health care provision for children. It is feared that medical provision will ignore socio-structural problems which severely marginalise the attainment of holistic health.

■ Influencing policies affecting health

School nurses have the ability to influence the way the school nursing service is delivered, and the potential to provide quality proactive and effective health services (HVA/UKSC 1992). However, their expertise can be wasted, and they can become frustrated and demoralised, when their role is perceived to consist only of routine tasks of health surveillance and screening, which, though of some use, do not address the priority health issues of school-aged children or of the wider community, particularly when the issues are caused by sociostructural inadequacies.

The Polnay Report (British Paediatric Association 1995) contains a detailed review of the literature on the school entrant examination and on school health in general. It concluded that the yield of significant new physical abnormalities at this examination is generally small, as anything of note had usually been detected by the pre-school health surveillance activities of primary care personnel. The third Hall Report (Hall 1996) suggests that nurses who work in the community should carry out less universal screening and more targeting of specific health care needs so that the nature of health care intervention is more proactive and preventive, and can be focused on those groups which currently are affected by unequal provision.

■ Management responsibilities for future service development

The development of market strategies in health care strongly indicates that there is a need for school nurses to be involved in 'commissioning contracts'. A detailed profile previously discussed could be an informed basis for the purchase of services to meet the needs of school populations (Health visitor Association and UKSC 1992). Commissioners of health care have a responsibility to assess the health needs of their population and to purchase health care to meet those needs (Royal College of Nursing 1993). Working in new and innovative ways, and meeting the challenges presented by commissioning, will enable school nurses to achieve a paradigmatic shift in the focus of their practice from the provision of care to the facilitation of 'care of the community'.

In this way school nurses could influence commissioners to contract for a comprehensive school health service through the construction of a national framework for the school nursing service which could include guidelines on minimum standards of care permissible. This national framework could then be complemented by services tailor-made to serve the specific needs of local populations. Thus school nurses could advise purchasers on a safe and appropriate service, on standards to be achieved, and on methods of monitoring and evaluating the care of school communities. In this way school nurses could make an important contribution to the achievement of primary health care.

The reorganisation of primary care services, including the extension of the responsibilities of professionals to include preventive strategies in the process of their work, is an important feature of recent NHS reforms; for example, GPs have been encouraged to adopt a leading role in primary care by including health promotion and preventative interventions in their services. To facilitate change, general practitioners were enticed by financial incentives to become fundholders and therefore purchasers of those services deemed appropriate for their patients. Extra payments were provided for preventative care in specific targeted areas.

Thus GP-led primary health care teams have become the focus of primary care services and in many instances are providing the greater part of child health care. How school nurses relate to these teams is of very great importance if they are to make a specific contribution to primary health care for children. School nurses must have knowledge of health service organisation in order to promote school health services, and to ensure holistic and equitable health service provision which takes account of both social as well as medical needs of the communities the serve. In short, school nurses should seek to play an increasingly high-profile role in community health care.

■ Current and future perspectives of school nurse practice

School nurses are the main health professionals to have contact with children of school age. Their potential for affecting the perception of children with regard to health issues is enormmous. They can deliver the right message in the right way to the right population at the right time. They can also evaluate their interventions. However, it appears that as both professionals and providers of a service school nurses are seriously undervalued at the present time, and this affects their potential to deliver a systematic, needs-related service which could make a significant contribution to public health issues.

In the new, post-Fordist organisation school nurses in the United Kingdom do not necessarily share a common role. Their professional qualifications may be as varied as their status and their grading Though most school nurses have had some form of post-registration education and training, there is no mandatory post-registration qualification prerequisite of school nursing practice (as is the case for health visitors and district nurses). Job descriptions vary from county to county and trust to trust. Access to equipment, resources and post-registration education is as varied as are working conditions. Whereas some schools make do with a cupboard and a corridor, others have a nurses' room with up-to-date facilities. Employment patterns for school nurses are highly varied also; for example, they may be employed by the NHS or by education authorities (who would decide their duties quite separately from NHS and nursing guidelines). School nursing may in some instances be an add-on bit to another role; for example in some areas health visitors also carry out school nurse duties. Many school nurses also work part-time hours, which means they barely have time to complete health surveillance activities, so that proactive health interventions are out of the question.

Increasingly, school nurses are becoming peripatetic, especially if employed by the NHS as opposed to the education authority. This can be disadvantageous, because the nurse is not based within the community she serves, but it can be of benefit, for example, where the school nurse serves the 'feeder' infant and junior schools plus the local comprehensive. In relation to this kind of model there is more continuity for the child and family; despite the numbers of pupils served, the nurse has a greater chance of knowing children as individuals and how their family dynamics are structured. Additionally, nurses have the opportunity to care for a larger section of the community. Unfortunately, at the present time there is a possibility that the number of pupils on caseloads is so great that any school nurse can do no more than those tasks dictated by her job description, for example heights, weights, vision and hearing screenings, immunisations and, if she is lucky, some school entry health reviews and subsequent health questionnaires. In this kind of scenario, where time and manpower is short, it is likely that the real health needs of pupils – as would perhaps be evident from the reviews and questionnaires – may never be addressed.

Employing authorities, searching for cost savings, may well leave vacant posts unfilled for varying lengths of time. The remaining practitioners feel morally blackmailed into completing 'number-crunching' tasks and quickly become stressed and demoralised. Enthusiasm and commitment to develop and deliver evidence-based practice may wane in the face of trying to cope with day-to-day chores.

> Thus it can only be concluded that although the government reforms appear to support a primary-care-led NHS and care in the community, all too often Trusts view community health services, which include the school visiting service, as a soft touch for cuts. (Carrell 1996)

School nurses should be an integral part of community health promotion campaigns to tackle significant modern threats to the public health for example poverty, unemployment, homelessness, social exclusion and marginalisation as well as coronary heart disease, substance abuse, HIV infection and Aids, and they should help spearhead national campaigns aimed at improving children's health and attempt to reduce the child accident rate and/or the undesirable teenage pregnancy rate.

■ Conclusion

School nursing is too good a community resource to allow it to dwindle to a collection of checklists of specified screening and surveillance procedures while the real health concerns of pupils are not addressed. Under current policy strategies there is a danger that all that is conveyed to school children is a negative view of health services when what is needed is to stimulate and sustain an enduring interest in health and lifestyle issues. Long-term national health goals will not be achieved unless we respond to the specific needs of young people. To this end, the government has produced a strategy, *Health of the Young Nation* (DOH 1996), but it will only be effective if social as well as medical needs are recognised, and professional autonomy is upheld.

Both the Court Report (DOH 1976) and the Warnock Report (HMSO 1978) highlighted the need for a strong effective and well-managed health service adequately resourced in both funds and personnel in order to give children a better start (Nash 1985). An adequately resourced, educated and focused school nursing service will do just that, provided that school nurses are allowed the professional autonomy they require to provide the service that they know is essential for the health of a young nation. An adequately resourced, educationally aware school nursing service could play an important role in bringing about change.

Chapter 11

Professions and community nursing

Anne Kelly, Gaynor Mabbett and Renata Thomé

■ Introduction

This chapter provides a 'snapshot' of how the roles and services of various specialties of community nursing are affected by changing policy. It is presented in three parts: the first discusses the role of the health visitor or public health nurse, the second the role of the district nurse or home care nurse and the third the emergent role of the nurse practitioner which, it is suggested, possibly represents an independent reaction to perceived patriarchal oppression of nursing by the medical profession. It is concluded, that the 'way forward' for community nursing is the development of autonomous nurse-led services which will work in partnership with GPs and other professions.

■ The professional practice of health visiting

From a historical perspective the profession of health visiting has traditionally occupied a somewhat hybrid position within the profession of community nursing, because the focus of its professional practice has embodied both medical and social domains of health care. Formal health visiting expanded in the early years of the twentieth century, having emerged as part of the philanthropic response to situations of extreme poverty and deprivation in communities. It appears that as expansion of the profession took place a dichotomous orientation of professional interest may have developed. A focus on medical type interventions and reactive care typified the public image of the role, but the private and subjective interpretations of the role still focused to a large extent on social welfare concerns and may have always been at variance with the public image.

There can be no doubt that the developing health visiting profession, strictly governed by medical officers of health, was strongly influenced by a patriarchal medical profession, which had adopted the concepts of Cartesian dualism. These concepts, according to Turner (1992), were based on the principal assumption that there is no significant interaction between mind and body. Therefore these two realms were seen as separate and distinctive disciplines. 'The body became the subject of the natural sciences including medicine, whereas the mind was the topic of the humanities or cultural sciences' (Turner 1992:32). This division of the medical sciences allowed medical practitioners to treat the problems of the body, with minimal reference to social or psychological causes of defects. Other carers were expected to adopt a similar view. Thus, given that the dominant metaphor of biomedicine was that of the body as a biochemical machine, and that of the patient being the owner of the machine, who brought it for repairs when it failed to function, it was not surprising to recognise that all health professionals could be conveniently lumped together as monitors of machine performances. Health visitors were delegated a special place in the order of these events: their role was to provide an early warning system of non-functioning in the private sphere of the home, so that the public spheres of work and duty were only minimally disrupted. This role might be compared to that of the overseer of factory workers, whose job it is to identify and remove unsatisfactory workers from the assembly line, so that their part of the product does not contaminate the finished article.

In the real scheme of things, however, many health visitors appeared to maintain the philanthropic altruism of the pioneers of their profession. Thus a spirit of welfarism continued to permeate the professional education, training and practice of health visitors, and the profession maintained its interest in structural causes of ill health. This brief overview and analysis of health visiting practice argues that although a dichotomy regarding the public and private images of health visiting has persisted, in recent times emphasis on welfarism in health visiting practice has re-emerged. This has happened despite the fact that the specific skills of health visitors are in danger of being negated by the demands of medically orientated purchasers, and a market-driven service (Symonds 1997). The extent to which this characteristic of interest in social welfare is allowed to dominate professional interventions may, unfortunately, still be affected by the patriarchal dominance of the medical and managerial professions (see Chapter 7), However, according to McClelland (1996), the profession is showing definite signs of being more self-directive in relation to identifying need and undertaking social intervention.

■ Historical perspectives of the health visiting role

McClelland (1996) remarks on the invisibility of women in social history. Similarly Hogreffe (1975) observed that it is difficult to obtain first-hand evidence of women's social and economic lives, unless they comprised the 'great or the good'. In terms of the health visiting profession there can be no doubt that such a situation applies. Lewis (1980s) for example notes that in relation to health care, while policy-makers were interested only in mortality statistics and the moral responsibilities of individuals, mothers concentrated on socio-structural concerns such as the need for housing, fertility control and employment. With these concerns at the top of their agenda mothers welcomed health visitors as they perceived that the profession gave their concerns more status. Condemnation of the profession appeared to be the remit of intellectuals who, exercising high moral and '*laissez-faire*' principles, refuted the right of the state to interfere with the rights of the individual (McClelland 1996).

Unfortunately, because the history of women and their work in the public and private spheres has mostly been recorded by men it remains invisible, and attempts to expose the real nature of events merely rely on subjective interpretations of historical events and records. For these reasons functionalist views of health visitor activity may be more prevalent than the real nature of their interactionist activity.

■ Various viewpoints

Origins of health visiting practice are usually located in the formation of the Manchester and Salford Ladies Sanitary Reform Association in 1862, which was a response to the appalling public health status of the day. Early practitioners were described as middle-class philanthropic volunteers, but in 1867 'respectable' working women were officially employed to teach hygiene and mental and moral health and to provide social support for working-class mothers (Report of Inter Dept Committee 1904). Official speculation on these events usually comments on the fact that middle-class 'do-gooders' were unsuccessful in their work, because they failed to communicate with mothers; in particular, their methods of communication (namely leaflets) were unsuitable for their illiterate clientele. Alternative, more common sense historical perspectives are, however, rarely discussed – such as the fact that the severity of situations encountered by early health visitors called for more extreme, intense and practical measures than leaflet distribution.

Other accounts of the health visiting profession echo similar dichotomous viewpoints to those already mentioned. For example, Symonds (1991) suggests that health visitors might be depicted as 'busybodies', intent on extending the public sphere of state control into the private sphere of the home, in order to improve the health of the nation's children. Davies (1988) has mixed views regarding the origins and intent of the service; both philanthropic and 'inspector' images are invoked, but it is conceded that efforts to reform behaviour were invariably based on friendly persuasion and a desire to improve the 'lot' of women. Dowling (1973) substantiates the view of Davies (op.cit.) by describing how the true forebears of health visitors, the 'bible women' employed by local missionary societies, were forced into welfare work by the extreme deprivation they saw around them. McClelland (1996) also supports the view that prevailing social conditions encouraged early health visitors to fight for improvements for all women across the social divide.

Images of the origins of the health visiting profession are therefore diverse; there is a lack of consensus as to whether the role is that of a 'busybody', a social welfare worker, a 'policer', or a 'friend' of mothers. Neither is it clear how health visiting became a branch of nursing, except that many health visitors were coincidentally nurses, and eventually all health visitors were based in public health departments under the control of doctors (Dingwall *et al.* 1988).

■ More recent perspectives of the health visiting role

While the typical orientation of other practitioners in health care has been towards cure or regeneration of the body-machine, the aims of the health visiting service are located in broader concepts of health, which incorporate prevention and well-being. Health visiting has adopted a proactive focus on health care, as well as a reactive orientation; thus it recognises the social as well as the biological aspects of well-being. Basch (1990 : 204) defined this perspective of health care in the words of the Primary Health Care documents of the WHO as

> Essential health care based on practical, scientifically sound, socially acceptable methods and technology made universally accessible to individuals and families in the community, at a cost the community can afford. It forms an integral part of the country's health system, is the central function and main focus of overall social and economic development of a community; and it is the first level of contact of individuals, families and the community with the national health system, bringing health care as close as possible to where people live and work. Thus the characteristics of such interventions constitute the first elements of a continuing health care process.

From this perspective, the Cartesian style of medical interventions is exposed as not being as effective as previously thought. According to Illich (1976 : 20–1) improvements in life expectancy over the last century have often been the result of social interventions rather than medical advances. Improved housing, nutrition, public services and cleaner environments play a more important role in preserving a healthy population than do medical interventions.

Whereas it may have been the case that as social health improved with the 'rolling in of the state', the necessity for health visitors to be immersed in social welfare concerns declined, nevertheless this aspect of the professional role did not sink into oblivion. The Jameson Report of 1956, (MOH 1956) for example, defined the main function of a health visitor as that of a health educator, and the 'rediscovery' of poverty in the late 1950s and 1960s presented health visitors with a challenge to resurrect their social welfare role. In response the Council for the Training and Education of Health Visitors (CETHV) was established in 1962 (Owen 1983), its remit being to establish higher educational standards, and to ground the epistemological knowledge base of health visiting in the social as well as the medical sciences. Health visitors remained in the employment of local authorities until the National Health Service Reorganisation Act 1974, and therefore had the freedom to exercise the social and public health aspects of their role. Following the 1974 Act, health visitors were employed by area health authorities, and became 'attached' to medical practices. For the second time in their history Cartesian logic was emphasised through patriarchal control, this time by general practitioners. This development might well be interpreted as a serious setback to the profession in terms of its struggle to maintain equilibrium in the social as well as the medical area of health. As an additional setback, the 1973 Act in adopting the recommendations of the Mayston Report (DHSS 1970) placed a greater emphasis on management of the health visiting profession. Thus health visitors were subordinated for the first time to hospital nurses with no experience of the community, or its needs. This subordination led to constraints on the expanded professional role of health visiting, which led to increasing conflict between the CETHV and other nursing institutions who wished to control health visitor practice and their training. In a bid to strengthen the position of health visitors the CETHV (1977) attempted to clarify the distinctiveness of the role of health visiting by defining the principles which underpinned its practice; these were:

- The search for (physiological, psychological and social) health needs at individual, group and community levels.
- The stimulation of an awareness of health needs.
- The influence on policies affecting health.
- The facilitation of health-enhancing activities.

Analysis of these principles reveals the facilitative nature of the profession, its continued focus on social rather than medical orientation of health, and the political nature of its orientations. Attempts by the CETHV to protect the identity of health visiting were overpowered, however, by the goal of other nursing institutions who were seeking to professionalise at all costs. Thus the Nurses, Midwives and Health Visitors' Act 1979 brought the health visiting profession as well as all other branches of nursing under the control of the United Kingdom Central Council (UKCC), a statutory regulatory body for the nursing, midwifery and health visiting professions governance.

It is interesting to reflect on the willingness of government to curtail the social interventionist style of health visiting practice at a time when the WHO (1978) declared the need for enhancing primary health care. In retrospect, however, the burgeoning emphasis on *laissez-faire* policy and a rising interest in global capitalism may have had much to do with these events.

■ Current aspects of the health visiting role

In retrospect the Nurses, Midwives and Health Visitors' Act (1979) was an achievement for the professionalising movement of all branches of nursing. The act has generated a larger professional base, and has made progress in equating the governance of nurses, midwives and health visitors with that of doctors in key respects of autonomy, registration, specified training and standards of practice (UKCC 1992, 1994). All nurses now have the opportunity, if the

UKCC continues to support its professional aims, and chooses the right professionalisation strategies (Davey and Popay 1993), to define the specific goals of their practice unambiguously. Glazer (1974) suggested, that true professions, if they aspire to professional status, must apply science, which consists of cumulative empirical knowledge about the means best suited to achieve chosen ends. The health visiting profession therefore has the greatest opportunity in its history to clearly define its ends, the preventive and social welfare aspects of its practice.

In 1993, the Health Visitors' Association publicly declared that 'The day to day work of health visitors with individuals and communities equips them to identify the grassroots issues that affect health' (Health Visitors' Association 1994).

The profession is concerned with international evidence on inequalities in health which reveal that people who live in disadvantaged circumstances have more illness, distress, disability and shorter life spans (Benzeval *et al.* 1995). Prevention of such injustices is seen as a legitimate aim of the health visiting profession. The intention of the profession to fight injustice was made clear in the professional publication *Action for Health* (Health Visitors' Association 1994), a response of the profession to the challenge of the Heathrow Debate (WHPF 1993) (a paper which invited the nursing profession to make decisions on strategic issues governing their future). In this response the HVA made the objectives of the profession clear; it was stated unequivocally that health visiting is firmly located in public health and that it is committed to identifying factors which adversely affect health at both individual and population levels. For this reason the health visiting profession states its intention to work collaboratively with other agencies, in order to encourage policies which prevent disease and promote better health.

■ The public health role

Williams (1985) suggested that the time is right for public health interventions, since modern-day epidemics are preventable, public and corporate business companies are concerned about escalating medical care costs, changing demography is pressurising health resources, there is a growing disenchantment with current health systems, and inequalities in health are maintaining undesirable levels of mortality and morbidity. In Williams's view, strong public health leadership is needed to provide direction for the development of a health care system in which prevention of dysfunction and disease are primary concerns. The specialties of public health and community health nursing have major roles to play in bringing about the new order; there is a great potential for a new 'flowering' of these respective specialisations. Potential for development is dependent, however, upon the extent to which leadership in public health nursing is able to prepare and support nurses. It is argued that the future of nursing in community-based practice will be determined by the extent to which the profession takes seriously a population-focused approach to practice. Thus it becomes important to distinguish between public health nursing or health visiting and other community health nursing roles.

Although community health nursing is defined as working with individuals and clients, while keeping the community perspective in mind, the major objective being the health of the community. Public health nursing is defined as having 'a focus' on public health sciences; specific characterisations are:

1. Its focus on populations that are non-institutionalised.
2. Its predominant emphasis on strategies for health promotion, health maintenance and disease prevention.
3. Its concern for the connections between the health status of the population and the physical, biological and sociocultural environment.
4. Its use of political processes to affect public policy as a major strategy for achieving goals.

Thus public health nursing practice or health visiting can be seen as a systematic process by which:

- The health and health needs of a population are assessed in collaboration with other disciplines in order to identify sub-populations at increased risk of social deprivation, as well as illness, disability or premature death.
- A plan for intervention is developed to meet those needs, which includes effective use of resources available and those activities which will contribute to health and its recovery.
- A health care plan is implemented effectively, efficiently and equitably.
- An evaluation is made to determine the impact of intervention on the health of the population.

To achieve these ends the health visiting profession will make use of the fact that they have a special legal position, and their own register, which was protected by the Nurses, Midwives and Health Visitors Act 1979. In order to facilitate public health practice the profession will rely on the principles of practice (CETHV 1977) which were re-evaluated in 1992 (HVA/UKSC 1992). There are already many empirical examples of health visiting successes in improving the 'public' health.

■ Constraints to change

Since the *Health of the Nation* paper was published in 1992 (DoH 1992), hopes for the revival of good public health strategies have remained high. However, the internal market in health care remains a continuing threat to the implementation of such strategies. NHS managers are intent on making cuts in community health services, as a means of reaching their 3 per cent efficiency target laid down by the government and achieving waiting list targets for institutionalised care. This strategy makes a mockery of WHO reforms and signifies a lack of government concern for the 'health of the nation'.

In addition, the future of the NHS is still being contested between those who want to see the health service run for profit and those who defend the NHS as the core of the welfare state. The strategies of profiteers are placing many stresses upon all professionals who work in the community. Worst of all is the recognition that the most vulnerable of client groups are bearing the penalties of undesirable strategic planning.

There are, however, counter trends and strategies at work. For the first time in a number of years regions are increasing numbers of health visiting students. This is a sign that those responsible for the delivery of primary care recognise that a shortage of health visitor professionals can limit primary health care service delivery. It is also evidence of the efficiency of the professions' political influence on decision-making at government level. More significantly, there is evidence of public as well as professional emphasis on the need for quality care rather than cost-cutting. The health visiting profession is determined to move from the uncertainties of today towards a new agenda, one that places at its heart the health of the nation, and the delivery of proper preventive care for all members of society (Health Visitors' Association, 1994). If this is the strategic aim of the profession, can anyone doubt that the private focus of individual practitioner care will be any different?

Health visitors are hopeful that at last they will be allowed to expose the true nature of their profession! This hope is also shared by the members of the profession of district nursing, who perceive that they have much more to offer than is currently recognised by purchasers of services.

■ The district nurse/home care nurse

The traditional elements of district nursing illustrate a breadth of role and function for the district nurse; they incorporate relatively complex, sophisticated assessment and evaluation skills as well as seemingly simple practical skills and tasks. The precise nature of the district nurse's role is, however, currently subject to a number of forces including professional, social and political pressures which do not necessarily result in complimentary effects regarding professional status

■ Professional pressures

Recently the NHS has attempted to move from a sickness to a health-focused service following international trends (WHO 1985). If district nurses are to secure health gains for local populations then they will need to examine different methods of working including collaboration with other members of the primary health care team. Bryar (1994) suggests that community nurses need to develop specific skills in order to achieve a new professional focus, which represents a shift from the individualistic to a more collective perspective while concurrently maintaining an intervention role. These skills include the ability to assess a community's health needs by working with the community and using public health data, health promotion skills and the targeting of services. Such a position is congruent with the Ottawa Charter's philosophy (WHO 1986) of enabling, advocating and mediating in relation to health choices. These role attributes necessarily require a relatively high degree of critical appraisal and informed decision-making by practitioners.

However, operating within a medical model requires a relatively lower degree of practitioner autonomy, because individuals are directed to comply with pre-scribed instructions, which has the effect of making their role more reductionist and task-oriented. The literature supports these conclusions and suggests that district nursing practice is currently predominantly medically oriented and mini-mally oriented to health promotion (Gott and O'Brien 1990). In consequence, practitioners are less able to respond independently, in keeping with the health-oriented approach. The greater weight or value ascribed to medical intervention by district nurses amounts to a virtual exclusion of a health-promoting role for a majority of district nurses. Ross (1990) suggests that the main reason for this perceived deficit is that district nurses are constrained within their practice by a management ethos which supports a task-oriented, target-driven service. District nursing therefore finds itself in a dichotomous position. The day-to-day culture imposed by medicine and management promotes reductionist approaches, while simultaneously professional and educational pressures point to virtually opposite philosophies and values in relation to health and holism. Such a system seems to be designed to facilitate target-driven, outcome-determined, prescribed care packages. In short, the system supports an individualistic perception of health and illness which is counter to that envisaged by the WHO Alma Ata declaration (1978) and to professional inclination.

■ Social and political pressures

A number of demographic trends, including an increasingly ageing population, more single-parent families and more people living alone, have affected needs and demands in health services. A consequence of the NHS and Community Care Act (1990) has been a differentiation between health and social care needs. Many activities associated previously with district nursing and health care tend now to fall within the remit of social care, for example giving patients a bath, helping them out of bed to dress, or helping to put them to bed. Specific health care activities include assessment and evaluation of need by district nurses and increasingly the management of quite sophisticated technological methods of care, such as the use of Hickman lines and nursing patients post-operatively. Schemes such as 'Hospital at Home' illustrate the increasing variation and complexity of nursing activities undertaken by district nurses in the community. In practical terms, these ways of working lead to a focusing of the district nurse's input which is directly analogous to a medical model, better described by McDonald (1993) as the 'engineering model'. Also, since time and input is focused upon particular (illness-related) interventions with the patient, time available for broader health-related practice is compromised, as is time for working with other family members or carers. (Additionally, care is becoming more fragmented with a number of different individuals and/or professionals such as home care assistants and private agency personnel visiting homes where previously the district nurse alone visited and undertook all the care required.) Managers and GPs have encouraged throughput of patients in line with meeting targets and conforming to policy initiatives, in other words the commodification of care. This is likely to lead to mechanistic, fragmented ways of working which are counter to the principle of holism.

This fragmentation of care is occurring in an environment undergoing unprecedented changes in terms of skill mix and the staffing of services, brought about by post-Fordist models of health care organisation. The Value for Money Unit (NHSME 1992) suggests a skill mix of 26 per cent staff at G or H grades and 65 per cent at D and E grades in the district nursing service (1992). This formula is based upon a task analysis of district nurses' work and ignores the professional focus on the importance of collective and preventive intervention; it is, therefore, significantly limited in respect of the breadth of function or role of the district nurse practitioner (Royal College of Nursing 1992). The skill mix review of district nursing occurred at a time when there were new challenges for those working in community nursing. These were the demographic trends referred to above, GP fundholding, increased day surgery and early discharge, as well as new demands from a better-informed public. Conclusions of this review typify the utilitarian approach adopted by service providers, and the lack of consultation with district nurse professionals regarding the holistic processes of care provided. In addition to these insults to professionally led service provision, consumerism has characterised recent times, as evidenced by government enthusiasm for producing charters which outline standards and expectations for the public. The Patient's Charter and changes in primary health care initiated by the 1990 GP contract have been reinforced with a focus on the primary-care-led NHS. In relation to the practice of district nursing, practitioners are constrained by such charters, because they set limits of 'time and motion' and these are capable of marginalising the real quality of care which can be offered to clients in the community. All of these challenges demand a highly skilled district nurse, who is capable of juggling professional and organisational responsibilities. The team leaders in district nursing are therefore faced with compromise and new ways of working. The role is becoming less interventionist, with a reduction in direct patient care and more responsibility for delegation, teaching, facilitating and auditing.

A criticism levied by district nurses of current situations is that their role as clinicians is being compromised, with administrative elements becoming more prominent. Clinical activities such as bathing and applying dressings are being undertaken by support staff, and there is an emerging body of evidence which suggests that although this may save resources in the short term, in the longer term care is compromised and costs are increased (Bagust *et al.* 1992; Helt and Jellinek 1988; McKenzie *et al.* 1989; Øvretveit 1992; Pearson *et al.* 1987; Prescott 1993).

Apart from strategic assaults on issues of professional practice, assaults of a different nature are also affecting the professional status of future recruits to the profession. Reduced numbers of district nurses will have an educational impact, since pre-registration nursing programmes (Project 2000) aims to prepare nurses in both community and hospital. The numbers of students in community settings has increased at a time when appropriate supervision is made even more difficult by new demands and role changes for district nurses, in addition to a manufactured shortage in professional numbers.

■ Hard inputs

The quasi-market ethos of the reformed NHS requires that health commissioners and providers, including GP fundholders, secure the health needs of local populations, contract the relevant services and evaluate the care provided. These activities are set against a background of meeting 'policy targets' in ways which are proven to be clinically effective (Welsh Office 1995). The dichotomy referred to earlier between task-orientated medical-style provision and holistic care is reaffirmed by these arrangements which lend themselves to a quantification of discrete, clearly measurable outcomes of nursing interventions. These forms of data are more likely to be of interest to GP fundholders, who may direct district nurse employees to work purely in a task-oriented way in order to achieve personal targets. Since 1 April 1996 GP fundholders have been able to buy the services of the district nurse directly from the health authority and may, as a result, be more prescriptive regarding expectations of patient care. Some of the work of district nurses is concerned with 'hard inputs' such as giving injections, dressing wounds and pressure sore care. Such activities lend themselves to quantitative investigation, that is, they are clearly amenable to numerical classification and analysis. Therefore, they are well suited to target-driven approaches and means of evaluation. However, interventions of these kinds are only a minute aspect of the process of care which is provided by the district nurse. There is no recognition of the many facets of professional knowledge, skills, attitudes and experience which are integrated into a deceptively simple task-orientated intervention.

The target-driven ethos is further enhanced by policy initiatives such as *The Health of the Nation* (DoH 1992) and *Caring for the Future* (Welsh Office 1994). These propose that health gain is achieved through the attainment of relatively precise targets which focus on behaviour change – for example, the numbers of people who give up smoking. In an endeavour to meet these targets district nurses are increasingly giving health education advice, but in this instance their interventions often appear to be 'victim blaming', because they and other health care practitioners are constrained from offering an easy health choice in many circumstances, by structural and social deficits. Specifically, in areas characterised by poverty, poor housing, or environmental limitations, where illness and disease are more prevalent (Townsend, Davidson and Whitehead 1988), district nurses are distinctly uneasy about constraints on their professional autonomy to make intervention. In such circumstances district nurses are inevitably constrained to adopt individualistic approaches, aimed at changing the individual's behaviour. This compromises the broader, community-oriented approach, and places the practitioner in a dichotomous situation. This situation enhances the tendency for 'victim blaming', when it is obvious that communities are lacking the wherewithal to be able to adopt responsibility for their own needs.

■ Soft inputs

A large part of the district nurse's work (much of which is concurrent with task-based activities such as giving injections and so on and therefore is overlooked) involves interventions such as counselling, education and social support ('soft inputs'). These elements and their impact upon both efficiency and effectiveness may be difficult to quantify, but they have been shown to have significant impact on health status (Benzeval *et al.* 1995). Similarly, health education activities with patients and families are often opportunistic and interwoven with other aspects of care, so that quantification becomes difficult. Additionally, evaluating long-term behaviour change in terms of it's relationship to health education is extremely problematic, because many complex and disparate variables may be involved between the provision of the service and the outcomes. However, the importance of these 'soft inputs' should be evaluated, given the confirmation that such elements significantly affect care-and health-related outcomes (Benzeval *et al.* op. cit.). The complementary nature of qualitative evidence (often generated in a 'bottom-up' fashion) to quantitative evidence (often 'top-down') is highlighted by Goodwin (1992). For example, caseload profiles combined with community health profiles (each including users' views) provide a more realistic basis for action than reliance on one particular form of evaluation such as epidemiological data. Consideration of evidence arising from both types of source should enable district nurses to delineate their unique role and contribution to health and social care. This in turn should inform purchasers, as well as the public, of the benefits of utilising district nurses in preference to other occupational groups to provide care in a primary-care-led NHS (UKCC 1994). An obvious conclusion here is that district nurses should have the opportunity to design specific methods of data collection more relevant to the nature and focus of their work.

■ Under fire

In addition to those aspects already discussed a number of other elements have been shown to compromise the district nurse's role. These include both managerial pressure from above to undertake more administrative functions and pressures from professional bodies to continue educational activities to diploma and degree levels. Concurrently, then, the clinical role is pressurised in terms of increased expectations and demands from a variety of sources. Those discussed include WHO strategy, new health care policy, service managers and purchasers, a better-informed public and GP fundholders. The tendency to submit health care delivery (including aspects of district nurses' work) to quantification may also pose a threat to district nurses' responsibility for the quality of care. Hennessy (1994) cites activity measures as an example: 'These are very basic and do not reveal any information on the quality of the process or the outcome of activity.' For this reason, district nurses are often frustrated by the imposition of their use.

■ The way ahead

If district nurses are to adopt role attributes which include audit, team management, health promotion and supervision elements, as well as maintaining a degree of clinical practice, they will require appropriate preparation to give them confidence to assert their professional authority. Realisation of this situation has prompted the professional body for nursing, the UKCC for Nursing, Midwifery and Health Visiting, to make changes in standards of educational preparation for the district nursing role.

The Specialist Practice Award (UKCC 1995) outlines discrete standards for education and practice in district nursing. These clearly relate to a broad role encompassing the above attributes, and differentiate district (specialist) nurses from Project 2000 diplomates by virtue of their 'expert' status rather than merely their practice within a speciality (Hunt and Wainwright 1994). Additionally, district nurses are cited as one of two groups (the other being health visitors) who may be required to prescribe limited medicines, dressings, appliances, creams and ointments Crown Report HMSO (1989). This illustrates increased autonomy of district nurses and represents a further development in the specialist role of primary health and community care provision.

To provide effective care district nurses must work collaboratively with other agencies and individuals, including patients and carers. Shared learning has been a feature of community courses for a decade or more, but the groups involved have been made up of health service personnel (district nurses, mental health nurses, learning disability nurses, school nurses, occupational health nurses, practice nurses and health visitors). If the divide between health care and social care is to be bridged then the inclusion of other disciplines such as social workers will be required in future educational programmes. The assumption made is that shared learning will better inform team working in primary health care, and ultimately it will ensure better standards for the public. These ideals are promoted by the UK Centre for the Advancement of Interprofessional Education, whose purpose is to encourage collaboration in education related to health and social care.

The recent policy initiative *Making it Happen* (DoH 1995) supports the combination of a health-promoting approach with an interventionist role. This mirrors the position advocated by Goodwin (1992) above and represents an apparent ideal interrelationship between an understanding of the macro view, which best informs individual interventions (the micro level), as well as purchasers and providers. However, this 'ideal interrelationship' will require district nurses to adopt a more political stance. To increase political bargaining power, district nursing perspectives must be heard by strategists and authoritative bodies. These include trust boards, commissioning authorities, total fundholders, advisory committees, government departments, and professional bodies. Additionally, recognising that much political weight may be attributed to the views of the public, district nurses might exert political influence through communication with community health councils or voluntary representative groups. Some groups of community nurses, tired of the passivity of the community nursing profession in relation to furtherance of their holistic role, have already undertaken innovative if somewhat controversial action. Nurse practitioners have adopted the political stance that well-qualified trained nurses have a right to increased autonomy in the execution of their role.

■ The nurse practitioner

Nurse practitioners are a relatively new arrival on the primary health care scene in the United Kingdom. To understand and define the role of the nurse practitioner it is important to gain an understanding of how it evolved in this country. However, given the limited space available it is only possible to touch on aspects of the fascinating debate taking place around the development of this role.

A few isolated nurse practitioners, usually trained in the USA, started to develop the role in general practice in this country. Using the US experience as a role model, they were the pioneers, who saw an opportunity for nurses to work in a different, more accountable role in primary care. No account appears to have been taken, however, of contextual differences which might occur within the different locations of practice and education, nor of debates which preceded the UKCC's document of post-registration education and training for 'specialist' community nurses.

At about the same time as pioneers introduced this new role, changes in primary care, particularly the GP Contract (NHSME 1992), brought about an explosion in the work of general practice nurses. Their role changed from that of treatment room nurses to working in screening clinics and health promotion, taking on some of the tasks which would previously have been carried out *ad hoc* by general practitioners. Thus it might be said that in many ways nurses were encouraged to embark on a role that clearly relieved general practitioners of more mundane tasks.

To view this change in a fair context, it is necessary to realise that the political and policy changes in health care implemented in the last decade, such as the

Community Care Act and the introduction of a market economy into the NHS, including fundholding, have altered the work of all primary health care workers. The administration and monitoring of chemotherapy, minor surgery, more extensive diagnostic facilities and other work previously carried out in hospital has come into the remit of the primary care team. This shift in work patterns has therefore blurred some of the boundaries between traditional nursing and medical roles. General practice nurses seized the opportunity they saw for clinical advancement and took on some of the routine aspects of patient care. Consequently aspects of work previously seen as the job of the general practitioner were delegated to the nurse.

It must be pointed out, however, that this was not the general case. Many general practice nurses felt ill-equipped educationally to fulfil this new role, and a number of short courses therefore sprang up to address specific clinical interventions such as for asthma, diabetes and cervical cytology. These courses were helpful, but they fragmented nursing care and did not really address the issue of a full and integrated training for nurses wishing to take on more responsibility and work as more autonomous practitioners.

In 1990 the Royal College of Nursing, nurse practitioner course was designed to address the 'gap' identified in nursing education provision, and gave a focus to the full development of a new role in primary care nursing. The course acted as a watershed in the development of the nurse practitioner role in the UK, giving nurses the opportunity to underpin their expanded role with a sound educational foundation. It also gave nurses an opportunity to organise, and begin to formulate the definition and role boundaries for this new role. The development of an educational programme specifically aimed at nurse practitioners has helped to further the role and has given it the impetus to become organised, where previously nurse practitioners tended to be isolated. These developments have not, however, escaped criticism, some of which is discussed in the conclusion of this chapter.

■ Nurse practitioners: evolution

The nurse practitioner role originated in the USA in the 1960s, a period of rapid social change. Loretta Ford, the founder of nurse practitioner education in Colorado, saw in this the opportunity for risk taking innovation, quick action and dynamic change (Ford 1993). Nurse practitioners were initially meant to fill the 'care gap' left by a shortage of physicians, especially in rural areas and in paediatric care. However the role expanded rapidly to other areas in primary care such as the care of the chronic sick and economically disadvantaged. There are now some 25000 nurse practitioners practising across the USA. For a fuller description of the role development in the US see Bowling and Stilwell (1988).

In the UK the emergence of the nurse practitioner role must be firmly linked to the pioneering work of Burke-Masters (1988), who developed the role in the British primary care setting amid much opposition and conflict. Both these nurses worked in a role well beyond the boundaries of traditional nursing in Britain (Stilwell 1988b). Opposition came both from nurses and from medical practitioners, each believing that the role encroached on their territory.

Barbara Stilwell started the first educational course for nurse practitioners in the Institute of Advanced Nursing Education at the Royal College of Nursing (RCN). At present the RCN is recruiting an average of eighty students per year and there are a number of franchised courses developing in other areas, so numbers attracted to this development role are rising steadily. The RCN training course was initially designed for nurses working in primary care settings. However, increasingly nurses working in the acute sector are using the title of nurse practitioner without having followed any formal training course. This rapid expansion in the use of the title makes it difficult to determine the numbers who legitimately hold this title, and clouds the debate as to the definition of the role.

■ The nurse practitioner title

The definition of the role and the use of the title of nurse practitioner remains controversial in this country. In the USA recognised courses and licensing exams define the role clearly in legislation. In the UK there is as yet no such clarity. Any trained nurse can take the title of nurse practitioner whether or not she has undergone any further formal training.

The UKCC PREPP (Post Registration Educational and Professional Practice) document failed to address the issue of nurse practitioners (UKCC 1994), for reasons which are difficult to ascertain; perhaps it was felt that by ignoring this new emerging role it might become absorbed in the already existing roles, such as that of general practice nurse. The latter, as seen by the UKCC, shares many of the competencies and much of the role description of the nurse practitioner as defined by the RCN. In the view of the professional body, recent changes in the scope of professional practice offer all nurses the opportunity to practice an expanded role. To differentiate the case of one particular group is to detract from the status of all others. Protagonists of the role suggest, however, that the differences lie in the extent and level of decision-making, problem-solving and autonomy exercised by the nurse. The UKCC is presently conducting a consultation exercise to explore the role and its place in the specialist and advanced nurse debate.

This development follows the first official RCN statement on the role and scope of nurse practitioner practice. The RCN defined the nurse practitioner as a nurse who has undertaken a specific course of study of at least a first degree (Honours) level and:

• Makes professionally autonomous decisions, for which they have sole responsibility.
• Receives patients/clients with undifferentiated and undiagnosed problems, and make an assessment of their health care needs based on highly developed

nursing knowledge and skills not usually exercised by nurses, such as physical examination.

- Screens patients/clients for disease risk factors and early signs of illness.
- Develops with the patient/client an ongoing nursing care plan for health with an emphasis on preventative measures.
- Provides counselling and health education.
- Has the authority to admit or discharge patients/clients from their own case-load and refer them to other health care givers as appropriate (RCN 1996).

The statement goes on to define the type and broad content of the educational programme that would lead to a nurse practitioner qualification.

This definition focuses on the autonomy of the role as well as the ability to diagnose, prescribe and treat. Many community nurses would identify themselves and their current role within this definition. The difference lies perhaps in the content and context of treatment as well as the extent of autonomy. However, the specialist practitioner role identified by the UKCC (1994) is based on similar educational requirements and attributes. Nurse practitioners still argue, however, that their practice has a different knowledge base as well as using problem-solving skills and reflective practice (Stilwell 1995).

The American Nurses Association's (ANA) definition of the role of the nurse practitioner offers a further dimension:

> Nurse practitioners have expanded nursing boundaries by creating an additional model for delivery of nursing care to the public. They have also incorporated selected medical services into professional nursing practice and have helped to change the relationship between nurses and physicians from dependent to interdependent with mutual referral and consultation. (American Nurses Association 1987)

Nurses are using specific tools which are usually the territory of the medical profession to enhance their nursing practice and have, by doing so, altered the traditional doctor–nurse relationship. This aspect of the nurse practitioner role is interesting and highlights the 'grey area' between the practice of medicine and nursing, an area of whcih many of us are fully aware of but which few have publicly acknowledged. Gibbon and Luker (1995) touch on this briefly when discussing the development of 'nurse clinicians'. They see the development of the nurse clinician or nurse practitioner as 'one route for nurses who wish to develop and expand their clinical skills' (Gibbon and Luker 1995 : 166).

■ Community practice or individual focus?

Nurse practitioners, like their medical colleagues, are sometimes seen as working within a very narrow individual focus, leaving out the community dimension of care. Nurse practitioner educational programmes in Britain do, however, contain a community orientation; profiling skills and the sociological aspects of health are an integral component of the educational base of nurse practitioner students. Many nurse practitioners also appear to be working in a population-centred way. Inevitably their attachment to a surgery will determine the extent of their community involvement and the work does tend to be targeted to certain client groups. This latter acknowledgement may be detrimental to the provision of equitous care, that is care which meets every individual need, and limit the potential of nurses to affect policies relating to health care provision.

The nurse practitioner role is new; it could have a lot to offer the future development of the nursing profession. There are obvious opportunities to further clinical skills and expertise, offering more choice for clients. Exciting possibilities present themselves in challenging traditional approaches to client–nurse, and nurse–doctor relationships; in particular the role may be seen to provide opportunities for real teamwork to take place, maximising the skills of all professionals involved in the delivery of health care. The main pitfalls to be avoided are the reinforcing of existing inequalities of access, and the creation of further disabling hierarchies within the profession. As Loretta Ford said, the development of the role of nurse practitioners is an idea whose time has come (Ford 1993). The role is at a developmental stage in Britain and it is up to nurses to shape the opportunity it presents to improve client care. The debate remains open.

■ Conclusion

From the contemporary observations of three branches of community nursing it is obvious that health visitors, district nurses and nurse practitioners are frustrated by restrictions on the scope of their professional practice. In particular, well-educated and competent practitioners perceive that others, namely more power-ful male professions, male-dominated policy-makers, and managers are interfer-ing with nurse-orientated patterns of care. In the case of health visitors this interference is perceived to curtail a social welfare community development approach, and public health interventions. As a result, health visitors perceive that there are many variations in the individual levels of health status. Health visitors are aware that barriers to the execution of their professional role can create increased long-term expenditure on health care.

District nurses are frustrated by the fact that they are constantly prevented from combining a rehabilitative, interventionist role with a health-promoting approach. There is also awareness of the fact that failure to recognise the importance of the process of professional care interventions by district nurses is resulting in purchasers wasting resources on a task-orientated service. It is perceived that such a service will only provide short-term resource efficiency.

Nurse practitioners have 'grasped the nettle' of carving a new niche in the market; they are marketing a professionally autonomous role, an ability to diagnose health need and plan care, as well as the technical skill to undertake various levels of intervention previously recognised as the domain of the medical profession. The example of action taken by the nurse practitioner lobby may have much to offer the future development of nursing. However, the dangers of this development lie in the potential for nurse practitioner services to be seen as a 'skilling up' process to enhance the proletarianisation process of medical practitioners, to exacerbate traditional patriarchal control of the profession, and to maintain biomedical emphasis on curative rather than preventative interventions.

Laying aside the current friction between community nurses and restraining policies and procedures, it is obvious that the profession has much to offer if it is allowed to contribute the full extent of its professional competence to the planning and delivery of holistic health care. To achieve their rightful place in professional society community nurses might benefit from an increasedly political stance to ensure recognition of their status.

Chapter 12

The community psychiatric nurse and primary health care

Pat Davies

■ Introduction

This chapter is primarily orientated around a study undertaken within two health authorities. It attempts to understand and analyse how community psychiatric nurses (CPNs) develop working links with general practitioners (GPs). First comes a brief background of the CPN's changing role, followed by a brief explanation of the research methodology. Findings of the study are presented, and are orientated around (1) Why GPs refer patients to CPN's and (2)an exploration of the CPN's power relationship with the GP. Finally consideration is given to the CPN's role in the light of legislation introduced.

■ The changing role of the CPN

The CPN's traditional role is well documented. Its origin occurred in the 1950s when the phenothiazine group of drugs were introduced to treat hospitalised schizophrenics. These drugs were major tranquillisers and dramatically changed the care of the mentally ill. The role of CPNs therefore was to follow up and to give support to the people who had been discharged from hospital on drugs (Roberts 1976; Sharpe 1982, Leopoldt 1979). It could be argued that in many ways people still view the role of CPN's as a 'follow-up function'. The nurse is expected to work in the community, but is attached to the institution and receives referrals from the consultant psychiatrist. There is no chronicled evidence in past literature that suggests CPNs have ever been involved with primary health care teams (PHCT). Relevant literature speaks of the members of Primary Health Care Teams PHCTs being GPs health visitors and district nurses. (Gilmore *et al.* 1974; Lamb 1976).

One reason for this, Kratz (1980) suggests, is:

> Then in 1977 a DHSS circular about nursing in Primary Health Care Teams stated that: 'Where nurses with a special knowledge of care of a particular illness or type of patient (e.g., the mentally ill) work with the patients and

families in the community and liaise with and advise members of the primary health care, it is essential that they maintain their expertise and therefore desirable that they should be based within their specialist field' (e.g., hospitals).

Conversely, many argue that CPNs would be well suited as members of primary health care teams. In 1961, a Government decision was taken to run down large mental hospitals and to provide care for the mentally ill in the community settings. Hence it was thought to make more sense for CPNs to be situated in primary health care rather than in hospitals, so that they could intervene prior to admission of the mentally ill, rather than after (Wing and Olsen 1979). Early preventive care would, it was thought, be likely to enhance the effectiveness of treatment. Although this policy decision was taken more than thirty years ago, the transition period has been slow. Research undertaken in the 1970s and 1980s indicated that there was a desire to have CPNs based in primary care, but it had not yet happened in many places. Leopoldt (1979), Shaw (1977), Sharpe (1982) and Dyke (1984) all found that GPs thought it would be beneficial to have CPNs attached to their practice as members of the primary health care team. Similarly, CPNs were reported to think the same:

> It's crazy when you think of how many GPs there are in the area and how often they need the psychiatric service. They should be able to get on the 'blower' and say – I've got this chap or lady, I'd like you to pop in and see her. (Shepperdson 1987 : 27)

When attached to primary health care teams, CPNs have the opportunity to be in contact with people before psychological problems become too disabling (Sharpe 1975; Brooker and Jayne 1984; Skidmore and Friend 1984; Clist and Brant 1986). Scott and Robertson (1985) reported that when GPs referred patients to CPNs over half the problems were resolved within three months, and only a limited number of patients required to be sent for further psychiatric investigation.

One of the greatest advantages of the proposed change is that when CPNs are attached to primary health care teams their role often becomes predominantly characterised by a 'family and social orientation' (Dixon 1985). In addition, the role of CPNs expands to include: formal and informal assessment of patients' mental health, the implementation of preventative, educative and specific therapy programmes, supportive visits and a consultative service to other related and voluntary services (Pope 1985; Dixon 1985; Morrall 1989).

Dixon (1985) believes that the primary health care team is an ideal base for the CPN, especially in terms of primary and preventative work. Whereas mental illness as opposed to mental health has been the traditional concern of the psychiatric nurses, community psychiatric nursing is adopting the concept of preventative care and health education. New forms of practice are expanding their interest into the social settings of everyday life, and are concerned with structural issues which have the potential to disrupt psychological health.

In order to determine the extent of 'preventive need' the author set out to determine why general practitioners referred people with psychological problems to CPNs.

■ Research methodology

The research methodology for the study was qualitative in nature, using the principles of grounded theory to analyse the data, Information was collected using semi-structured interviews which were audio-taped. Grounded theory helped to validate information collected because the data was analysed as it was collected. The researcher was able to test theories with respondents as they emerged from the data.

The sample was drawn from one rural area in Mid-Wales and an urban area in the (English) Midlands. Although the two areas studied had different patient populations and different socioeconomic situations, the institutional frameworks and the inter-professional socialisation remained the same. A total of 30 CPNs and 12 GPs were interviewed. In addition 14 health visitors and 14 district nurses were also interviewed, but the findings from these two professions are not used in this chapter.

■ Why GPs refer to CPNs

A sample of GP referrals was drawn from two health authorities, one rural, the other urban. In all 30 generic CPNs (all CPNs who worked with adults aged 18 to 65), 14 health visitors, 14 district nurses and 10 GPs were interviewed. Although information was collected from four different disciplines, only the data relevant to explain the CPN's working relationship with GPs will be used for this chapter. Data was collected by using semi-structured interviews.

The author was interested in why GPs referred people to CPNs. The reason continuously given was that of time. During surgery visits GPs did not appear to have time to talk to patients. Typical comments from GPs regarding the reason for referral were: 'You don't know what is coming through the door and if someone comes in pouring their heart out, you can fall half an hour behind time . . .' (rural area). In order to determine the extent of 'preventive need' the author set out to determine why general practitioners referred people with psychological problems to CPNs: 'Most patients who come to us with anxiety, we deal with ourselves, which means sitting down and letting them talk about it, but that depends on how pushed we are for time; that is the most important factor . . .' (urban area). And 'Sometimes people need a lot of counselling, that I haven't the time to do . . .' (rural area).

These findings compared with those of White (1986), who also reported that lack of time was the main reason why GPs referred patients to CPNs. There has been a time, however, when GPs had an alternative to talking to patients. Brown and Ginnberg (cited by Goldberg and Huxley 1980) reported that in the recent past the majority of patients who required psychological help consulted their GPs hoping they would have an opportunity to discuss their problems. Unfortunately they received only a short interview and a prescription for a psychotropic drug. Now that drugs that treat anxiety-related problems are an unpopular remedy, GPs are left to consider alternatives. As Illing *et al.* (1991) found, GPs are under pressure to 'do' something when consulting with a client. Clearly GPs want to offer an alterative to medication. CPNs, therefore, working in primary health care appear to be a useful alternative.

It was interesting to explore the concept of time held by GPs. Specifically it was important to understand if GPs simply made referrals to CPNs because they did not have time to talk to patients, or whether there were more sophisticated reasons underlying the decision making. Some GPs explained it like this:

> You need help with patients who are not so psychiatrically disturbed, but need a lot of time to explain to them what is going wrong. They can see they are sad or depressed, but feel that they can't do much about it. (urban area)

> I don't like the psychiatrist because if a patient needs ongoing psychotherapeutic care he won't do this. I like Sue (the CPN) because she has time, she can see them weekly or twice weekly or whatever. She is very gentle, she allows them to talk and she actually works their problems out with them. I don't think that is what the psychiatrist is into. I think they are into making psychiatric diagnoses and then dishing out the pills. (rural area)

> Where the whole family has interrelated problems, or where the carer is suffering more than the patient, then it is useful for someone to go into the home. Especially where the home and the family dynamics are part of the problem, for example, where there is a young adult, who has had problems with relationships and his family. So it is not just the problem, but the way he relates to his parents and they to him. That is not the sort of think I can sort out by talking to one member of the family in the surgery. Someone needs to go in the home and see what it is like and be prepared to go back, and back again. That is one of the most useful things a CPN can do. (urban area)

> Sometimes I feel a problem is beyond my depth; I can use the CPN as a thermometer, for an assessment . . . . I may be getting confusing and conflicting ideas. a patient comes in and says I am feeling depressed, but he is laughing and is quite happy. He may show some symptoms of depression, like loss of appetite, loss of interest in sex . . . This is where the CPN can help to clarify the situation. I find myself lacking sometimes, to eek out the minor details and the differences in symptoms. There are times when I can't get a clean knife edge as it were, and this is where I find the CPNs very useful. (urban area)

Thus it could be argued that GPs refer to CPNs because they do not have time to talk to patients. As illustrated by the GPs' comments, it is not simply a matter of time, but CPNs are useful when patients are difficult to treat in a medical way, that is by making a diagnosis and prescribing treatment. The specific reason for referral, it appears, then, would be that GPs don't have time to sort out patients' intricate concerns, which are based on family and social problems. This new role of CPNs, as identified by GPs, matches the description previously cited (Pope 1985; Dixon 1985; Morall 1989).

It is therefore interesting to consider if GPs use CPNs as an aid to diagnosis, or for the delegation of unwanted time-consuming tasks, or whether the working relationship between these two professionals is based on equality and collaboration, that is whether GPs treat CPNs as professional equals. This point will be dealt with later in the chapter.

GPs appear to have a particular problem in treating people who present with vague psychological problems culminating in illnesses, such as anxiety and depression. These illnesses are not serious enough to warrant consultation by the psychiatrist, nor indeed admission to hospital, but often they are time-consuming and difficult to diagnose and treat. GPs, it would appear, are often unable and unwilling to give effective therapy, so in many instances it is CPNs who apparently can solve this dilemma to some degree.

■ An exploration of the CPN's power relationship with the GP

Historically, nursing has been subordinated to medicine. Well-known sociologists such as Freidson (1970a) believe that from the physician's point of view the need has been for someone (the nurse) who could be relied on to carry out his orders in caring for a patient in his absence. Later, Strong (1979) made similar observations. He suggested that the nurse's role was more like that of a personal secretary to the doctor. The doctor became heavily dependent on the nursing staff, and the absence of a regular nurse was cursed by every doctor, for things kept going wrong and nothing was in the right place when the nurse was not available.

Similar working relationships can be found in the primary health care team. Dingwall (1976:35) described the situation like this:

> They [the GPs] saw themselves as a spider sitting in the middle of a web which they organised and controlled. Other health workers would only relate to the doctor on an unequal basis. Their skills merely duplicated those of the general practitioner in a partial fashion, and could be exercised only under his direction.

Hannay (1980) believed that the state of this leadership implies a hierarchical system in which one commands, and another obeys, and that the history of the medical and nursing professions has created the myth that the doctor, in terms of authority, is always senior to the nurse.

In recent years nursing has striven to become a more autonomous work force and to move away from medical dominance, that is they have made concerted efforts to move from the less autonomous positions of the semi-professions and to achieve enhanced professional status. Wright (1985) says that this move has made slow progress and it is only now that nurses are developing a clinical career structure rather than an educational or managerial one. He argues that to stand on a par with medicine nurses in a leadership role must be seen as credible practitioners. It was interesting therefore to explore in more detail the relationship between GPs and CPNs. As mentioned earlier, the debate centres on whether GPs delegate work to CPNs or collaborate with them in planning patient care. Precisely, the question asked is whether the relationship between GPs and CPNs is one of superiority or equality.

CPNs who were interviewed in order to answer this question stated that some GP's referred to them, but others did not. It was interesting to appreciate why it was that when CPNs informed GPs of their role, and suggested that they were available to receive referrals, some GPs chose to use the service offered but others did not. One way this situation could be explained was to view it through concepts of power and status. Kelvin (1969) suggested that one of the major sources of inequality is derived from the structure of a group in terms of the roles of its members. The concept of role, by itself, however, is insufficient, because power and status are integral parts of roles. In theory, there is no reason why one role need be more important or influential or more highly valued than any other, but, in practice team membership is frequently inequitious. A number of reasons may account for this phenomenon. It could be said that status is the value attached to a role by society, and power is the extent to which the occupant of one role may influence or determine the behaviour of the occupant of another.

In connection with 'status' and 'power', French and Raven (1959) presented a taxonomy of power in an attempt to explain its complex social basis. Their taxonomy is as follows:

1. Expert power, based on the perception that a person has some special knowledge or expertise.
2. Legitimate power, based on the perception that a person has a legitimate right to prescribe behaviour for someone.
3. Reward power, based on the perception that a person has the ability to mediate rewards to someone.
4. Coercive power, based on the perception that a person has the ability to mediate punishment on someone.
5. Referent power, based on a person's identification with someone else.

Using this taxonomy, it is possible to construct a framework that helps to explain the working relationship developing between CPNs and the GPs. In the remainder of this chapter, therefore, expert, legitimate and reward power are briefly explored. The strength of expert power varies with the extent to which knowledge or perception is attributed to a person within a given area. It is probable that in most instances society evaluates expertise in relation to perceived knowledge as well as against an absolute standard (French and Raven 1959).

The findings of this study show that CPNs can occupy this expert power base. GPs on their own admission in this study said they were generalists. Therefore by inference they are lesser experts than CPNs. Handy (1976), however, says that expert power is comparative, hence not all GPs viewed CPNs as being experts, possibly because GPs viewed CPNs as being in a lower status group and not as co-experts.

The traditional dominance of medicine over nursing has clearly given GPs legitimate power; a possible reason for this phenomenon was provided by White (1986), who comments on the fact that GPs have direct access to the public while in most cases nurses do not. This gives the medical profession a greater influence over the public, and performance and development. It is therefore GP's who make the initial diagnosis of psychiatric disorder, which leads them to decide to refer (or delegate) patients, choosing thereby to recognise the CPN's expertise.

In this study GPs were the reward-givers. CPNs described how they were allowed access to rooms in health centres and had access to patient case notes. These rewards were not given automatically; CPNs had to earn them. They earned them by caring efficiently and effectively for GPs' time-consuming patients. It would appear that CPNs got more rewards the more referrals they accepted and dealt with competently.

> We have a coffee and just wait for whoever we want. This seems to be linked with how much work is offered from certain individuals. I suppose what I am saying is that the health centres that seem to offer the most work are equally the ones who make it the easiest. The ones that are less accessible are the ones with the least amount of contact and offer the least amount of work. (rural area).

An analysis of the working relationship between CPNs and GPs therefore reveals a situation where GPs are the major power holders. This power relationship puts CPNs into a potentially vulnerable situation, because they have been conveniently recruited into a labour gap that is ill defined and convenient for GPs. The new role for CPNs as it is currently defined and organised by GPs appears to construct for CPNs a traditional handmaiden role.

This chapter has put forward a theory to explain the new working relationship between CPNs and GPs. It is for individual practitioners to consider the accuracy of this theory, as it is suggested that it applies equally to the relationships of all community nurses with GPs. If these findings are correct then the future of CPN work and probably the work of other community nurses requires scrutiny. The Community Care Act and the drive for GPs to be fundholders will have a serious impact on their role and professional status if the findings of this research are ignored. Implications of ignoring current trends in relation to the professionalisation of community nursing will be considered in the next section.

■ Developments in community care: what are the implications?

Legislation (DoH 1991) has brought CPNs a new challenging role, but the power and status embodied in this role is questioned. The Community Care Act and policy relating to GP fundholding both ask the question of who will hold the power in relation to the delivery of community services. The Community Care Act places the power firmly in the hands of social services. It is they that are responsible for acting as coordinators for community care. Local authorities must now ensure that there are suitable multidisciplinary and cost-effective assessment procedures for patients. In mental health, local authorities are clearly identified to carry the lead responsibility in collaboration with medical, nursing and other workers (Butterworth 1989). Turner (1989) and more recently Tronbranski (1995) point out that a crucial aspect of new community care strategy is collaboration between disciplines, but Turner raises the question of whether social services perceive community nurses as partners or as an ancillary force.

The other development that has greater implications for CPNs and has already been touched on is that of GP fundholding. In this scenario, GPs purchase services such as hospital treatment and community nurses from providers. It could be argued that buying the services of hospital consultants and nurses strengthens the GPs' position in the power stakes and that they remain the ultimate power holders. Although the value of the CPN's role is crucial, because of the preconceptions of doctors it may not be developed. Firstly, CPNs' expertise may not be recognised, especially when caring for those with 'minor mental health problems'. Indeed White (1991) reports that preliminary studies have taken place to investigate the functions of practice nurses and the role they might play in the treatment of depression. Additionally Naughton (1993) reports that over 25 per cent of GP fundholders brought private counsellors into their surgeries, and Monkley-Poole (1995) revealed that 55 per cent in his study employed counsellors. Naughton suggests that this should send alarm bells ringing in CPN quarters, because the counsellor role might also supplement community psychiatric nurses. It is therefore important that CPNs market their expertise. The move to put people with mental health problems out into the community is their opportunity to sell their expertise to GPs. In fact, Monkley-Poole argues that the key role for CPNs may be the administration of neuroleptic depot injections, a role predominantly belonging to CPNs prior to working with primary health care teams. This task-orientated, GP-defined role may seriously reduce the effectiveness of the CPN professionally, particularly as it is focused on technological interventions rather than on holistic care.

GPs who buy CPN services may interpret that they have in fact employed them; although this is not the case, the attitude of the GPs may be a serious threat. Studies undertaken of practice nurses who are employed by GPs reveal that this group of nurses are in a vulnerable position as far as education, professional supervision and performance review goes (Martin 1994). Practice nurses lack the means for improving their knowledge and skills and must rely on the GP purchaser to direct their work. Therefore, it might also be argued that if this is the case for practice nurses then relationships taking place between the GP and the CPN will be based on delegation rather than collaboration.

Finally, Armstrong (1993) argues that traditionally only 10 per cent of people who have mental health problems have been referred for secondary care. GPs have often considered themselves well able to treat those with depression and anxiety. This situation might well return in a market-orientated environment. If this is the case then it could be argued that CPNs' services may not be purchased, because, in view of budget conservation, it might be more convenient for GPs to treat time-consuming patients themselves. Thus it is essential and advantageous for CPNs to clarify their own boundaries of power and autonomy. They have been conveniently recruited into a labour gap that is ill-defined but which, in relation to GP requirements, it is convenient for CPNs to fill. If CPNs are not sufficiently aware they might easily remain in a marginal handmaiden role. There is no doubt that CPN's have a role within primary health care, but they need to advertise their skills and demonstrate that they can give value for money if they are to achieve rightful status within the primary health care team.

New legislation introduced in April 1996 known as the Mental Health (Patients in the Community) Act 1995 gives designated CPNs the power to insist that certain people with mental health problems will attend a specified place for treatment or be required to live in a specified place. While this legislation allows for more supervisory powers, it could be argued that it may be contrary to collaborative patient care because the enhanced power of the CPN may be resented. Time will indicate how this Act effects the role of the CPN with patients and work colleagues; however, if the community psychiatric nurse is to claim a rightful place in society, then an awareness of factors likely to undermine status and professional judgement is essential.

Chapter 13

Professionals and the voluntary sector

Robert F. Drake

■ Introduction

This chapter discusses the impact of 'market strategies' on charitable agencies, and the way these strategies affect relationships with statutory health and social welfare organisations. It is concluded that professionals need to be aware of changes in the voluntary arena, and the fragmentation of voluntary services. Specifically, the divide between traditional charities and those of disabled people is identified, and a shift in the location of intervention from specialised services to the pursuit of rights and social and environmental change is seen as desirable.

■ Background

In seeking to create a marketplace in health and social services, the Conservative administrations of the 1980s and 1990s encouraged competition within and between voluntary, statutory and commercial organisations. In the statutory sector an artificial divide was introduced between the purchasing and provision of services, and a plurality of agencies (public, independent and charitable) was invited to bid for contracts (Newman and Clarke 1994; Flynn 1994; Le Grand and Robinson 1984). In this chapter I assess the impact of these policies on charitable agencies, and I explore the implications for their relationships with statutory health and social welfare organisations.

The British voluntary sector has always been structurally amorphous and diverse in its interests (Houghton and Allen 1990; Handy 1988; Brenton 1985). However, charities have often been regarded as fulfilling two main purposes: first, the provision of auxiliary welfare services, and second, the representation of the views of consumers or clients. These expectations were voiced, for example, in the strategic statement on the funding of the voluntary sector published by the Welsh Office, in which it enunciated three main roles that charities were expected to perform:

- To represent the interests of service users in the planning, management and delivery of services.

- To promote the acceptance of disadvantaged people in their communities and to encourage others to work alongside such people so as to maximise their opportunities for dignified and fulfilled lives.
- To directly provide (*sic*) a wide range of services to maximise user choice and promote innovation and best practice. (Welsh Office 1991: app. B, para. 4)

As will be seen in this chapter, all these functions are, for different reasons, now under scrutiny. First, some disabled users of services are insisting upon the right to undertake their own representation, and demand separate places around the planning tables. Second, seeking social acceptance for disadvantaged people merely emphasises the fact of deprivation rather than exposes its (social) causation (Barnes 1991, 1990; Barton 1989). Thirdly, the political emphasis upon enhancing the role of voluntary agencies as service providers brings them, potentially at least, into direct conflict with the professional domain, and (again, potentially) diminishes their ability to take a critical and independent stance with respect to the planning and development of social welfare.

■ The changing circumstances of the voluntary sector

□ 1. Pressures towards service provision

Though there are some exceptions, many traditional voluntary agencies receive statutory funding (from both central and local government) in order to employ staff, rent premises and buy equipment. For example, Broady (1989) has shown that intermediary bodies (County Associations of Voluntary Organisations) in Wales receive 90 per cent of their total revenues from the Welsh Office. In the past, the conditions under which grants were given meant that voluntary agencies enjoyed wide discretion in the formulation and implementation of their work. In recent years, however, their degree of dependence upon statutory monies has rendered charitable groups vulnerable to political pressure applied through the funding mechanism. By concentrating the availability of finance upon some activities rather than others (service provision has been accentuated but political comment has been rigorously circumscribed (Charity Commission 1994)) agencies have been forced to choose between accepting public finance in order to secure their infrastructures and eschewing statutory funds so as to safeguard their independence.

Leaving aside questions as to whether voluntary groups actually have the capacity to run mainstream services (see for example allegations of serious failures in homes run by the Cyrenians and Mencap – Timmins and MacKinnon 1995; Timmins, 1995), it remains the case that under the new contractual arrangements charities have faced mounting pressure to adopt a commercial ethos and evolve into major suppliers of services. This pressure is made all the more acute by the fact that an agency may find itself in some jeopardy where the loss of grant aid is not compensated by the awarding of a contract (Mabbott 1992).

There is an irony here in that charities were once considered the watchdog of the statutory social services. Now, however, the roles have been reversed and the Social Services Inspectorate has been charged with the responsibility of monitoring voluntary sector subcontractors. The upshot of all these changes is that agencies are finding it harder to acquire funds for those more sensitive activities – such as campaigning – normally associated with their functions as pressure groups. Furthermore, first indications suggest that the impact of these trends (away from relatively 'free' money towards 'strings attached' funding) has been exacerbated for some groups by the significant fall in general charitable donations occasioned by the advent of the National Lottery (Frean 1995a, 1995b).

☐ 2. The representation function

In addition to the financial pressures that have resulted from contemporary social policies, traditional charities are also under attack from the British disability movement. Disabled people themselves are challenging vigorously the assumed right of the predominantly non-disabled leaders of the voluntary sector to speak on their behalf (Derbyshire Coalition of Disabled People 1989; Greater Manchester Coalition of Disabled People 1989). The legitimacy of their concern is corroborated by quantitative evidence that details the absence of disabled people from positions of authority in the traditional voluntary sector.

Briefly, a study of 149 social welfare charities in one British county revealed that only 18 (12. 1 per cent) agencies employed any disabled people at all, and in only 4 (2. 7 per cent) agencies did disabled people form more than half the work force. In only 33 (22. 1 per cent) of the 149 agencies were disabled people in the majority on the governing body, and these groups received far less statutory funding than the traditional charities led by non-disabled people. In just 15 (10. 1 per cent) groups did disabled people occupy posts as press and publicity officers, and a mere 14 (9. 4 per cent) agencies had nominated disabled people to represent them on planning committees and other public bodies. (A full account of the research is given in Drake 1992, 1994, 1996.)

The disability movement argues that in circumstances of the sorts described above it is illegitimate for traditional charities to claim to represent disabled people's views, whether this be on service-planning panels, in the media or in consultation with government. In order to establish their own lines of communication, many disabled people have founded their own agencies and the British Council of Organisations of Disabled People now has in excess of 90 member groups representing some 300000 disabled people (Oliver 1996; Hasler 1993; Shakespeare 1993; Morris 1991).

At the heart of these two issues (service provision and representation) stands a fundamental clash of principles. The dispute is at its sharpest over the use of terminology. From the traditional medical perspective, *disability* has been understood as an individual attribute. People are disabled by their physiological or cognitive impairments.

The disability movement challenges the validity of this conceptualisation, and sets against it an entirely different definition of disablement. While accepting that individuals may have physiological or cognitive impairments, *disability*

is the disadvantage or restriction of activity caused by a contemporary social organisation which takes no or little account of people who have physical impairments and thus excludes them from the mainstream of social activities. (UPIAS 1976: 3–4)

Oliver (1990) exemplifies the difference between these two understandings of disability by contrasting the approach of the 1986 OPCS survey of disabled adults which asked (for example) 'Does your health problem/disability make it difficult for you to travel by bus?' with his own alternative question, 'Do poorly designed buses make it difficult for someone with your health problem to use them?'

Clearly, the medical or 'personal tragedy' perspective locates disability in the individual and so seeks to modify human beings by 'rehabilitation'. Accordingly this model has given rise to specialised, ameliorative interventions in segregated settings such as hostels, day centres and residential homes. By contrast, the social model proposed by the disability movement highlights the disabling propensities of 'non-disabled' society through its promotion of attitudinal prejudices, physical obstacles and social barriers.

Even more fundamentally, this debate not only questions the definition of 'normality', but also confronts the locus and objectives of 'care' practice in both the statutory and voluntary sectors. Hitherto, the focus of those concerned with disability has been centred on the impaired individual, and the epithet 'normal' has been reserved for human beings who exhibit no medically classified physiological or mental impairment. The disability movement identifies a different focus of intervention, namely, society as a whole. Here the word 'normal' is used to indicate a society socially and environmentally configured to serve all its citizens irrespective of their personal physiology. 'Abnormal', in this sense, describes a society built in such a way as to exclude certain citizens from public life purely on the basis of their anatomical state or cognitive processes (Oliver 1990; Abberley 1987; Borsay 1986).

From the perspective of the social model of disability, then, change must be located not in individual human beings, but in the norms, values and structures of society itself. Adaptations must be carried through at the environmental, rather than the personal level. The idea that we live in a disabling society has gained much political ground in recent times. The Civil Rights (Disabled Persons) Bill 1994 (HMSO 1994), introduced into the House of Commons by the Labour MP Dr Roger Berry, was drafted substantially in sympathy with the principles of the social model. The authors of the Bill sought to extend civil rights and equality of opportunity to disabled people, and equip them with legal powers to combat discrimination and exclusion. Though the Bill enjoyed all-party support, it was lost when the government took fright at the estimated costs of its implementation (Blakemore and Drake 1996).

■ Implications of change

□ 1. Implications for the voluntary sector

For charities, a number of implications follow from the pressures outlined above. First, there has been a fragmentation of the voluntary sector itself (Drake and Owens 1992). While the larger, more traditional charities have identified opportunities for growth in the new policy ethos, groups led by disabled people have sensed danger in too great a dependency on the state and have responded more warily to the siren call of the contract culture.

Second, the desire of government to promote a mixed economy of welfare has emboldened traditional charities to see themselves in a new light. As early as 1981 Leat *et al.* (1981 : 1) discerned that voluntary organisations were showing a 'new audacity, identifying themselves in the national debate as a permanent and indispensable part of the welfare scene'. The national voluntary bodies in England, Ireland and Wales all indicated general approval for an enhanced voluntary sector role and the development of partnership with the state (Wales Council for Voluntary Action 1989; Northern Ireland Council for Voluntary Action 1987; National Council of Voluntary Organisations 1980). A number of well-established charities such as Age Concern and the Community Development Foundation have accepted the realities of the new, market-orientated environment. Some have welcomed partnerships with the statutory sector (Payne 1984) and many are well positioned to bid for contracts (Anderson 1990; Williams 1990; Kunz *et al.* 1989; Gutch 1989; Fielding and Gutch 1989).

Third (and here I acknowledge a fair degree of overlap), traditional groups have emphasised the development of contractual services, whereas other agencies (most of them *of* rather than *for* disabled people) have followed very different agendas. Their priority has been to promote the campaign for anti-discrimination legislation, to lobby for access to public buildings and to militate for the redesign of public transport. For these groups, the goal has not been to build improved services designed to give disabled people a 'surrogate' life away from the everyday social world. Instead they have aimed to achieve attitudinal, structural and political change within the community itself so that disabled people can no longer be excluded (literally *by definition*) from 'normal' society (Barnes 1991; Brisenden 1986).

Fourth, in affirming the medical model, traditional charities continue to separate disabled people not only from the mundane world but also *from each other*. In so doing, charities retard the development of a common consciousness among disabled people: an awareness that exclusion and oppression arise not from impairments but from the contours of society (Abberley 1987).

In summary, the fragmentation of the voluntary sector has resulted in many agencies becoming increasingly professionalised – in effect, adjuncts to the state. With their need for government funding and their adherence to the medical model, traditional charities continue to stress their service-providing role, and they target their 'products' at particular groups of people with specific impairments. However, other groups led by disabled people themselves remain focused on the acquisition of rights and the affirmation of citizenship.

☐ **2. Implications for health and social welfare professionals**

At the beginning of the chapter I proposed that the statutory sector viewed charities as performing two main functions, the provision of auxiliary services and the representation of consumers. The evidence adduced so far in this chapter invites health and social welfare professionals to review their understanding of the roles and purposes of voluntary agencies within the contemporary social policy environment. There are several questions to be raised here.

First, it is clear that in the name of choice the government's ambition has been to develop a keener edge between statutory and voluntary sector service providers. Professionals in the statutory agencies may increasingly come to regard their erstwhile voluntary sector colleagues as competitors for a limited number of service contracts. An example of the effects that may follow from this kind of change in status can be found in the area of housing policy. The state's involvement in the direct provision of housing for rent diminished throughout the 1980s as a result of the 'Right to Buy Act' (the Housing Act 1980). The government was predisposed to transfer the public housing role performed by local councils to the private sector and to housing associations in the voluntary sector. Though there are particular constraints (for example, some professional staff exercise specific legal powers and fulfill specialised duties), the government has desired a similar transfer of responsibilities in the field of social services.

Second, in the light of these shifting roles and responsibilities, how legitimate is it for the statutory sector to continue to view voluntary agencies as being the voice of the clients they may now – or in future – serve on a contractual basis? This question becomes especially acute where a client wishes to complain about services received from the voluntary group which purports to be his or her representative.

Third, the statutory sector has hitherto rather taken it for granted that charities are the collective voice of disabled people. However, disabled people themselves increasingly refute this assumption and demand to be heard, speaking on their own behalf. There is growing research evidence that disabled people enjoy little power within the traditional voluntary sector and exert minimal influence over what is done in their name (Drake 1992, 1994, 1996; Hevey 1992; Sutherland 1981). Accordingly, it becomes increasingly dubious for the statutory sector to treat the voices of traditional charities and disabled people themselves as being one and the same thing. There are distinct differences in the aims and objectives of the two.

Fourth, those who advise on, and provide, statutory funding must reconsider the purposes of such monies. If the arguments that proceed from the social model of disability are accepted then it follows that finance should be diverted away from traditional charities offering segregated service provision, towards pressure groups aiming for social and environmental change, disabled people's rights, and the promotion of disabled people (on their own terms) in society at large. The support here is for voluntary action that confronts discrimination, and for voluntary groups in which disabled people exercise authority.

■ Conclusions

In this chapter I have argued that Conservative social policy has determined a more directive use of public funds *vis-à-vis* the voluntary sector. Two central strands are apparent. First, the government has encouraged the replacement of grant aid with contractual arrangements. Second, the emphasis has been on making money available for service provision.

In response to these moves, some traditional charities have been attracted by the lure of more secure funding and have set aside worries about the maintenance of their independence. Other groups, especially those *of* disabled people, have been less willing to divert their attention away from rights issues based on a philosophy of social rather than individual change. Yet other groups have attempted to accommodate these diverse pressures by compartmentalising the different functions of their organisations.

For the sake of clarity I have portrayed current trends in voluntary action as a bifurcation: professionalisation on the one hand and protest on the other. After pointing at the outset to the amorphous nature of voluntary action, it is appropriate to offer a *caveat* to the general analysis. Clearly, not all agencies fall happily into one of the two camps described above. A few traditional agencies have made genuine attempts to redistribute power, sharing authority with their consumers. For example the mental health charity MIND has obliged its local branches to ensure that a minimum of two service users or ex-users have seats on the management committee of each local association (Beresford and Croft 1993; Gordon 1991; Croft and Beresford 1990; Barker and Peck 1987). Equally, some groups of disabled people have been ready to cooperate with statutory agencies in the reorientation of services (Derbyshire Coalition of Disabled People 1985). There are many shades and nuances in between.

I have argued that health and social welfare professionals need to be aware of these fundamental changes in the voluntary arena, changes that command a far more sophisticated view of the relationship between the two sectors than has obtained hitherto. I have outlined the main planks of that more subtle analysis: the impact of politically directive funding; the dominance of the medical model in service provision and development; the fragmentation of the voluntary sector and, in particular, the need to differentiate between the voices of traditional charities and those of disabled people; and finally the location of intervention, away from specialised services that are based on (and reinforce) the artificial categorisation of impairments, towards the pursuit of rights and the promotion of social and environmental change desired by disabled people themselves.

Part II

Summary

This part has attempted to deconstruct the changing social world of professionals who work in the health and caring services. It is apparent that the consequences of 'rolling back' state provision have caused professionals much concern and have challenged them to critically assess the service that they provide.

In many instances it would appear that reassessment is leading to innovative and new ways of caring, but it is still apparent that professional carers sometimes have to work in the divide created between the myths of rhetoric and reality of current directives for policy implementation.

Yet the total picture of change is not so bleak, although there are many constraints; committed professionals appear to be seeking to redress current imbalances in service provision through their concern for consumer rights. Practically, they acknowledge that to 'resume normal' service they must seek to mediate excesses of current policy changes in their organisation; the excesses of managerial strategies; alleviate the injustices in care provision and the abuse of marginalised groups of service users, and seek to ensure that consumers and their carers are fully informed about the process of change and its limitations. In so doing professionals may enhance their professional status and precipitate community development for health.

The way ahead will pose many challenges; these are discussed in Part III.

PART III

Care for communities

Introduction

In Part III we turn our attention to the objects of care – the communities to be cared for. The main theme to be pursued is that of the *diversity* of groups deemed 'in need' of community-based care and the importance of understanding the needs which may be 'hidden'. The uncovering of unmet needs is a facet of community-based care which is understandably often neglected by those who are daily working within reduced budgets and under pressure just to hold the line on a day-to-day basis. As we have argued in Part II, the professional care givers are under enormous pressure from changes in the internal organisation of the health and social services. This pressure is the background to the following chapters, which focus upon the needs of different groups and the necessity of a more proactive approach by health care and social workers in the assessment of need.

The chapters in Part III focus on two main issues and on specific needs of diverse groups; first, there is the use of language in the organisation of community care services and of the way in which 'community care' has become a code in the popular culture for chaos and danger on the streets; the second issue to be discussed is the way in which poverty has become almost a taboo word in the assessment of need. The group which forms the majority of the recipients of community-based care is, of course, the 'elderly' population, and their needs for care and housing are analysed with reference to the diverse nature of this group. Finally, we turn to the often neglected area of ethnicity and community care policies. The diversity of minority ethnic groups and their specific needs must be placed within the framework of care *for* all communities.

■ Constructing a 'reality'

The social construction of reality has been the dominant theme of this book, and in Chapters 14 and 15 we focus upon the way in which the use of language can both construct a 'reality' and at the same time obscure an understanding of lived experience.

David Rea (chapter 14) returns to the theme of the organisation of community care within the framework of the internal market, but with a difference (chapter 14). He argues that the 'market' so often referred to by managers and policy makers in the health and social services is, in fact, a myth. Myths however play a very important part in a culture, because they embody fears and aspirations and serve to guide actions and underpin beliefs and policies. The phrase 'community care' itself has become a coded way of referring to the perception by the press and other cultural agenda-setters of a breakdown in the care services for the mentally ill. This mixture of myth, metaphor and the demonisation of the 'mad on the streets' is discussed by John Wilkinson in Chapter 15. He also focuses on how rhetoric about 'empowerment' and 'choice' can obscure the relationship of power which underpins the delivery of services to mentally ill people.

Although the construction of the 'mad' as a danger on the streets may be a part of populist tabloid myth-making, nevertheless many people 'recognise' a reality in the perceived 'danger'. There have been much-publicised killings and suicides which have been linked to people being released from institutional care into an underfunded and inadequately equipped community-based service, and concerns which this situation has prompted has caused a change in mental health policy. Thus announcing that new 'homes' are to be provided for people suffering severe mental health problems, Stephen Dorrell, the previous Secretary of State for Health, referred to the necessity to provide a wider 'spectrum of care'. But as Nicholas Timmins (1996) illustrates, the 'sums don't add up'; the numbers in need of places offering 24-hour residential care have been assessed at approximately 5000, which would cost between £450 and £600 million, yet the government has allocated an extra funding of only £100 million for 1997. Interestingly, the two major organisations which represent the interests of mentally ill people, MIND and SANE, both criticise the new policies for different reasons. MIND argues for a system of after-care services to be put in place rather than an increase in institutional care, and SANE expresses great concern over the shortage of beds in long-stay hospitals (Fletcher 1996 : 4). This divergence illustrates the differences of needs and interests *within* the group often classified merely as '*the*' mentally ill.

■ Poverty – the ignored reality

In Chapters 16 and 17 the existence of widespread poverty among families is focused upon as a primary need to be addressed within a system of community-based care. Mark Drakeford in Chapter 16 argues that poverty 'dominates the landscape of social welfare practice', that which so far however lacks a coherent strategy to address its impact. He argues for a more proactive approach by workers to combat the devastating blight of poverty on an increasing number of communities. In Chapter 17 Matthew Colton *et al.* argue that a more proactive practice needs to be employed by workers in definitions of children 'in need' under the Children Act. The writers see poverty as not only assuming nineteenth-century proportions in some areas but also being relegated to the margins of definitions of 'need'.

If poverty was 'rediscovered' in the 1960s, then it can be said to have been disinterred once again in the 1990s. Recent reports of poverty in Britain have received great publicity in the press. A report in *the Observer* (Hugill 1996 : 18) reported that the 'gap between rich and poor in the UK is as wide as it is in

Nigeria'. The report goes on to quote a GP in inner-city Bristol as saying 'We are dealing with crises, not prevention.' In a similiar vein *The Independent* (1996 : 2) reports that 'Britain is the most unequal country in the West'. The report goes on to quote the words of a single mother, that 'Most of the social workers are disgusted by the way I live,' revealing that the division between workers with the poor and the poor themselves has not changed very much this century. Health care professionals such as health visitors as well as social workers have opportunities to work in the front line in anti-poverty strategies but are often not encouraged to do so by practice guidelines issued by health trusts and social service departments. These two chapters offer a way forward in the recognition that poverty has been marginalised and ignored by policy-makers.

■ Older people and their lives

Chapters 18 and 19 focus upon the group which contains the majority of recipients of community-based care – older people. Both chapters show that there is a wide diversity within this group and that a homogenity based upon age does not exist. Robert Drake in Chapter 18 argues for a more central place for housing policies in the long-term care of elderly people in the community. The importance of staying in one's 'own home' must be paralleled by the realisation that an older person's home may be a cause of worry and distress to them if they are not fully supported by housing policies.

In Chapter 19 Bill Bytheway and Julia Johnson illustrate how the role of 'the carer' for an elderly person is also a social construction. Both chapters recognise that poverty is also a common experience (but not a universal one) for older people, especially women.

■ Ethnic diversity and inequality

In the final chapter Ken Blakemore looks in depth at the diverse groups which constitute the minority ethnic communities in Britain and their varying needs and experiences. He pays particular attention to the inadequacy of policies which attempt to ignore cultural and ethnic diversity in the delivery of community-based services.

Two recent reports have pinpointed the necessity to carefully define the needs of different minority communties and to recognise a diversity of experiences. The survey by the Office for National Statistics (1996) revealed the extent of the discrimination suffered by the Asian and Afro-Caribbean communities. But even here there was a diversity between groups; 'black' and Pakistani/Bangladeshi people had the highest unemployment rates (24 per cent and 27 per cent), but Indians had approximately half the rate of these two groups (12 per cent) which was slightly above that of the 'white' population (8 per cent). Just over half of Afro-Caribbean children live in single-parent households, while South Asian groups (Indian, Pakistani and Bangladeshi) have a much higher proportion of married couples than any other group, including the 'white' population.

The definition of an overall label of 'white' for a wide number of divergent communities has had the effect of making inequalities *within* this group relatively invisible. As mentioned by Ken Blakemore, the Irish are the most vulnerable group within this 'white' category. As John Haskey has recently reported (1996 : 1373), people born in Ireland (both Northern Ireland and the Republic) make up the largest minority group in Britain and suffer poorer health than any other group. Mortality and morbidity rates for first-generation Irish people exceed those of all residents of England and Wales (approximately 30 per cent for men and 20 per cent for women). A report on the patterns of mortality among second-generation Irish men and women showed a similiar pattern (Harding and Balarajan 1996). This report showed that socioeconomic differences were not significant, with Irish men and women experiencing higher mortality across social classes, although the Irish community remains largely in the lower social economic groups. This final chapter argues for a recognition by care services of the diverse needs, and the potential for the cultural strength of minority ethnic communities themselves in the organisation of care.

The overall theme of this final part is to set out the definitions and needs of the diverse and heterogeneous communities which themselves have been socially created.

Chapter 14

The myth of the market in the organisation of community care

David Rea

■ Introduction

This chapter argues that 'the market' for health and social care is best understood as a metaphorical device. Metaphors refer by virtue of 'social and intersubjective' mechanisms (Boyd 1993 : 524), so they do not simply refer to or describe reality: they create or influence it by conditioning understandings of the social realities to which they apparently refer. Because 'the market' is used metaphorically without referents, its use requires and allows it to be mythologised as an autonomous and powerful social agent. Using research evidence from mental health services, this chapter is intended to demonstrate how this myth has distinct effects on organisations where managers and others lack any agreement of what a market should look like. The first section of the chapter examines the variety of available interpretations of 'the market', and aims to show how 'the market' is an over-burdened metaphor. Next, the chapter examines the nature of care as a unique commodity. Then, using empirical illustrations, the chapter examines the implications of using this metaphor in defining organisational purposes and in creating organisational identity through the establishment and negotiation of boundaries. Finally there will be a discussion concerning the dilemmas resulting from adopting competitive or collaborative strategies in relation to other parts of the service that have acquired a separate status.

■ Defining a 'market

The idea that health and social care should be organised like any other commodity – through a market – has widespread international support. Nevertheless, such forms of care differ from other commodities in that expenditures on most commodities are regarded positively as a contribution to national wealth while expenditure on health and social care is regarded as unwarranted – as a barrier to international competitiveness. In a belief that 'the market' can curtail costs while ensuring 'appropriate' use of scarce resources, a variety of structural changes have been introduced, dubbed 'internal markets' (Enthoven 1985), 'quasi-markets' (Le Grand, 1990), or 'planned markets' (Saltman and Von Otte 1992). None of these terms is satisfactory, but all serve to indicate that health and social care is not provided through 'real' markets. Any notion that there are 'real' markets to imitate is, of course, misguided because all markets are planned markets (Polanyi 1945) and 'free markets' are an idealisation. Even the *freest* of free markets are regulated through property rights, contract laws, limited liability, patent laws, consumer and environmental protection, planning legislation and the prevention of collusion and of monopolies. Markets are supported by economic management, state purchasing and a plethora of cross-subsidies. Indeed, state welfare offers a wealth of opportunities for cross-subsidy because private corporations (medical equipment, pharmaceuticals, insurers, building contractors and so on) and private individuals (physicians, consultants and others) compete for business funded through taxation. Once we recognise that there are degrees of regulation, the so-called 'introduction' of markets can be viewed as part of a more general strategy of deregulation associated with the New Right and public choice theory (Buchanan 1969, Burrows and Loader 1994, Glennerster and Midgley 1991; Hoggett 1990; Niskanen 1971; Wolf 1988).

However, because idealisations are used in science for their explanatory or persuasive value, 'the market' confers on economics a scientific understanding of the social world. It allows description and allows economic behaviour to be subjected to calculation and analysis. But 'the market' is without figurative referents, because there is no unanimity on such fundamentals as to what a market is or what its effects are. It defies attempts at technical definition.

Given that organisations are commonly defined as discrete entities, united by a purpose, the use and importance of 'the market' metaphor is clearly distinctive. 'The market' implies a multitude of discrete, self-interested entities yet still results in organisation. It therefore undermines conventional views of organisation in that purposes are not defined centrally or shared. Used *within* organisations, 'the market' metaphor implies a radical relocation of authority so that individual units trade with each other. Each is concerned to maintain its financial viability and is forced to regard other elements of the organisation as competitors and/or as valued customers or suppliers. This creates a tension between the overall profitability and authority structure of the organisation and that of its component parts. The introduction of an 'internal market' results in the creation of a network of service providers and purchasers. Within provider organisations, separate trading units are established ('directorates' within health service trusts), responsible for their own financial budgets and for the planning and delivery of services. So, an 'internal market' implies a devolution of authority to autonomous provider units.

The authority structure is further threatened because the legitimacy of central authority has never been widely accepted. So, use of 'the market' metaphor is not only an alternative to bureaucracy: it poses a challenge to service providers, to the professions and to collegial forms of organisation (Johnson 1972).

The mental health directorate I use in this chapter to illustrate the effects of 'the market' can be seen as an organisation with particular definitions of itself, its purposes, and its problems. Only some of these are arrived at by adopting 'the market' metaphor. Others originate in professional, legal, managerial and political definitions of the organisation. It is the interplay between these and 'the market' that creates a unique dynamic. A mythologised 'market' is used metaphorically to affect compliance to organisational goals and to define goals in ways that stress 'choice' for consumers' priority and quality, rather than (professionally defined) effectiveness.

■ The power of 'the market' as a metaphor

Once located spatially as a place where people met to trade, 'the market' has more recently been associated with the development of capitalist economics, where it is represented as a mechanism in which supply and demand adjust to reach equilibrium. 'The market' is said to be superior to all other forms of organising human activity because it coordinates activity and allocates resources effectively and efficiently. It is not coercive, but voluntary. It is flexible. It encourages innovation. These claims are advanced regardless of the coordination problems and transaction costs that may outweigh the benefits of markets (Bartlett 1991, Dietrich 1994).

Drawing upon images of medieval fairs, souks and horse trading – scenes of lively social interchange – and partly from political economy, 'the market' serves as a powerful metaphorical device to remake national governmental authority structures. It is a metaphor used to justify inaction where any interference in market relations is portrayed as an unjustified incursion on basic human rights. However, 'the market' is an over-burdened metaphor in several respects. For instance, it can denote extreme levels of competitiveness or, more generally, reciprocal relationships (variously regarded as collusion or as collaboration). The interpretation given to such relationships is socially constructed, embedded in economic and political theory, and dependent on judgements concerning notions such as 'the public interest', 'efficiency' and 'social cohesion'.

While there is no unitary concept of 'the market' (for it has also been represented as brutal, arbitrary and unjust) 'the market' is generally portrayed as a structure standing in opposition to hierarchical control. This is because 'the market' engages people on a voluntary or contractual basis and is associated with freedom and democracy. This is vital when 'the market' is compared with authoritative hierarchies or the relationships characteristic of state provision and state regulation. Power is devolved down to the multiplicity of decisions taken by consumers. The idea that consumers are sovereign is a powerful political ideal. Consumers judge what is in their own best interest and are allowed to act accordingly in an unfettered market. They are entitled to expect sole use of the purchases they make. Under such circumstances, producers of goods and services voluntarily enter 'the market' with innovative products, at prices that are attractive to consumers and competitive with other suppliers. If they fail to respond to consumer demands, they are forced out of 'the market'.

Under these circumstances, state provision or regulation of markets is justified only where it is thought that 'the market' will fail. In health care, market failure is expected for the following reasons:

1. Professional occupations are organised to allow the sharing of information and knowledge, restriction of their numbers; and self-definition of acceptable technical and ethical practice.
2. The capital investment of modern hospitals means they cannot be closed down without huge loss.
3. Consumers are apparently unable to choose a healthy lifestyle and to avoid hazards.
4. Sole benefit and costs cannot be guaranteed because everybody stands to gain or lose health from the activities of others.

For these reasons, many governments have sought to introduce 'internal markets' rather than allow private health care to operate in a deregulated or privatised market.

For the New Right, however, market failure occurs only because governments and professions have failed to allow 'the market' to function freely. In viewing 'the market' as a dynamic social process, however, the New Right has added a further indeterminacy to the available meanings and significance of 'the market'. Here the activities of a relatively small number of entrepreneurs is significant, even allowing them some degree of monopoly power as a reward for effort and investment. While orthodox economics portrays monopoly power as distorting 'the market' and preventing thereby the efficient allocation of scarce resources, the New Right argues that the primary purpose of 'the market' is the stimulation of innovation through competitive pressures and adequate rewards. Here, also, 'the market' is seen as allowing the 'language of price' to function so that consumers can signal their wishes to producers.

This provides an argument for the introduction of a pricing system in health and social care, regardless of market failure. Their argument is that only a price mechanism – however artificial – can ensure that comparisons are made. These comparisons act internally to examine the efficiency and effectiveness of particular organisations and externally to examine the use of social investment on health and social care as opposed to other economic activities.

Within commercial organisations, the 'language of price' argument has encouraged 'demergers' and 'unbundling': the creation of new forms of organisation held together by contractual structures and information technology, rather than by ownership of the whole enterprise exercising hierarchical control. Within public services, the metaphor has similarly been used to encourage contractual rather than control relationships. It implies a customer focus, value for money and quality service (Tuckman 1994). This is despite the requirements of public accountability and central government policy that may make 'the market' incompatible with state authority, accountability and bureaucratic structures.

'The market' denotes a crucially different relationship between users and providers of health and social care. The next section examines the role of consumers in health economics and the practical difficulties for health and social care delivery that have then ensued.

■ On care as a commodity

'The market' relies on an assumption of 'consumer sovereignty' whereby people behave as self-interested rational agents able to choose between alternatives. Consumers are then assumed to have 'unlimited demands'. This, confronted with 'finite resources' is sometimes described as the very reason for economics (Culyer, 1992:7). The use of 'the market' metaphor implies a strategy of converting patients and clients to consumers (Mooney 1994:160; Rea 1989) that might present a radical threat to a situation where patient and client perceptions of needs are dominated by professional opinion and the availability of services.

However, it is far from clear whether patients and clients will respond to the redefinition of their role as 'consumers'. People generally choose to not think about the hazards and risks to life they take. Many delay seeking help, underestimate their need, and even deny that anything can be done. Demand for care is governed by perceptions of their condition relative to their age and circumstances. Their expectations are also framed by the availability of services and their knowledge of them. When vulnerable through sickness, people choose to hand over the responsibility for choice to the professions (Moody, 1994: 18–20).

Furthermore, people come under considerable social and legal pressure to accept treatment. Pregnant mothers, sick employees, immigrants, criminals and children are all subject to treatment that is near-compulsory or is required in order to obtain social benefits. In mental health services this compulsory element to treatment is justified further by a discourse of dangerousness (as Wilkinson argues in chapter 15).

Given the difficulty of 'patients' becoming 'consumers', demand for health and social care can equally be associated with the demands of the state and for employers to have a healthy, undistracted work force. 'The market' then requires radical revision. In the UK the government's response has been to attempt to enrol professionals both as agents of the government in limiting expenditure and as agents of patients/consumers in selecting alternatives (Butler 1993:62–3; Glennerster *et al.*, 1991; Opit, 1993).

In mental health this is matched by user-led initiatives which are taken more or less seriously by health care management and professions (Brandon 1991; McIver 1991; NHSME b and c 1992; Rogers *et al.* 1993; Wykes 1994). So 'the market' is a metaphor that some potential 'consumers' may find useful. However, the overall constraints on expenditure mean that any ability to influence overall provision and their own treatment remains questionable. Britain's 'internal market' is restricted to the demand side of finance: the supply of money remains under budgetary restraint. So markets have not been extended to permit consumers to determine expenditure levels, nor to determine any particular type of provision.

Within the overall health care programme budget, the responsibility for deciding on budget allocations is placed with so-called 'purchasers' of care. Acting on behalf of patients rather than directly influenced by them, purchasers have responsibility for assessing local needs and deciding priorities. Any desire they have to work on behalf of endusers is likely to be governed by overall policy and financial constraints.

The role of providers is equally questionable and it is to their position in 'the market' that this chapter now turns.

■ The role of provider organisations in 'the market'

The next three subsections illustrate the profound effects that 'the market' has on a provider organisation, a mental health directorate. It examines its effects on the provider's (1) identified purposes, (2) internal and external boundaries, and (3) external relationships.

□ Organisational purpose

Purposes are a defining characteristic of any organisation, however loosely its objectives are agreed or articulated. The introduction of 'the market' required purposes, the scope of its activities, to be redefined and for alternatives to be excluded. However, professional practice and government policy affected the ability of the directorate to define autonomously its market strategy. Policy required a focus on people with previous episodes of 'severe mental disorder', rather than, say, short-term traumatic disorders of bereavement or stress.

This is at odds with the demands of 'the market' as it was understood, as when a proposal for a cross-department cancer support team was rebuffed by the clinical director as 'at the softer end of the market'. Other instances were related to discussions over the following:

- Whether the directorate should support local GPs who wanted to offer counselling services.
- The support given to local voluntary agencies aiming to reduce tranquilliser use.
- The provision of an eating disorders service.
- The directorate's investment in IT and training.

Activities were also affected by the trust. Service developments were discussed in relation to the risks faced by the trust when costs might not be covered and when competitors might emerge to threaten financial viability. On a more mundane level, whenever the directorate discovered that activity levels were exceeding previous levels then the budget would be overspent. This occurred, for instance, whenever consultants changed their prescribing practice, when outside agencies changed their pricing structure, when GPs began referring drugs and alcohol patients to the directorate's in-patient services, and when consultants filled out their forms incorrectly. So the business manager would then be required to investigate whether the cause of the overspend was within their control and, if it was not, to seek extra contractual payments from the purchaser in recognition of the extra business they had been forced to accept. The directorate has to live with considerable uncertainty while negotiating with the purchaser for acceptance of each case, and financial uncertainties also affect the directorate's ability to plan for existing services.

Moreover, the provider has no immediate right of exit from the market. The provider cannot wait for the purchaser before accepting the work. Refusal to offer a service will risk exposure to legal complaint. Despite the use made of 'the market', the organisation of health and social care is as constrained by legal responsibilities and bureaucratic structures as before.

Nevertheless, 'the market' involves an explicit focus on the forms of work to be undertaken and the appropriate level of activity in each. Some anticipate that this implies the demise of bureaucratic control (Hoggett 1990), but here 'the market' remains a metaphoric device rather than an actuality. Organisational purpose is thereby determined as a result of historic practices, policy guidelines, legal requirements and negotiation with purchasers. However these negotiations, while conducted 'as if' they were in a marketplace, are framed partly as an enquiry and justification process. Service developments are framed in terms of policy requirements, rather than in any expectation of securing extra finance from provision of a better service.

■ Organisational boundaries

'The market' requires that boundaries between various economic entities need to be negotiated and defined, even if this goes no further than the creation of separately definable trading units within the one organisation. The boundaries are not spatial, but concern issues such as:

- Trust versus directorate responsibility.
- Strategic autonomy in service provision and development.
- The terms under which negotiation takes place.

These boundaries, while consistent with the purposes of new organisational entities, may be inconsistent with policy. This is particularly the case in mental health care services, and national policy acknowledges this difficulty in speaking of the need for a 'seamless service' between the various component organisations (DoH 1989; DoH/SSI 1991 : 81).

However, these boundaries are not 'fixed', except during negotiation processes that also determine their duration and purpose. Negotiated agreement implies imply no permanence. The trust originally established its community services under separate management but later community mental health services were amalgamated within the mental health directorate. Then, in time, the management of services for people with learning disabilities were also moved in with the directorate.

The fluidity over autonomy is illustrated most dramatically by debate over the replacement of a building containing 50 acute beds, plus another 50 for psycho-geriatric patients, at the centre of the community-based services. Board members and senior management of the Trust were instrumental in securing the agreement of the purchaser in funding its replacement. Subsequently, the directorate's management was changed and was then able to convince the purchaser of another service model that would not require any central building. However, the trust's management and board were committed to the rebuilding process, had obtained planning permission, and still retained overall responsibility for funding the service and for service development.

So, while the directorate is supposed to take responsibility for control of its budget and for delivery of the service, its separate status and autonomy remains negotiable at even mundane levels. Budgets are derived from an annual business planning cycle in which needs and service development plans are presented to the trust. The trust has then taken savings achieved by the mental health directorate to fund overspends by other directorates. Clearly, this is acts as a disincentive to achieving savings but it also undermines 'the market' principle that each entity should maintain the financial viability of its own business. In short, the legitimacy of 'the market' can be overruled by the trust's bureaucracy.

The autonomy of the directorate may seem merely a matter of the trust's management control structures. 'The market' implies a great deal more separation than that, however. The issue here is that the directorate has to compete in a market for custom. It has to compete against other mental health services, of course, but market players compete in 'the market' against all alternative uses for a customer's money. Here, mental health services have to compete against medical and health care services with the trust. Given their near-monopoly locally for mental health services, the trust's other services are the most important competition. Professionalised bureaucracy takes precedence, despite use of 'the market' as a metaphor to provide incentives, allocate work, determine service levels and the search for efficiencies.

■ Competition and collaboration

While markets can incorporate degrees of collaboration or collusion, the usual assumption is that 'the market' is governed by competitive pressures. Use of 'the market' and the competition it implies presents several problems because a considerable degree of collaboration is necessary.

Until the community-based services were merged with the directorate, they were regarded as competitors. This came to be regarded as unhelpful because of the cooperation required. Costing mechanisms were relatively crude and did not encourage collaboration. A higher discharge rate from the hospital could make for greater overall efficiency if community-based services could provide care more cheaply but adversely affected the acute unit's income. Moreover, reduced occupancy rates tell against it in measures of efficiency and increase the costs per patient because the remaining patients had higher dependency.

Nearly two years into the process of creating an 'internal market', the general consent among the directorate's management was that internal contracting arrangements had been divisive. In relation to the CMHTs, the contractual focus was on a 'customer focus', which, in effect, tended to play down the relationships between each team that were required of a multidisciplinary approach. Contracts tended to ignore the services 'we provide to each other'. Britain's internal market is largely determined and regulated by central government and does not allow providers to establish contractual terms that acknowledge their various roles in provision.

■ Conclusion: the power of 'the market'

This chapter has argued that 'the market' is best described as a metaphor intended to effect behaviours and relations within organisations that remain instruments of the state. So 'the market' is used where consumers are not purchasers, where competitors may determine budget margins, where success in winning business actually increases costs but not income, where investment is too high to be placed at risk and where barriers exist to both entry and exit, where health is a social and economic issue rather than simply an individual's, where cost containment rather than expansion is socially desired, where occupational regulation is firmly established and predates market regulation, where legal obligations override market opportunities, and where professional and commercial interests are subsidised by (at least) the stability offered them by state-regulated financing of health care.

'The market' therefore does not replace existing structural arrangements but is effective in defining organisational purposes, identity and relationships. These processes of defining, negotiating and understanding create the new organisational reality, rather than an actual market. Metaphorically, 'the market' offers a challenge to control structures and to medical dominance over what are suitable cases for treatment because it relies more heavily on customers, payers, or purchasers as arbiters of the service offered. For organisational actors and managers, 'the market' provides additional methods of ensuring compliance to organisational goals. These goals can be redefined as being user-led, patient-centred or consumer-focused, without any reliable mechanism for knowing what users, patients or consumers demand of the service.

Chapter 15

Danger on the streets: mental illness, community care and ingratitude

John Wilkinson

■ Introduction

This chapter aims to trace the social construction of mental illness as a menace which is 'out of control' since the introduction of community care policies, and how this image is 'carried' by the Press into our mainstream culture and social reality. It also addresses the ethical debate on 'justice' and 'caring', and how the politics of mental health pressure groups often offer contradictory views of the public perception of mental illness within this debate. The ambiguity of the rhetoric of 'enablement' is discussed in relation to the provision of care and the way in which it is often employed by professionals. Another interesting consideration is whether the mentally ill person in receipt of care should be cast as exhibiting 'ingratitude'. This question is addressed, and finally an alternative model of 'acceptable' care is suggested.

■ 'Community care' – the coding of mental illness

We look first at the ways in which the vision of 'the mad' has been set up by the popular and quality press in the specific identification of mental illness and danger with care in the community as a policy. Mentally ill people are often conflated with other groups such as homeless people, and all of them seen as social dregs. This is reminiscent of the visceral dread evoked by the medieval figure of the leper who brings death and destruction to all he meets. Both groups, but especially the mentally ill, are seen as 'waste': that is, they give nothing to society because they do not actually belong 'in' society; they are migrant 'waste'. Migrant waste is pollution; that is, waste which is not securely warehoused. Such pollution functions in advanced Western society as the 'return of the repressed', the 'dregs' who haunt the streets. The image as applied to mentally ill people is remarkably pervasive and is linked to a discourse of the 'erosion of the social fabric of British society'.

The Press plays a major role in this discourse of panic over the collapse of British society, but it would be a mistake to see the identification of sufferers of mental illness as 'the mad on the streets' as just another hysterical outburst from the tabloid Press in their belligerent quest to identify agents of this social collapse. A cursory survey of the quality press over a period of just one week in 1994 illustrates the wide-ranging nature of this image. I illustrate this point with reference to three articles, one from the political Right (the *Sunday Times*) and two from the social-democratic centre (*Weekend Guardian* and the *Guardian*).

The chief 'Opinion' article in the *Sunday Times* of 22 May 1994 (Amiel 1994) addressed the increase in 'crime, blood and guns' in British society. This classic rending-of-the-social-fabric document by Barbara Amiel identifies the social elements responsible for the 'changing of the rules' which has affected 'a social consciousness that permeates the entire society', and has provided 'an unspoken understanding', which, translated, means that 'England was a happy society' before! (Exactly *when* before is unspecified.) Amiel writes:

First we have to think about what caused the rules to change. Here are some of the reasons:

1. the dismantling of the authority of the family;
2. the abandonment of the religious ethic and our failure to replace it with much else;
3. the emptying of mental hospitals;
4. allowing two thirds of a sentence of the courts to be disposed of by a capricious and unpredictable parole system;
5. the political policies and social pressure for women to go into the labour force thus diminishing the roles of both mother and father in the family;
6. immigration policies that allow the uprooting of large ethnic groups to places where they have no culture or roots and social policies that favour separateness rather than assimilation.

These seemingly disconnected elements combine into a totality of image. This is how a discourse is carried: the sewing together of fragments of ideas, policies and practices to constitute the whole as an offence against the natural order of things. It is interesting to note that in this list of the structured order of society, which includes the family, law, religion, royalty, gender and racial identity, sanity occupies an important place. Amiel is cautious in identifying the blameworthy. Elsewhere in her article she gestures at bureaucrats, politicians, and that favourite target, social workers. Nevertheless, it is not difficult for the reader to translate from her once-removed villain (the state), to identify those she regards as responsible directly for the destruction of the social fabric through their violence. These are young men undisciplined by the traditional family (and whom she describes elsewhere as 'young mutants', thereby excluding them from human and social identity), irresponsible mothers, blacks and the mentally ill. Black people and the mentally ill occupy a similar position as outsiders in this symbolic order. Alongside the abstraction of the family and the law, black people and the expelled denizens of mental hospitals are startlingly identifiable and material actors.

Identification is, of course, relatively difficult where the mentally ill are concerned. Black people, specifically males, are visible, all too visible as a threat to this order. By contrast, the mentally ill represent a lurking menace, invisible until they leap from the bushes, audible only as the footsteps pursuing the victim down the perilous inner-city streets. Again, what might sound an extravagant account has permeated the press, to the extent that reference to such a menace is deployed as a sign to ensure the reader's complicity with the author's view when setting out a contentious argument.

An article in the *Weekend Guardian* magazine of 28 May 1994 affords an especially pertinent example. This is an extended interview with the American anti-rape campaigner, the lawyer Catharine MacKinnon, by Catherine Bennett (Bennett 1994) – the kind of interview which is concerned not so much to elicit the views of the interviewee as to expound the interviewer's opposite position through ridiculing the interviewee in counterpointed commentary (but not to her face). The mockery of MacKinnon's obsession with pornography as the root of all evil, and of her interpretation of penetrative sex as innately violent, is highly entertaining, even if the tactics leave a bad taste; but Bennett cannot withhold an aside which identifies humorously the social threats which *she* recognises as she goes about her daily life:

> MacKinnon's case against pornography rests on her assertion that it saturates all our lives and it is clearly a constant source of chagrin to her that we can't all feel the same. Myself, I find pornography repulsive, from Page 3 downwards, but I feel less directly threatened by it than by stray dogs, dangerous driving and 'care in the community'.

These social threats are united by their common unpredictability and random violence and underlying all three agents is the unconscious and condensed phrase 'stray dogs'. For there can be no doubt that 'care in the community' here refers to the mentally ill, even if, in terms of numbers, elderly persons are affected to an infinitely greater extent by community care policies than are mentally ill people. It is unlikely that Bennett fears she will be felled by a Zimmer frame as she ascends the ramp to the public library. No; mental illness where unbounded by the walls of the asylum has come to figure the invisible, the unpredictable danger in the streets. To this extent only has the mentally ill person retained the leper's grace – that he or she embodies the threat of the 'acts of God' which is the sole attribute God now retains: the potential for unanticipated, meaningless violence. The outcome of the policy of mental hospital closure, still ritually if less than whole-heatedly approved as a humane and decent policy, starts to figure as a sign of the limitations of torn social fabric, where best intentions come into conflict with nature, nature being understood as British common sense.

Five days after Bennett's article, The *Guardian* published a harrowing account, headed 'Liberation of the Damned' (Smith, 1994), of the advent of community care on the Greek island of Leros, 'Europe's most notorious mental home'. The first words in this account of the results of work by 'teams of young and dedicated psychiatrists' are given by a local dignitary:

> We have paid a very severe price housing this hospital,' sighs Michalis Bolulafendis, the feisty president of the local hoteliers association. 'Psychologically and socially the effects have been traumatic, just when we want to change our island's bad image, they start letting the patients out on the streets and even worse, begin settling them in tourist areas. There are many of us who are so afraid we daren't go out.'

It is no coincidence that these words echo so precisely the complaints of well-heeled London concert-goers at the distasteful spectacle of the homeless who congregate in the vicinity of the city's chief arts complex. The underlying figure is of the disgorging of waste across an island whose image of amenable nature, attractive to tourism, is thereby polluted; and a significant contrast between such waste matter and the economically active citizen is marked by the adjective 'feisty', connoting directed energy, which appears precisely in order to conjure up its negative in the mentally ill population, ascribing to it an undirected and potentially violent pervasiveness.

In 1996 a front page of the *Independent* (7th March 1996(b)) illustrated perfectly this connection between 'community care', violent death and madness, the family and the legal system (see Figure 15.1). This portrayal of mental illness as a danger both to the community at large and to those who care in the community must be set in the context of a larger concern with the opposing ethics of justice and care. These two concepts can be seen to inform the whole debate on 'care in the community'.

■ Concepts of justice and care

It has been argued in Chapter 1 that care has been socially constructed as being a 'natural' female attribute and responsibility. It could be argued that this gender bias is present in many moral and psychological theories of care, such as Kohlberg's (1976, 1978) which place the concept of an abstract justice above all considerations, a point made by Gilligan (1982). Other writers argue that the hidden assumption that care will fall to women to perform is internalised by them and that women actually negotiate with this given role in their lives (Puka 1993; Tronto 1993). It is evident in both Gilligan's and Kohlberg's work that the concepts of both justice and care can be said to have an individualistic orientation. Gilligan argues that care is embedded not just in one individual but in a whole set of interrelationships with others in a similar social and cultural position as, for instance, between a group of white women. This however becomes problematic when care has to be extended towards other groups which do not 'belong'. On the other hand, a theory of justice is based upon a more universalist

Care in the community

He went berserk and stabbed his mother 43 times with a 12-inch Bowie knife When his 11-year-old brother tried to intervene, he stabbed him 25 times before clubbing them both with an iron bar. Later, he said: 'It was inevitable'

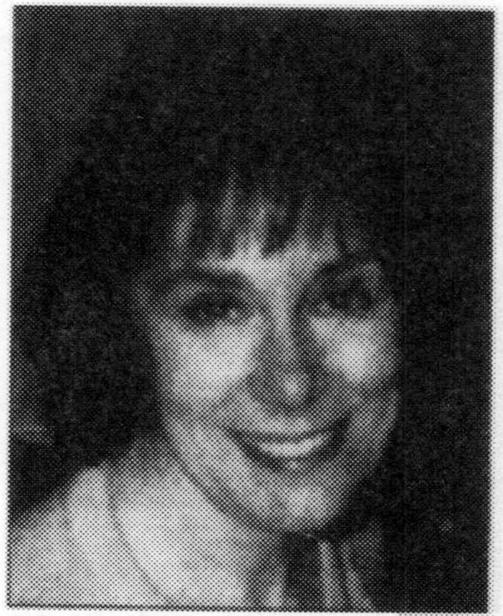

GLENDA COOPER

A judge yesterday highlighted how the Government's 'care in the community' policy had turned into a nightmare when a paranoid schizophrenic discharged himself from hospital and a month later stabbed his mother and young brother to death in a frenzied attack.

At Nottingham Crown Court Anthony Smith, 24, pleaded guilty to manslaughter with diminished responsibility and was ordered to be detained in Rampton secure hospital indefinitely.

The judge, Mr Justice Latham, sought a review of the circumstances in which he received "care in the community", saying that the case presented "the nightmare that those who care for people with schizophrenia must fear".

Smith was diagnosed as a paranoid schizophrenic in July 1995 and had been a patient at Derby City General Hospital for less than a month before discharging himself and returning home with the approval of his consultant Dr Sarah Barrett. At home he stopped taking medication.

A month later, after an argument with his mother, Gwendoline, he said he had "just gone berserk" and stabbed her 43 times with a 12-inch Bowie knife. When his 11-year-old half-brother David tried to intervene he stabbed him 25 times before clubbing them with an iron bar.

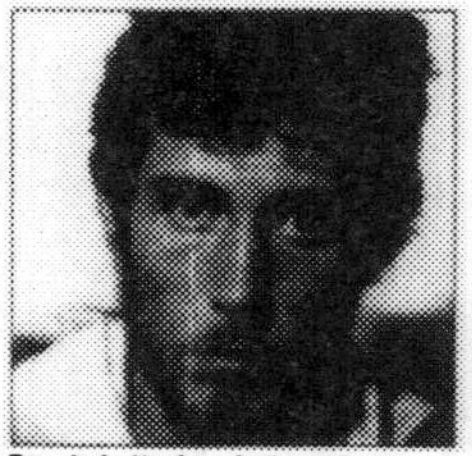

Smith cleaned the knife, showered and changed his clothes. He then left a note on his brother's body, saying: "I am sorry David, I love you," before locking up the house and handing himself in at his local medical centre. He told staff there: "It was inevitable".

Ordering Smith to be detained indefinitely, the judge said: "This is a case where the circumstances of this young man's release into life community, and perhaps more importantly the circumstances of the care that has been given in the community, are to be looked at with great care."

His adoptive father, Peter Smith, said yesterday: "I knew something was going to happen from what I was learning about the illness. There was nobody else to help, it was down to me. I had nowhere else to turn. I don't want this to happen to somebody else, to some other family.

"I have nothing to say to [Anthony] any more. I have said what I wanted to say and that is it. As far as I am concerned ... I have lost both my sons.

Southern Derbyshire Health Trust said an inquiry would be held into the case but that an internal review had found "no major breakdowns" in the care given. Dr Barrett, who is now on maternity leave, will not face disciplinary action.

"[Anthony] Smith was keen to return home and the consultant felt that he was ready to return to an environment where he had lived safely for 23 years, providing he took medication regularly and agreed to out-patient follow-up," said a spokesman. "The acts committed were totally unexpected."

But Jayne Zito, of the Zito Trust, said the case left the Government with "blood on its hands". Mrs Zito, whose husband, Jonathan, was killed by schizophrenic Christopher Clunis in December 1992, said: "We would hope the inquiry goes one step further to show where there has been negligence in the care. How can they say there has been no major breakdown in care when two people have been killed?"

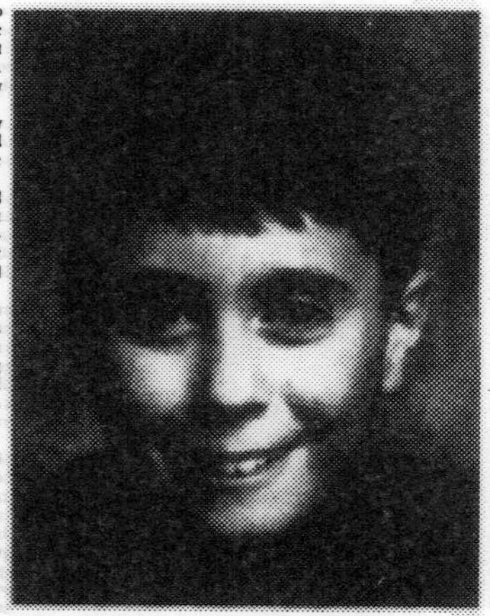

Frenzied attacker: Anthony Smith

Victim: Smith killed his mother Gwendoline after a row

Victim: Half-brother David, stabbed 25 times

Figure 15.1 Newspaper linkage of 'community care' with violent death

view which aspires to universally applicable rights which override an individuals' personal beliefs and preferences. A concept of community care which relies upon specifically personal interactions runs the risk of determining the limits of care and withholding care from those who do not 'fit'. Therefore a theory of care has either to pay heed to the ethics of justice, or else to extend the responsibility of care beyond the borders of a community. An example of the latter view is to be found in Dalley's (1988) radical feminist critique of community care policies, which she regards as hopelessly complicit with a sexist construction of care. She argues powerfully for the abandonment of such policies (for which she reads unpaid and oppressive women's work) in favour of the collective organisation of care. The term 'collective' she adopts in order to avoid the pejorative connotations of 'institutional' care. In this reading, this would extend to provision for the family in terms of childrearing and the feeding of the collective; it refers to the socialisation of the means of reproduction as well as to the means of production, and looks forward to the provision of public restaurants and nurseries as have feminist radicals at least since the bolshevik revolution.

While the academic debates around the concepts of care and justice shed some illumination on the politics of mental health in the community, it is striking that the debates say little about what it means to be the object of care, that is to be the cared-for. Often it does indeed appear that for the object of care either a stark choice or an involved contradiction is apparent: they are cast, on the one hand, as the recipient of care, to which the appropriate response would be gratitude; on the other, they are viewed as a (potentially) free social agent, who is required to make a range of choices, *as if* they were a fully empowered member of society requiring no care, *in order that* should become this fully empowered member requiring no care. The latter option is underpinned by an ideology of the relations of care, which insists that if they fail to act (as if they were a fully empowered agent) then they become undeserving of care, while acting as if fully empowered – that is, no longer in need of care. Care in this connection may be little more, of course, than attendance at a day centre during specified hours; as Prior observes, 'the tendency to view the directed and synchronised activities as fulfilling some kind of therapeutic or beneficial aim can be found just as readily outside the hospital as within it' (Prior 1993: 171) and is just as much a pretext for surveillance and containment.

There is a faint echo here of housing policy – that if evicted by a local authority an individual may be deemed to have made themselves 'intentionally homeless' and therefore undeserving of rehousing. This approach is not entirely fortuitous; as we will see, the homeless and the severely mentally ill fulfil an important common function in delineating the boundaries of community. The identification of 'the homeless' with 'the mentally ill' discharged from long-stay hospital wards is a tenacious myth that is not easily dispelled despite evidence to the contrary. For as Thompson (1993) states,

> Despite adverse publicity about mentally ill people 'roaming the streets',
> official fears that many are ex-long stay psychiatric patients appear to be

misplaced. Current research indicates that less than 2 per cent have been in psychiatric hospital for a year or more and 68 per cent have spent an average of less than *three months* (my emphasis) in a psychiatric hospital at any one time. (Thompson 1993:27).

■ Justice

The complexity of the contradictions embodied in the person of a sufferer from severe mental illness may be further illuminated by reference to the most influential of current justice theories, that of John Rawls (Rawls 1972). The rights and responsibilities attached to a member of a just society are necessarily compromised in the interests of care, because rights and responsibilities can only be attached to and entertained by a fully rational being. Consequently children, for instance, both enjoy a restricted range of rights and face limited responsibilities, and fall into the sphere of compensatory care. The same would apply to those affected by severe learning difficulties. (There is of course a major question, both individually and collectively acute, as to the extent to which both children and those with learning difficulties are actually excluded from full social being by socially imposed disability rather than by any inherent irrationality and unreliability – a question which arises, for instance, in the status of a child's evidence in court.)

The adult sufferer from severe mental illness, however, occupies a curious position in respect of rational social being, and its attached rights and responsibilities. They cannot be regarded either as at a stage on a developmental pathway towards full social being, with restrictions warranted in the interests of their attaining full developmental status, or as fixed at an early point on the developmental pathway (as with severe learning difficulties), with a presumed lack of potential for further progress. First, their presumed irrationality may be amenable to therapeutic intervention in order to restore them to full developmental status. Second, following psychiatric diagnosis, their rationality is deemed always susceptible to relapse into irrationality. Third, their irrationality is fitful, with the textbook psychiatric indicator of 'lack of insight' not having a definitive status as a sign of psychosis, either positively or negatively. Fourth, it is notoriously the case that reading the signs of irrationality is a culturally determined practice, with ample evidence now published of the effects on psychiatric diagnosis of racism or sheer cultural ignorance (Littlewood and Lipsedge 1982; Frosh 1989).

■ Community care – enablement and disablement

Care being a compensation for an ineligibility to enjoy the full range of adult social rights and responsibilities, it follows that for the politics of disablement as represented through some user organisations care has implicity become defined as the contrary of enablement. Enablement can be defined as that set of political practices which challenges conferred ineligibility and its resulting social disablement. Thus the construction 'community care' stands exactly for 'social disablement', through a sleight of hand in which social responsibility is rejected for a myth of the organic community and enablement is substituted for the myth of care, where care seals and contains the cared-for in their place of exclusion. The model shown in Table 15.1 may illustrate more clearly this dichotomy between the formal and the informal structures of meaning.

Table 15.1 Codes of alternative meanings in social care language

Community Care/Social Disablement

Enablement/Rehabilitation

Ingratitude/Failure of recipients to respond to care or enablement

Care/Compensation for deprivarion of full adult rights

Packages of care/Distribution of services.

Competent self-help/Recipient constructed as fully responsible
citizen

The model illustrates the potential for the actual inversion of meaning. In this way enablement becomes rewritten as proposing the individually targeted supply of compensatory goods and services (material benefits, skills training, therapeutic services and information) to sufferers from mental illness.

In its final reduction, 'enablement' becomes an effect of the delivery of a 'package of care', with the individual under the moral obligation to respond through full entry into an implicit contract. Only in this way can the individual be transformed into a responsible social actor. This process effectively 'splits' the individual into fragments, their many needs parcelled to different members of the multi-disciplinary team. But at the same time, the person retains the potential for full citizenship rights and obligations.

■ Ingratitude

There is a further twist, however, failure to fulfil the terms of the contract implicit in community care marks the mentally ill person as ungrateful. He or she has failed to take advantage of the services offered. This mark of ingratitude associates the mentally ill person with the black person in a racist society – ingratitude, indeed, is linked closely with irrationality, unpredictability and danger. This can be read in the major pejorative construct of the mentally ill person, as represented in the popular journalism already discussed. The mentally ill person uncontained by care represents a threat to the natural, civilised order which has nurtured him or her, as the black person represents a threat to the natural civilised order which has adopted them. 'Natural' in this sense is defined as the social order to which people are expected to conform. Those who do not can be seen as ungrateful in their rejection of the care provided by that social order. Such an offence against the social order tends to be read in terms of ingratitude for care, it being deemed 'natural' to be grateful for care as one is obviously grateful to one's mother for bearing and nurturing. People who do not articulate or show gratitude to mothers are often referred to as 'unnatural'.

Within this definition, the mentally ill individual is one whose ingratitude is shockingly apparent in the nakedness of its denial of family obligations. This ingratitude haunts the literature of carer organisations, even at its most measured; for instance, the pamphlet *Schizophrenia: The Forgotten Illness* issued by SANE (an acronym for Schizophrenia A National Emergency), while couched in the main in dispassionate scientific language, refers repeatedly to the particular distress which schizophrenic individuals visit on the family, giving the impression that the nation is the family writ large: 'They may involve their relatives in their persecutory symptoms, become difficult, antagonistic, abusive or even threatening towards them'; and: 'This may call for great calmness and restraint by the family and possibly separation of the sufferer from them ...' (SANE 1993). In the heart of the home lurks the nightmare child who will not grow up, and whose response to care is unpredictable and violent ingratitude. This is not at all to deny or downplay the distress experienced by those close to a person with severe mental illness; the irony is that this 'unnaturalness' and 'ingratitude' within the natural order is paralleled by an assignment of the mentally ill as outsiders.

Little wonder, then, that people with severe mental illness come to internalise this social view of themselves as violent and polluting agents, even as they contest the category to which they are so assigned. Thus the author found members of a MIND organisation in West Glamorgan, who were considering the transfer of acute treatment resources to a general hospital, to be preoccupied with the fear that their own presence would literally kill physically ill patients through causing them heart attacks. Their demand was explicitly for segregated services which would render themselves safe for the general public when acutely ill – even though not one of those involved had a history of violence during episodes of illness. This ran alongside an equally striking pride in the mutual support which membership of MIND afforded, and contrasted with the irregularity of the support received from family and erstwhile friends.

Such a split reflects precisely the rationale advanced for the Independent Living Movement among those physically disabled, with its 'increasingly dominant view that disability is not merely socially constructed, but socially created as a form of institutionalised social oppression' (Oliver 1990: 119), within which the victim is blamed and comes to blame themselves for that oppression and to regard it as natural and reasonable. The development of self-help strategies is proposed as a response to this bind. Care when associated with the commitment to self-help may cease to be a mechanism which compensates for exclusion or which aims to restore the individual to the status of the fully responsible citizen. For care as delivered through community care services will always be resented, in so far as it locates the cared-for as no more than the site of a lack – as lacking human rights and dignity, categorically as less than a full citizen, economically as useless, symbolically as waste and therefore lacking the potential for conversion into value. Care of this kind both infantilises and denies the privileges of infancy, because its characteristic is that it is never there when needed, only when scheduled. The kind of dependency it enforces is a cruel one, in which the good is offered and snatched away in the same movement, its withdrawal always being ascribed to a lack in the cared-for (no motivation, no initiative, failure to take advantage of what is offered); no wonder the politics of radical users' groups deploys the term 'care' pejoratively!

However, to follow this logic as far as it will go, towards an advocacy of separatism and the proposal that care delivered through formal, professional mechanisms is fatally blighted, would be not only a counsel as much of despair as of hope, but also would lay upon those suffering from mental illness an intolerable burden and obligation. Indeed, through implicit acceptance of social hostility towards those disabled on whatever account, it would revert to an exclusionary social policy, whereby those afflicted would withdraw themselves rather than await legalistic confinement. Self-help can only be a choice for those in a position to recognise its benefits; in practical terms, the person who falls ill has an immediate need for care and (sometimes) treatment which cannot and should not be curtailed or withheld, and to enjoin self-help is merely to translate onto group level the same double-bind which faces the individual in the therapeutically reinforced programme of 'enablement'. Thus it was that when working in an inner-city resource centre I experienced at first hand the indignation of users who had been required to 'empower' themselves through taking responsibility for all aspects of the centre's management and day-to-day activities; 'So what are these social workers and CPNs paid to do?' was their often heard (and justified) complaint.

■ Towards a model of 'acceptable' care

In reverting to the initial question of the experience of the subject of care, the urgent task, is therefore, to articulate a model of acceptable care – that is, care which follows a kind of natural logic through recognising its foundations in the course of maternal nurturing. This would entail an understanding by the carer of the dynamics of envy, and an explicit commitment towards the issuing of formal care into mutual help (a term preferable to self-help), a dynamic analogous to that of the passage from the paranoid-schizoid to the depressive position. Some inkling of the style of care required can be gleaned from a remarkable article by Tom Kitwood (1990), which reviews the effect of styles of care on the course of an illness regarded conventionally as determined exclusively by physiological process, but which Kitwood demonstrates to be affected profoundly by what he terms a 'malignant social psychology' mediated through poor care. Analysing the characteristics of care which seems to inhibit the course of dementia, he identifies three positive qualities:

Good care giving requires a person to 'be there' for the other in a way which far transcends commonsense... High levels of empathy and imagination are required, as also a kind of flexibility of thinking that sits loose to literal, concrete interpretation. It requires a person to slow down inwardly, and to cultivate a kind of inner quietness, so that messages given by the sufferer may be attended to without distraction.

... to be a person is to have the status of a sentient being, to be recognised as having a value, and to hold a distinct place in a group or collective of some kind.

The third quality, I would suggest, applies exactly to a mutual-help group such as the MIND group whose benefits were so appreciated by its members (p. 216). What is striking about the first two qualities is their consonance with the Kleinian concept of 'maternal reverie', which describes the mother's receptiveness as a container for the infant's anxieties and fears, a presence which entails a kind of hovering attention (Bion 1970), allowing the mother to receive the infant's envious projections without the damage which would result in the infant's catastrophic experience of themselves as damaging to her on whom they are dependent. This quality of containment is transferred during the course of adult life onto other persons and onto the groups and institutions within which we have our being, and the effects on an individual's internal life of reiterated designation is that which causes damage could hardly be expressed more vividly than by those who envisage themselves as the bringers of death into the hospital.

The implications of this for the style of community care can only be gestured at in this chapter, but crucially it could be argued that the whole panoply of 'packages of care' distributed among a range of services and professionals is fundamentally antipathetic to good care, and that the mechanisms of key-working and care coordinating represent little more than an impotent recognition of the inherently antitherapeutic power of such a system of care delivery. Abstracted surveillance in the tracking of those at risk is an extrapolation from maternal reverie which can only result in furious resentment, given its unamenability to the needs of the sufferer. This is a container which would attend to everything, but take nothing return in for true care and permit no reparation for damage. In short, we may need to look again at the potential of the well-trained 'good carer' or even of the 'good institution'. There could be a link to material encouragement (but not an obligated membership), for mutual-help groups to be accorded far more power, responsibility and resources than the tokenistic 'user involvement' which are boasted of in a thousand policy statements but which have no discernible effect on actual practice.

■ Conclusion

This chapter has attempted to deconstruct the image of the supposed danger to society which is threatened by the policy of care in the community for those suffering from mental illness. The fact that there have been a series of sensationalised and tragic cases involving recipients of such care should not distract us from the essential image of 'waste' and 'pollution' on the streets which has been powerfully constructed. I have also addressed the problematic enactment of ideals of 'justice' and 'caring' and the significance of these concepts for the practice of the delivery of care. The rhetoric of care must be carefully analysed, especially when it is delivered via a stated objective of 'enablement'. This term is also, I suggest, in need of rigorous deconstruction. Is such a policy objective of 'enablement' merely a camouflage for the reduction of human rights and the curtailing of resources? Indeed, is the delivery of 'care' itself a means of surveillance and control? These are questions which need to be addressed if a truly 'caring' system is to be constructed.

Chapter 16

Poverty and community care

Mark Drakeford

■ Introduction

In this chapter, I begin with a brief justification of the premise that the management of poverty by the social security system is oppressive in nature and practice. The argument I suggest is that poverty on a large scale forms the inescapable background to the work of community care practitioners. Indeed, I suggest that, in some important ways, the typical working practices and frameworks of community care – purchaser–provider splits, assessments, community care managers and so on – make these factors all the more acute. Having established this essential context, I then go on to consider ways in which social welfare services might respond, suggesting a model and a set of working practices which, it is argued, provide a defensible and worthwhile way of working, even in these troubled times.

■ Poverty in policy and practice

Poverty dominates the landscape of social welfare practice. Fifty years after the implementation of the Beveridge Report, one of his five giants – want – has grown to produce hardcore and lasting impoverishment. The social security system, far from being a safety net, has come more to resemble a hunting net in which individuals and families are unhappily corralled. Treated with suspicion and contempt by those responsible for the net, they are nevertheless trapped within it and unable to escape its meshes. In ever-increasing numbers they turn to social-welfare workers for help. This pattern applies as much in community care work as in any other part of the professional field. Despite the rhetoric of 'empowerment' or 'anti-oppression', the response which services offer to individuals in this position is all too often geared to confirming them in, and reconciling them to, their unhappy situation. Alternative models do exist, of particular relevance to community care, which might hold out some hope of acting otherwise.

■ Policy

The world which community care workers and their clients inhabit is the product of policies carefully planned and deliberately pursued. Theorists debate the extent to which governments 'control' the way policies are provided and implemented or are at the mercy of what Harold Macmillan, answering an interviewer's question about what shaped his actions, described as 'events, dear boy, events'. Paul Wilding, for example, in an overview of public sector policy during the 1980s, concluded that even the ideologically driven Thatcher administrations had proceeded by 'a process of shuffle, test and stumble' (Wilding 1992 : 10). In the field of income maintenance, however, it is clear that a series of guiding principles, adapted and amended over time, have amounted to a qualitative shift in the operation and impact of government policy. Two central ideas have produced a particular impact upon poor people, and specifically those who come within the ambit of community care.

First, governments since 1979 have espoused a clear belief that in order to make the rich work harder they must be better rewarded, while in order to make poor people work at all they must be weaned from the luxury of over-lavish state benefits, while their resolve to seek employment must be sharpened with the carrot of necessity and the stick of an ever more restrictive and stigmatising administration. J. K. Galbraith (1989) captures most elegantly the enduring belief among governments that:

> there is something economically damaging about help to the poor. It destroys morale ... It seduces people away from gainful employment ... the case is made and believed. There is something gravely damaging about aid to the unfortunate. It is perhaps our most highly influential piece of fiction.

Bill Jordan and Jon Arnold (1996) characterise the resulting British system more forcefully as one in which the income maintenance system has been 'criminalised ... trapping claimants in roles of resentful, excluded supplication' (p. 38) and in which 'government policy in every sphere treats the poor as calculative criminals, and devises its rules and procedures accordingly' (p. 40). The result has been a worsening in real terms of the position of the poorest in our society. According to the government's own figures, since 1979 the bottom 10 per cent has seen its income after housing costs drop by 14 per cent, (House of Commons 1993), whereas the top 10 per cent has experienced a real-terms 62 per cent explosion in their incomes through a combination of pay increases and tax advantages (Quick and Wilkinson 1993; Oppenheim 1994; Hills 1990).

Second, and particularly during the tenure of the last Conservative Secretary of State, Peter Lilley, social security policy became driven by the fear that spending on income maintenance had grown too fast for the economy to be able to sustain, a position which was seen to be set to worsen sharply because of the 'demographic timebomb' of an ageing population supported by fewer and fewer economically productive people (for a useful setting out of both these arguments see Lilley's own *Mais Lecture* (1983)). While the premises upon which this approach is based are open to convincing challenge (see, for example, Hutton 1995; Oppenheim 1994), they have produced a direct policy outcome: Firstly, the Job Seeker's Allowance has been set to cut the value of insurance-related benefits (while increasing the level of contributions) and to introduce a series of eligibility constraints which would extended the demands upon claimants to 'prove' that they are 'really' looking for work and penalise them more harshly and more capriciously should they be found wanting (see Venn 1995 and CPAG 1994 for further details).

At the same time, the replacement of Invalidity Benefit by Incapacity Benefit has extended the assault upon the 'jobshy' (*Conservative Party News* 1994), an already well-established target, to the malingering, a characterisation of the long-term sick which any government has previously proved wary in making. Now, in the words of Lilley, the changes have been needed to ensure the 'weeding out of those who are not genuinely sick'. Incapacity Benefit both is less generous than Invalidity Benefit and treated less favourably in other ways – for example, by being made taxable, which Invalidity Benefit was not. In a genuine departure in income maintenance policy, benefit claimants will thus be treated less favourably than some groups able to afford tax-deductible private health insurance. Incapacity Benefit will also be more difficult to obtain. The 'all work' test which claimants will have to pass is variously estimated at producing a fall in 14 per cent of the number of successful applicants (Lynes 1994) or, in the government's own prediction, a reduction in the number of claimants of 70000 a year and a saving of £1.8 billion over two years (Barnes 1995; CPAG 1995).

For those people who characteristically come to the attention of community care workers these changes are clearly detrimental. They also contain a peculiar double jeopardy which threatens to worsen the lot of some individuals in particular. These are claimants who find themselves denied Incapacity Benefit, because, under the 'all work' rule, they will be found capable of *some sort* of work, but who also, because their personal and health circumstances are regarded as so limiting, will be deemed to be unavailable for work and so not entitled to Job Seeker's Allowance either. There is evidence of this having begun to happen even before the changes have been fully introduced. As Peter Raynor (1996 : 20) has suggested in the context of criminal justice work, 'changes in sentencing patterns *precede* legislation, on the basis of political statements which signal shifts in policy'. So, too, in the field of community care, government messages about attitudes towards people in poverty influence both the climate for practice and the outcomes of daily decision-making.

■ Practice

If this is the policy background, then the evidence that the practice agenda of social work and other social welfare agencies is dominated by poverty is overwhelming. By the end of the 1980, 90 per cent of new referrals to social workers came from social security claimants (Clements 1995). Two-thirds of all referrals were benefit-or housing-related and nearly one-third of these were to do with the Social Fund (Becker and Silborn 1990). Gill Stewart, in one of the major research programmes into the establishment and operation of the Fund, found that fully six out of ten clients in active contact with social services departments were said to be so because of self-referral for a Social Fund problem (Stewart and Stewart 1990). The National Association of Probation Officers, in a survey of its members, found that individuals 'commencing probation supervision were 8 times more likely to be unemployed and 2 to 3 times more likely to be long-term unemployed than the rest of the population' (NAPO 1993). Almost 80 per cent of the whole client population were dependent upon means-tested benefits, compared with 20 per cent of the whole population, rising to more than 90 per cent in major urban areas.

Evidence directly within the community care field is, because of its recent nature, more difficult to discover. It is also a concept which has escaped some of the more convinced writers in the field. A very recent, lengthy and highly congratulatory evaluation of the Darlington Community Care Project (Challis *et al.* 1995), for example, makes no mention of poverty at all. A useful exception is to be found in David Barrett's (1992) exploration of the experience of 'economically fragile' older people within the new system. Barrett points to the bifurcation of income maintenance policy in relation to older people. Here, in what Eric Midwinter (1991) of the Centre for Policy on Ageing has called 'a hideous dichotomy', occupational pensions and fiscal advantage will lift a significant proportion into relative security, leaving the remainder to survive upon the residual, resentful and rationed provision of the state. In a comprehensive review, he concludes that 'for older people living in poverty... the notion of choice must, indeed, be a hollow one, whether the person is in the position of being cared for, or is a carer' (Midwinter 1991:310). Barrett also reiterates, in this context, a finding which has been well established elsewhere (see, for example Glendinning and Millar 1992; Lister 1992). The poverty he discovered among 'economically fragile' older people and their carers was not equally shared among the different groups of people who come to the attention of social welfare workers. Women carry the burden of poverty in our society, through their often marginal relationship to the economy and because of the burden of care for dependants which government policy has forced back into the domestic sphere. Black people, too, because of their over-representation in unemployment and poorly paid, low-status occupations, are more likely than other groups to be at the sharp end of poverty and material deprivation (Amin and Oppenheim, 1992; NACAB 1991).

Economic fragility is the linking thread which characterises all the groups of people with whom community care workers come into contact. It is time to look in more detail at the response to that poverty which such workers provide.

■ Community care, poverty, policy and practice

At the start of this chapter, I suggested that the general response of social welfare systems to the impoverished state of their users has been insupportable. The idea that poverty lies outside the scope of what such services have to offer or beyond the ability of local teams and individuals to design and develop is highly integrated into a professional culture of pessimism. Yet it is assistance precisely in these basic areas which is most valued by clients and appreciated by them when it is delivered (see, for example, Stockley *et al.* 1993). Sadly, the policy framework within which community care has been developed appears more often designed to add to this paralysis than to challenge it. From the outset, it has been clear that behind the pieties of client choice lie the stark realities of resource constraint. Case managers, according to *Caring for People*, '*Should* take account of the wishes of the individual and his or her carer' but '*will have to* take into account what is available and affordable' (my emphasis) (Department of Health 1989).

Resources are finite; people are malleable – and the poorer they are, the more malleable they will need to be. Scarcely was the ink dry on the paper than the government moved to make it clear that 'needs assessments' were not to be carried out or recorded in such a way as to suggest that the discovery of need implied an undertaking that it would be met. Appearing before the House of Commons Health Committee, Herbert Laming, Chief Inspector of the Social Services Inspectorate, was questioned about Department of Health guidance which cautioned local authorities against recording assessment of need in a way which might 'raise unrealistic expectations on the part of users and carers' (House of Commons, Health Committee 1993a). Indeed, the advice appeared to suggest strongly that assessment of need might best be recorded so as not to link individuals and need in an identifiable way:

> If individual feedback is recorded, it should be borne in mind that, even though it might not form part of the user's assessment or care plan, it might still be accessed by users, under the terms of the access to information legislation, if the data identifiably relates to them.

The Committee's response was unequivocal:

> we recommend that clear guidance be issued urgently to local authorities on this matter and, if necessary, legislation be introduced to make sure that there are no inhibitions on the ability of social services departments and health authorities to make a full assessment of unmet needs. (para. 64)

Against this unpromising background, and in a period of ever more severe expenditure cut-backs, the results have been predictable. Large-scale purchasers – in the shape of cash-starved local authorities – shop where prices are lowest. Block contracts and undifferentiated provision becomes the result. A series of studies have found that community care assessments take a standardised form with needs having to be met against a standard list of available services:

> From our sample of contracts it is not at all clear that service users have more choice as a result of the process. Either the contracts replicated existing services or established a new service which then became the only one on offer. (Common and Flynn 1992, quoted in Davies 1994 : 11)

Or, in the words of one carer group interviewed by Hoyles *et al.* (1994 : 11): 'The theory of package is bunkum – there is a set list and if what you want is not there, it is not available.' Working within highly pressurised budgets, it was difficult for staff to switch from matching people to services to identifying needs. 'In most cases', the authors concluded, 'it was a matter of being offered what was available – the choice was to accept it or not' (Hoyles *et al.* 1994 : 17). More disturbing still are the findings reported by Ellis (1993 : 7), where the pressures on services produced a rationing complex among some groups of staff which clearly militated against any sort of needs-led service. Here it was not simply a matter of stereo-typical responses chosen from a limited menu but of a cast of mind in which the closer a worker was 'to resourcing decisions, the more conservative their practice appeared to be' (Ellis : 22).

Indeed, if there is a criticism to be made of the developing pattern of community care, it is surely this: budget inadequacies and cut-backs have been too easily accommodated into practice in a way which justifies and defends rationing, rather than protesting and campaigning against the effects upon individuals who have no recourse to funds of their own. Thus the High Court judgement in the case of Gloucester County Council – which found that resources could be taken into account when assessing clients' needs – amounted, in the words of Thompson and Dobson (1995 : 20) to 'a significant blow. In one stroke the judgement endorses cuts in services and kills stone dead the late Sir Roy Griffiths's philosophy, the essence of the policy, that community care be driven by need not money.' The point I wish to make is not to heap criticism upon an authority so affected by cuts that it felt itself obliged to remove services from what Clements (1995) characterised as individuals in their seventies with 'fairly severe disabling conditions', notifying them of that decision by letter. It is rather to protest against the reported reaction of the Director of Gloucestershire Social Services that the judgement 'reinforces good practice. It reinforces the power of local authorities to ration services' (reported in Thompson and Dobson 1995). People fortunate enough to share sufficiently in the wealth of a rich society are able to make their own arrangements for care and comfort. Those who in old age or disability are so poor as to have to rely on community care arrangements deserve better than to have their needed services withdrawn and that withdrawal defended in such terms. Their comfort is cold indeed.

In a world where resource constraint produces such unintended and perverse outcomes, it is those already afflicted by poverty or other disadvantages who are at greatest risk. Jadeja and Singh (1993) reported on the community care experience of a group of Asian elders at an inner-city Leicester day centre. The dominating factor in their lives was the extent to which they were considerably poorer than a comparison group of their white contemporaries. In community care terms it led to a double jeopardy. Flat rate charges for services bear most heavily on those with lowest incomes. Means-tested schemes result in those with least money themselves costing purchasers the most. For the Leicester group the question was directly raised: were they likely to get a worse service as a result?

Even in studies which are enthusiastically supportive of the policy and of particular examples of implementation, the practical nexus of individual poverty and limited budgets is clear: 'the general trade-off incurred is that the cheaper the type of community care utilised then the lower will be the corresponding quality of life experienced by clients' (Haycox 1995 : 104).

■ A way forward

This depressing picture of harassed workers, zealously protecting budgets, fending off requests for help or rudely shoehorning those whose claims cannot be avoided into a predetermined, choiceless, set of cheapest-available service, is deliberately exaggerated. What it does, however, is to highlight an approach to social welfare practice which remains dominated by professional perspectives and by a view of 'community' which is uniformly top-down. As a counterbalance to these powerful forces I offer instead an approach to working with people in poverty which puts that part of their experience at the forefront of practice and which places attempts to assist in those areas closer to the core of what social welfare services provide.

Three distinct strategies are suggested through which, even in these times, workers and agencies can move in this direction. The first, and in some ways the most obvious, is to consider the direct ways in which social welfare agencies, as powerful organisations in their own right, deploy their financial resources. Social Services Departments in England alone spent £6600 million in 1994–5. Transfer of resources and additional funding to meet community care responsibilities have been estimated at £1.8 billion in 1995–6 (Department of Health 1995). Working within impoverished communities such agencies are in a position – often ignored – to have an impact upon the economies of such localities. Decisions about employment strategies, location of offices, purchase of goods and services all contribute to a pattern in which services are either net contributors or net subtractors from the amount of money which circulates within a local economy. When an organisation needlessly develops recruitment policies which determine that its staff have to be drawn almost exclusively from outside such communities, when it locates these staff in large and remote office suites and when it uses its purchasing power to enrich far-off companies and corporations, rather than local firms and facilities, then it actually worsens the financial circumstances of those it is meant to assist. In contrast, decisions to invest these resources within such communities stands as a practical and principled symbol of determination to tackle the circumstances which produce such problems in the first place. Community care practice ought to be in the forefront of such an anti-poverty strategy. The replacement of large, centrally situated offices by a pattern of local and neighbourhood centres brings particular benefits to service users for whom mobility is a constant problem. A recruitment strategy which aims positively to include people with disabilities among social welfare workers not only enriches the quality of service but also helps to address the financial needs of a group which, according to the estimates of the Disability Alliance (1991 : 3), have a produced an 'income gap' of nearly £8 billion between the incomes of disabled and non-disabled people.

Such strategies are not new, either in the field of social welfare or in local authority practice generally. In South Glamorgan, for example, social work decentralisation has seen the breakup of a large, city centre office – at least two bus journeys from the parts of Cardiff in which most clients live – to a pattern of local and neighbourhood centres. The practice basis for this change is most often expressed in terms of partnership, accessibility and sensitivity to local needs. In economic terms, however, the change is also part of the council's overall anti-poverty programme, which positively encourages an alignment of spending and service-delivery decisions and the direct investment of resources within the most needy communities.

A second strand in a strategy for addressing poverty among community care clients lies in a refocusing of work in the basic business of welfare rights. The massive extent to which older people, in particular, continue to miss out on benefits to which they are entitled is well established (Oppenheim 1993). Yet, in a time of ideological and practical attack upon social security provision, a simple 'claim it' campaign approach, as in former days, is no longer adequate. Inter-vention with hostile systems which proceeds from a naïve belief in their basic helpfulness, or which places a premium upon the maintenance of 'good relations' between one worker and another or one bureaucracy and another, is certainly likely to produce unintended and harmful results. Instead, a more general integration of the 'determined advocacy' approach developed in relation to the Social Fund is required. This strategy has been widely adopted by organisations representing social welfare workers and managements.

The evidence of professional performance in this area contains some encour-agement. The central thrust of findings among the different research projects set up to investigate the impact and operation of the Social Fund the central thrust is to confirm the central flaws of the Fund itself while vividly illustrating the shocking impact of its deliberate shortcomings upon the lives of the most dis-advantaged clients. Against that background these studies (Becker and Silburn 1990; Stewart and Stewart 1991, and Craig and Glendinning 1990) also develop two further themes of particular relevance to the purposes of this chapter.

First, there is clear evidence of widespread and persistent effort of the part of social workers in pursing Social Fund claims, and general agreement that such intervention was likely to result in beneficial outcomes for their clients. The Joseph Rowntree Foundation, for example, reported that workers 'spend a lot of time and effort in dealing with clients' Social Fund-related problems: at least an hour had already been spent in 64 per cent of cases', producing a result in which 'interven-tion on clients' behalf seemed to be effective insofar as contact had been made by social workers in the course of 62 per cent of successful grant applications, while there was no contact in 53 per cent of those which were rejected outright' (Rowntree Foundation 1990). Currently, the scandal of the Social Fund, in its ritual humiliation and casual neglect of desperate people, remains. The lesson for community care practitioners has to be that in this, and in other social security encounters, determined pursuit of clients' interests has to be maintained in the face of, and in the expectation of, a deliberately hostile system.

Second, the surveys establish that clients themselves were appreciative of effort as well as results, or even where no results were forthcoming. The same Rowntree survey commented that 'clients often had low expectations and were easily pleased with very little'. In a smaller-scale local survey in the Northumbria Probation Service, a survey of practice on poverty issues found that 75 per cent of clients who had received such help from a probation officer rated that help as useful or very useful (Northumbria Probation Service 1994). Community care workers are involved in assisting their service users to make decisions which stretch into some of the most fundamental and intimate aspects of their lives. The trust and mutual respect upon which such decisions need to rest have to be properly rooted. For individuals whose circumstances are shaped by poverty, a willingness to make efforts on their behalf in this area provides a secure foundation for further work. That security rests on the demonstrated determination of workers to start from the perspective of their clients, rather than being driven by the exigencies of their employing organisations.

Finally, the third strand in this strategy is the one which, in many respects, has the closest relevance to pursuit of a genuine *community* care. If the position of poor people in our society is as bleak as the picture presented here suggests, then attempts to assist might best begin from looking at and learning from the experience of such communities. For, even within the most disadvantaged communities, examples already exist of local initiatives which can have a direct impact upon the financial circumstances of those impoverished families and individuals who live within them. These initiatives include: credit unions, debt redemption work, cooperative buying schemes, LETS schemes, self-build initiatives and cooperative employment arrangements. These initiatives are characterised by principles of self-government and cooperation. They are created and maintained by individuals within some of the most economically abandoned communities, drawing on a resourceful and skilful sense of enterprise which is based both upon resilience and determination, together with a clear-eyed understanding of the environment in which they live and the knowledge how best to bring about necessary improvement in it. Care of the economically fragile which is rooted in a real rather than imaginary notion of 'community' would begin with the experience of those who know how their communities work, and how they could be helped to work better. There is a real role for professional workers in linking their service users to these networks and helping to ensure that they obtain access to the direct benefits for their financial circumstances which would follow.

■ Conclusion

This chapter has argued for an extension of those same values to embrace a more direct understanding of the effects which poverty wreaks in the lives of so many who depend upon community care. There are things that can be done. Both workers and agencies have an obligation to get on with them. To return, as this chapter almost began, with a view from J. K. Galbraith (1989):

> There is, we can surely agree, no form of oppression in our society that is quite so great, no constraint of thought and effort quite so comprehensive, as that which comes from having no money.' Best practice in community care already encompasses those core social welfare values of respect, choice and partnership.

Chapter 17

Working with children in need under the Children Act 1989

Matthew Colton, Charlotte Drury and Margaret Williams

■ Introduction

This chapter opens by tracing the historical antecedents of the Children Act (1989). The immediate origins of the Act, its principles and its provisions in relation to children in need are then outlined. This is followed by an account, based on research, of the progress made in implementing the legislation. The factors which have impeded progress are then examined as a prelude to a discussion of possible ways by which to move towards needs-led services.

■ The Children Act 1989: origins, principles and provisions

In England and Wales, the idea that children are best brought up by their own families was given legislative expression in the Children Act 1989, which is widely seen as the most important child care law passed by the British Parliament this century. The new concept of family support contained in the Act is said to represent 'a quantum leap from the old restricted notions of "prevention" to a more positive outreaching duty of support for children and families' (Packman and Jordan 1991 : 323).

■ Origins

The narrow conception of prevention replaced by the 1989 Act had its origins in the Victorian welfare system of the nineteenth century. This system emphasised 'rescue' and 'fresh start', rather than prevention and rehabilitation. Parents were regarded as the cause of the problem, which meant that the solution necessitated permanently separating them from their offspring. Indeed, the concept of rehabilitation did not reach the statute book until the Children Act 1948 was passed following the Second World War. Together with the social welfare legislation of the 1940s, which reduced poverty and contributed towards full employment, decent housing and improved health, the children's departments established by the 1948 Act also provided impetus for preventive work. The Children and Young Persons Act 1963 extended the work of the children's departments from a curative rescue service to one whose role was to promote the welfare of children by working with the whole family. This goal was further pursued through the creation of unified local authority social services departments at the beginning of the 1970s.

However, the highly publicised, tragic death in 1973 of the child Maria Colwell – killed by her stepfather shortly after being returned to the care of her mother from foster parents – and research evidence suggesting that substantial numbers of children were being allowed to 'drift' in care (Rowe and Lambert (1973), fuelled calls for renewed stress on removing children permanently from their parents. The Children Act 1975 appeared to reverse child care policy and practice in the direction of removing children rather than addressing the social disadvantages which put them at risk in the first place.

However, an inquiry by the Social Services Committee of the House of Commons, published in 1984, argued that the stress on permanency had resulted in neglect of preventive policies and practices. The report also called for 'a major review of the legal framework of child care' (House of Commons 1984). In response, the government set up an interdepartmental committee which, in 1985, published a *Review of Child Care Law* (Department of Health and Social Security 1985a). The review concentrated on the need to enable parents to keep or receive back their children, and, together with the White Paper which followed (House of Commons 1987), paved the way for the Children Act 1989.

The case for increased emphasis on family support was reinforced by the findings of a series of research projects commissioned by the Department of Health (Department of Health and Social Security 1985b). Moreover, an inquiry into arrangements for dealing with child abuse in the county of Cleveland supported the view that measures were needed to safeguard the rights of parents (Department of Health 1988).

■ Principles and provisions

A number of key principles underpin the Act. For example, the concept of 'parental responsibility' has replaced the traditional emphasis on parental rights and duties. Thus, parents, rather than the state, are responsible for their children, and they cannot divest themselves of this responsibility (although others can exercise it for them in certain circumstances) except through legal adoption. Parents can be seen as 'consumers' who obtain a 'service' from the local authorities in time of need to 'look after' the child for a limited period. In this context, it may be argued that the new focus upon parental responsibility reflects a reinforcement of right-wing market values.

The focus on parental responsibility is confirmed by emphasis on a second concept: legalism in child care. One important factor in child welfare from the late 1960s on has been a number of criticisms, from both the Left and the Right, that social workers were authoritarian and, indeed, almost beyond the law. The Act has dealt with this by making social workers more accountable to the law, particularly where the exercise of parental responsibility by the local authority is concerned.

Recognition that parents may need a service from the local authority in order to fulfil their responsibilities has led to an emphasis on a third key concept: partnership. The concept of partnership is not actually mentioned in the Act, but derives from the *Review of Child Care Law* (DHSS 1985a). The *Review* argued that the focus should be on maintaining family links 'in order to care for the child in partnership with rather than in opposition to his parents, and to work towards his return to them'. Hence, partnership between parents and local authorities is promoted in the Act, previously restricted notions of 'prevention' are superseded by the much broader concept of 'family support', and local authorities have a general duty to safeguard and promote the upbringing of 'children in need'.

Under the Act, children are deemed to be 'in need' if they require local authority services to achieve or maintain a reasonable standard of health or development, or to prevent significant or further impairment of their health and development, or if they are disabled (s. 17, Children Act 1989; Department of Health 1991d). The terms 'health', 'development' and 'disabled' are further defined, but the Act gives no clear indication of what is to be understood by a reasonable standard of health and development, or by significant or further impairment.

Thus, it is evident that the definition of need contained in the Children Act is wide enough, potentially, to embrace all children who could be helped by the provision of services. This, along with the qualified language in which local authorities' duties are generally expressed, means in practice that local authorities have wide discretion in deciding what range and level of services will be provided to whom, by whom, and in what particular way.

■ The implementation of the Act

Research shows that uneven progress has been made by local authority social services departments in implementing the family support provisions contained in the Children Act. Some departments have made notable advances, while others have made considerably less progress, failing to make even modest headway in the face of the difficulties encountered.

Operational policies are obviously a vital component in the process of implementing of any piece of legislation. There is wide variation in the length, quality and content of the policy documents of local authority social services departments. The fact that some departments do not have written policies on key areas of the Act naturally raises questions about how the Act is being implemented. Although departments may be attempting to comply with the requirements of the Act through unwritten and informal policies, service goals are frequently not documented. A lack of formal goals will inevitably lead to inconsistency of service, an absence of effective monitoring procedures, and the possibility that goals will alter in an unplanned way (Colton *et al.* 1995, 1995b).

■ Needs assessment

If policies are to be effectively translated into practice, it is essential that guidance is provided for practitioners. However, such guidance is frequently lacking with regard to key areas pertaining to the assessment of need (Colton *et al.* 1995a, 1995b; Department of Health 1994a). As noted earlier, the Act does not say exactly how its definition of need should be interpreted. For their part, social services departments generally appear content to leave the definition of need, and hence the identification of children 'in need', to individual practitioners (Colton *et al.* 1995a, 1995b). As might be expected, inconsistent service provision has resulted, and has led to dissension in the social network of the families being served.

Moreover, in the absence of appropriate guidance, social workers have resorted to material formulated for use in child protection work. This has reinforced the imbalance between family support and protection (Colton *et al.* 1995a, 1995b), whereby child protection is given universal priority. Children at risk of abuse or neglect and those being accommodated receive highest priority. Children whose needs are already manifest receive priority above those whose problems are less critical but whose difficulties may worsen if ignored (Department of Health 1994b; Colton *et al.* 1995a, 1995b).

Social workers tend to define a child as 'in need' only if there are resources available to meet that need. In other words, the only children identified as being 'in need' are those who can presently be served. To complete the vicious circle, data on the number of children being served are used to estimate the number of children 'in need'. The Act does require that new assessment studies be undertaken, but such studies have rarely been implemented on the grounds that it is not worth while to identify children whose needs cannot be met. Estimates of the cost of meeting needs are rarely produced for similar reasons (Colton *et al.* 1995a, 1995b).

■ Inter-agency cooperation

In the United Kingdom, services for children and families are fragmented between several different local authority agencies, including social services, education, health, the police and probation services, youth services and the department of social security. Progress towards an interagency strategic approach to the full range of children's services has been disappointing except where it is mandatory. Various reasons have been cited for this: changes in agency structures and personnel, a lack of skill and resources, and agencies remaining fairly insular and wary of joint ventures (Audit Commission 1994; Department of Health 1994a).

Although relationships between practitioners from different agencies seem to be generally good, conflicts tend to occur where joint work is most common; for example, between social services, education and health (Colton *et al.* 1995a, 1995b; Department of Health 1994a). Difficulties centre around referral procedures, attitudes, lack of understanding of each other's roles, and disagreements over who should take responsibility for particular clients, especially where lack of resources encourages agencies to pass responsibility for clients to someone else. In the present economic climate, the cost associated with reaching agreement and implementing cooperative endeavours has also been a factor.

■ Partnerships

The principle of partnership has been generally accepted, but specific policies are frequently lacking and the level of implementation varies markedly (Audit Commission 1994; Colton *et al.* 1995a, 1995b). Although parents and older children in the study by Colton *et al.* (1995a, 1995b) generally felt consulted about decisions made regarding them, they drew a distinction between being consulted and actively participating in decision-making. For example, some felt that they were being used as 'rubber stamps' to give formal consent to decisions made by others in their absence.

An inspection of services to disabled children and their parents found that practitioners generally did not ask (disabled) children how they felt about decisions made about them, and their views were not routinely recorded on case files. This inspection did find some positive practice where social workers recognised parents' unique knowledge of their children, and involved them in decision-making (Department of Health 1994b).

The partnership element most lacking is undoubtedly information. This may reflect concern that disseminating information about services might lead to increased demand, which would outstrip resources. Parallel anxieties exist regarding complaints procedures about which service users usually know very little (Colton *et al.* 1995a, 1995b). Social service departments are encountering difficulties regarding the following: using complaints data to review service delivery, selecting suitable independent investigators, and acting within the required time scales for complaints and reviews (Colton *et al.* 1995a, 1995b; Department of Health, 1993).

Colton and his colleagues (1995a, 1995b) found that in spite of generally positive relationships with social workers, parents often felt that practitioners were ineffective at solving problems, particularly in areas of major concern such as truancy and drug abuse. Parents also felt stigmatised by receiving services. Isolation, which is an aspect of stigma, was a common theme. Parents and children typically considered that both the emotional support and the material help they received were inadequate. Children with siblings or friends in foster care frequently wanted to be accommodated themselves because of the perceived material benefits.

Another difficulty centred around the placement of children in foster homes close to their parents' home. Although this is obviously of benefit in the maintenance of family links, some parents felt that it enabled children to continue to demonstrate problematic behaviour, in the local school, in the family home and in the community. A related problem was the return home of accommodated children to parents who felt that they were still not ready to cope.

■ Cultural issues

Social services departments are attempting to comply with the requirements of the Act by formulating general policies to the effect that a child's ethnic, cultural, linguistic and religious needs will be considered when providing services. However, as with other areas of the Act, written policies of a more detailed nature are frequently lacking. No data are routinely collected on the linguistic, ethnic or religious background of service users. Indeed, little is known about the demography of local populations other than what is available from the Census (Colton *et al.* 1995a, 1995b).

Other identified problems include: language, exacerbated by a lack of translators; too few practitioners from ethnic minority groups; lack of awareness of ethnic needs; lack of resources for ethnic minority children; and problems in working with children from travelling families, whose unique lifestyle is rarely considered (Colton *et al.* 1995a, 1995b). Attitudes on the part of some service providers reflect the belief that culturally specific policies, and indeed services, need not be a priority when the cultural group that will benefit is relatively small.

■ Impediments to progress and organisation of services

Many of the problems that social welfare practitioners have encountered in operationalising need appear to arise from the incongruity between the all-embracing spirit of the Children Act and current political, economic and social realities. Therefore, the context of family support is now considered, beginning with the organisation of services.

A positive approach to family support entails the promotion of policies and practices aimed at helping children to enjoy in their own homes the kind of parenting, the freedom from suffering, the standards of living and the quality of community life which is considered reasonable for children in our society (Holman 1988). .

We are far from achieving such proactive policies and practices, largely because the basic contextual requirements for an effective system of family support are lacking.

According to Holman (1988), the localisation of services into small geographical units would increase the capacity of social workers to help families at an early stage of their difficulties and to enlist local resources. However, on the whole, social services departments have not adopted this approach. Rather, they have tended to pursue a reactive stance with an associated focus on child protection. This has contributed to the fact that need is still defined in terms of individual pathology rather than as a matter of social justice. It is worthy of note that social justice is a more expensive definition than individual pathology, since, in terms of social justice, whole communities rather than individual families may be defined as needy.

Family centres should play a pivotal role in community-oriented family support work (Holman 1988). However, services are not generally decentralised on a local neighbourhood basis, and family centres have so far not been given the pivotal role in the activities of local authorities that effective family support services necessitate (Colton *et al.* 1995a, 1995b). This is unfortunate, because the evidence suggests that small geographical units of localised services, with a key role for family centres, would make it easier to involve users in decisions about the kinds of services which are offered; they would facilitate participation by users in the actual delivery of services, and would reflect a conception of users which focuses on their strengths as well as on their limitations.

In short, services organised along the lines suggested would be more conducive to establishing a genuine partnership between social workers and services users. The presence of other facilities in the same centre, such as health workers and educational consultants, might also go some way towards providing integrated service and facilitating interagency cooperation.

■ Child poverty

A second precondition for effective family support services identified by Holman (1988) entails reducing inequality and social deprivation. The broad spirit of proactive family support enshrined in the Children Act 1989 can be effectively implemented only in a society which is moving towards the reduction of its vast inequalities and social deprivations. Yet it is plain that the United Kingdom of the 1990s does not constitute such a society. Rather than being a society that is moving towards a reduction of inequality, Britain has moved in the opposite direction over the past decade or so. Social polarisation has occurred (Bradshaw 1990; Halsey 1988), there is debate about the possible emergence of a distinct underclass (see Murray 1990) and levels of child poverty have increased (Bradshaw 1990).

Thus, to an extent unparalleled since 1945, the daily agenda for social welfare practitioners is dominated by the consequences which prolonged and deepening penury produces in the social fabric of society and in the lives of families and individuals (Colton *et al.* 1995a, 1995b). In this regard, senior officers in social welfare agencies might recognise that they themselves control resources and have the power to improve conditions in impoverished communities through their own spending decisions. With reference to wider anti-poverty strategies, the development of credit unions, cooperative buying schemes and bond banks will also have some impact upon the financial circumstances of disadvantaged groups.

Conflicting models of welfare

The increasing pressure on families has increased the demands placed on local authority social services departments. However, rather than increasing the capacity of social welfare practitioners to meet these demands, it would appear that central government policy has had the opposite effect. The trend towards reducing the role of the state in welfare provision (Johnson 1990) has contributed to a profound contradiction which social services staff are understandably finding it difficult to resolve.

It is plain that local authority social services departments in England and Wales are faced with a major dilemma. On the one hand, there is the Children Act 1989, which is widely seen as the most progressive reform of child care law this century. On the other hand, there are flourishing social policies, both inside and outside the child care field, which would seem to blatantly contradict the spirit of this reform. One commentator has observed that 'the language of "needs" contained in the 1989 Act, is usually associated with a collectivist model of welfare, and . . . sits oddly in our new residualist era' (Hardiker *et al.* 1991 : 356). Others have noted that noted that 'concepts like sharing responsibility between parents and the state, reaching agreements and partnerships . . . have a surprisingly communitarian or even collectivist ring about them . . .' (Packman and Jordan, 1991 : 315).

The 'collectivist' philosophy manifested in the Children Act cannot be easily put into practice in an increasingly 'residualist' social policy context. There is an inherent (where a basic minimum of groups) conflict between present resource constraints and the additional resources which are required if a wider definition of need is to be reflected in increased service provision.

Towards needs-led services

It is clear that the creation of needs-led, family support services requires a shift away from the existing overwhelming emphasis on child protection. This requires, first, that social services policy documents reflect the positive outreaching duty of support for children and families contained in the Act; and, second, that the procedures by which this duty is to be fulfilled are specified. Steps to be taken might include the following:

1. Social services agencies should discourage social workers from using protection material to guide them in the assessment of children in need by issuing alternative guidance designed to emphasise family support. This should preferably be done in cooperation with other statutory and voluntary agencies.

2. Budgeting arrangements should be reviewed. For example, in recognition of the Children Act trend towards fewer applications for care proceedings and fewer children in care, it may be possible to recycle resources trapped in capital costs and turn these into available revenue.

However, it is apparent that merely urging agencies to make better use of existing resources is not sufficient. Issues of a more fundamental nature must be addressed. Perhaps more than any other factor, poverty threatens the practical achievement of proactive family support services. Yet, for both policy-makers and practitioners, poverty appears to have been relegated to the margin of their concerns and actions. It is as if the only way of coping with the overwhelming fact of hardcore poverty – the product of increasing inequality – is to look the other way and act as though it were not happening. While understandable, perhaps, this response merely leads into a cul-de-sac of inappropriate and ineffective policy and practice. The successful implementation of the Children Act, and indeed, community care policy more widely, necessitates that poverty be placed again at the centre of the policy, practice and research agenda.

This does not imply that individuals and families who live in poverty should be transformed into 'welfare' clients in order to obtain services. Nor is it to suggest that there is any substitute for action at the national level to tackle primary poverty and to ensure that local authorities have the resources necessary to carry out their mandate under the Act. A comprehensive national strategy to tackle need is required involving employment, housing, wages, taxation and social security policies.

Nevertheless, there are three distinct strategies through which, even in these difficult times, social welfare practitioners and agencies in England and Wales can at least seek to make a direct impact upon the financial circumstances of their service users:

1. Policy-makers and senior officers within social welfare agencies can recognise their own status as major resource holders and the impact which their own spending decisions might make upon the impoverished communities with whom their organisations have almost all their dealings. Through patterns of employment, location of offices, choices concerning purchase of goods and materials, organisations have the capacity to invest within the human, physical and social fabric of such communities. As indicated, the organisation of service delivery appears incompatible with the concept of family support contained in Part III of the Children Act. Family support services should be decentralised on a local neighbourhood basis, and family centres should play a pivotal role in such services.

   Currently, however, it is difficult to escape the impression that local authority social services departments tend to operate in ways that are self-defeating, that seem bound to frustrate their efforts to develop effective family support services, and that appear inimical to their attempts to fashion an authentic partnership with parents, children and local communities: workers tend to be drafted in from outside the local area, operations are often directed from remote headquarters, and more appears to be sucked out of deprived communities in terms of simple financial resources than is invested in them.

2. Within social welfare organisations, a reformulation needs to take place in traditional welfare rights activities. To begin with, these strands need reaffirmation as part of mainstream work, rather than being located at the margin of organisational activity. Social workers have long been somewhat ambivalent in their attitudes towards income maximisation. At a time when the social-democratic institutions of the welfare state are under wider threat, and the policies of rationing and coercion are in the ascendency, a new style of intervention in this field has to be developed. A technocratic understanding of the labyrinthine ways in which the remnants of the welfare state doles out its remaining benefits is not sufficient. Rather, a more proactive approach is required, which recognises and seeks to redress the unfairness and discriminations within the system.

3. With regard to the wider anti-poverty strategies of local authorities, while the development of credit unions, cooperative buying schemes and bond banks are not solutions to primary poverty, they remain capable of producing an impact upon the financial circumstances of groups in poverty. Moreover, they do this in ways which build upon the extensive systems of mutual support which remain remarkably vigorous within the most disadvantaged communities.

Nevertheless, given the reality of limited resources, it is inevitable that difficult choices will have to be made with respect to defining and prioritising the different types and levels of need. Not only will the decisions finally reached reflect the current fiscal climate, but they will also be influenced by the skills and attitudes of service providers.

It may be argued that resources, attitudes and skills are interrelated factors. New skills, for example, can be achieved only through training, for which resources are needed; and existing skills may only be fully demonstrated if service providers are genuinely committed both to the kinds of services they are required to offer and to the people whose needs they are supposed to meet. In other words, operationalisation of the Children Act will be affected not just by the content of the Act, nor solely by the resources required for its implementation, but by its entire economic, political and social context.

■ Conclusion

This chapter has focused upon the new concept of family support which is contained within the Children Act. This concept is said to represent a quantum leap from the old, restricted notions of 'prevention'. However, uneven progress has been made by many local authorities in implementing the family support provisions contained in the Act. Research shows that difficulties have been encountered in the following key areas: agency policy, needs assessment, inter-agency cooperation, partnership with children and parents and cultural issues. The creation of an effective, needs-led family support service requires a shift away from the current emphasis on child protection, and we have argued that a new multifaceted approach is needed. This approach involves both organisational and practice initiatives as well as action at a national level to ensure adeqaute resources. Family services should be decentralised on to a locality basis and initiatives involving welfare rights work should also be employed. The most important issue to be confronted by policy and practice is that of primary poverty.

Chapter 18

The social construction of 'carers'

Bill Bytheway and Julia Johnson

■ Introduction

In this chapter we trace the dramatic history of this concept and attempt to explain how it has acquired its statutory status. There are two distinct threads to this history: that of pressure groups seeking to improve the situation of those looking after disabled and older people, and that of researchers and policy-makers who have been concerned to develop the policies and practices of service and support agencies. Both interest groups have focused primarily on the policies of central government and have frequently collaborated. Nevertheless, as will become apparent, their distinct interests have also generated tension in the course of the category of carer being constructed and promoted.

■ Constructing the 'carer'

In 1995 the Carers (Recognition and Services) Act entered the statute book: carers now have legal status. It is perhaps difficult to appreciate that, less than forty years ago, the term 'carer' was barely in the English language, and parti-cularly difficult for those many people who perceive themselves to be carers and who are indeed devoting themselves to the care of sick or disabled people. For people with such experience, the idea that 'being a carer' is a recent social invention will seem absurd. Yet people who were in the same situation in the 1950s would not have used the word 'carer' and, more to the point, would not have thought of themselves as distinctive in the sense of belonging to a special category of people. It is for this reason that we can think of the concept of 'carer' as a social construction, a category created through the interplay between individual experience and various interest groups – policy-makers, researchers and pressure groups.

The literature on care has grown rapidly since the emergence of this concept, and in this there is no ambiguity: 'the carer' is one particular person providing care for one other particular person. The care relationship so conceived is essentially asymmetric and one-to-one: A cares for B. In the development of care services in the community, policy has focused on the needs of B, the person receiving care. This means that the role of carer often appears in practice guidelines in taken for granted, not unlike that of 'the GP', an individual – not indeed necessarily always the same individual – who is always 'there'. Other people are incidental in the conceptualisation of this relationship and the multiplicity and reciprocal nature of many caring relationships are overlooked.

■ The emergence of the individual female carer

To a large extent, contemporary policy and research is being developed by people who graduated in the social sciences in the 1960s and the 1970s. Many current beliefs about the value of community and family can be traced back to Townsend's seminal text, *The Family Life of Old People* (1957). In the 1950s the term 'carer' did not figure in either research or policy but, in a chapter titled, 'The Family System of Care', Townsend created an image of how care was provided by relatives within the context of ongoing family life. He argued for the central importance of the *family* rather than *individuals* (that is, carers) in the conceptualisation of how care was routinely provided within the community. However, he made it quite clear that the responsibility to provide care in London families of the 1950s fell primarily on women, although he also emphasised that older women played an active part in the early adult lives of their children: they provided care as much as they received it. We return to this point later in this chapter.

Townsend also discussed the various roles of unmarried adult children and was particularly interested in the extent of co-residence among older siblings. Many women were of course unmarried or widowed because of the huge numbers of men who had been killed in the First World War. With time, many had taken up a caring or supporting role within their (extended) families but, in the 1950s, some in turn were beginning to need support themselves. It was in the context of such demographic trends and changing pressures that the National Council for the Single Woman and Her Dependants was formed to campaign on behalf of single women. As we will argue below, it is significant that this organisation, having begun by representing single women, a comparatively small group numerically, 'opened its doors' in 1982 to men and married women and renamed itself the National Council for Carers and Their Elderly Dependants. In our view, it is important to the history of 'the carer' that this organisation initially directed attention on one particular category of – largely middle-class – individuals: 'single women'. In so doing it challenged Townsend's more diffuse focus on care needs within the working class family.

■ The impact of feminism

The concern of the Labour governments of the 1960s and 1970s with social security and the financial welfare of chronically sick and disabled people led, in 1975, to the introduction of Invalid Care Allowance (ICA). This was intended to 'protect the current incomes and future retirement pensions of members of the labour market whose full-time employment was prematurely terminated by the care of elderly relatives' (Glendinning 1988:131). Arguably this was the first significant gesture made by central government towards people providing care. However, being focused upon the financial cost of leaving employment, it was not payable initially to married and cohabiting women who it was presumed would be at home anyhow (Baldwin 1994:187). After a long and active campaign ICA was eventually in 1986 to include them. It was only then that it could be construed to be a payment for care rather than a benefit to (partially) replace lost earnings.

In 1981, in the course of the campaign to extend the ICA to married women, the Association of Carers was formed. It defined a carer as 'anyone who was leading a restricted life because of the need to look after a person who is mentally or physically handicapped, or ill, or impaired by old age', and among its aims was 'to encourage carers to recognise that their own needs are just as important as those of the person they are looking after'. One year later, the National Council for the Single Woman and Her Dependants reconstituted itself as the National Council for Carers and Their Elderly Dependants. Although clearly competing with the Association for Carers to represent married women carers, it maintained its focus on the needs of the 'elderly infirm relatives'. The competition was short-lived, however, and in 1986 the two were merged to form the Carers National Association.

The campaign to extend ICA to all women politicised the issue of care and, as a result, the assumption that women 'naturally volunteer' to provide family care began to be seriously questioned. In particular, attention was drawn to how this expectation denied middle-aged women opportunities to gain paid employment, or to regain it when children had left home (Finch and Groves 1980). Responding to this concern, the Equal Opportunities Commission produced the first author-itative assessment of the unpaid and unacknowledged contribution of women to informal care. Following its own research, it concluded that:

it remains the case that families are expected to provide care for the vast majority of the handicapped, the sick and the elderly, and, as is demonstrated in this study, it is the closest female relative to whom the task of caring usually falls. (EOC 1980:1)

This report also provided another early definition of carers: 'those adults who are responsible for the care of the sick, handicapped or elderly' (p. 1). The author of the report suggested that the term 'carers' was not entirely satisfactory, but was 'probably the best available'. The conclusion that the task of caring fell on the 'closest female relative' implies that the EOC conceptualised care as an asymmetric one-to-one relationship, and that it saw individuals as the social unit that was primarily involved in the provision of care. The author, in noting that the majority of carers were women, added the words 'of course' and went on to explain that, because of this, the feminine pronoun would be used throughout the report. This, we would argue, was a crucial step in the feminisation of the concept of carer in the UK, one reinforced by the publication of Finch and Groves (1983) influential collection of studies of women and caring. Effectively, by definition, a male carer had become anomalous. But more significantly, so too had the idea that caring might be produced collectively by 'relatives' as part and parcel of ordinary family life.

The White Paper *Growing Older* (DHSS, Scottish Office, Welsh Office, Northern Ireland Office: 1981), reflecting the priorities of the newly elected Conservative government, issued the now famous decree that: 'care *in* the community must increasingly mean care *by* the community'. Far from confirming the importance of the role of the carer, this policy document did not refer to carers. Rather, it associated the concept of informal care with 'the community', not just the family but 'kinship, friendship and neighbourhood' (p. 3), although it acknowledged that caring 'may involve considerable personal sacrifice, particularly where the "family" is one person, often a single woman, caring for an elderly relative' (p. 37).

The government's conceptualisation and promotion of 'care by the community' was widely interpreted to mean 'care by women'. A series of research studies developed out of this and many reports and seminars were given titles such as 'Caring for the Carer'. In this way the term 'the carer' became established in the professional vocabulary.

In much of this research, carers were identified through the users of services. For example, the study of Charlesworth *et al.* (1984) was based on a sample of older people who had been referred to specialist services in two urban areas in the North West during 1979 and 1980: 'Wherever possible a principal carer was identified (following initial contact with the specialist service and an assessment by a psychiatrist) and this person was interviewed by a social scientist' (Charlesworth *et al.* 1984 : 8).

Through this procedure, a sample of carers was obtained, each caring for one of the older people in the initial sample. Likewise, the sample for the well-known and influential study of Nissel and Bonnerjea (1982) was located primarily through the health services and voluntary agencies in Oxford. There were many other similar local studies that identified carers through the users of formal services. This sampling strategy was appropriate at that time in that two widely expressed concerns were the adequacy of the support provided by the formal sector, and the suspicion that men were offered support more readily, and more generously, than were women. The effect, however, was to define carers as one more 'newly discovered' element in the system of support that surrounded service users: people living in the community who were already receiving health or social services. This dependence on the 'service provider route' meant not only that the ability of the researchers to generalise to all carers was limited (Twigg and Atkin 1994: 157), but also that policy began to be related to the apparent needs of such carers – needs that the service agencies that were already involved could and should be taking into account.

Overall, the extensive body of small-scale research undertaken in the 1980s reinforced the assumption that informal care is largely about the relationship between one carer, a middle-aged woman, and one dependent person – usually an older parent. It could be argued that the feminist critique, intended to expose the 'burden borne' by middle-aged women, only served to reinforce the expectation that, despite the apparent injustice, women would continue to provide the care that was required. As Arber and Ginn comment: 'caring has been portrayed primarily as work done by daughters for parents.... There has been little examination of the concept of caring, or questioning of the stereotype of "carers as middle-aged women" ' (1991 : 130).

■ The 1985 national survey

Many commentators concluded from the early research studies not only that women provided by far the greater partportion of informal care, but also that the contribution of men was negligible. In fact, the percentage of male carers in these samples ranged from 23 per cent to 41 per cent (Arber and Gilbert 1989 : 73) – certainly under 50 per cent, but not negligible percentages at all.

The first authoritative national survey of the population to address the question of care was the 1985 General Household Survey (Green 1988). On the basis of this, it was estimated that there were 6 million carers in Great Britain, of whom 40 per cent were male. Both statistics came as a shock to the policy world. In assessing these two statistics, it is important to consider the methodology that the General Household Survey used to define and identify carers. Carers were adults who responded positively to either of the following two questions:

Q1: Some people have extra family responsibilities because they look after someone who is sick, handicapped or elderly. May I check, is there anyone living with you, who is sick, handicapped or elderly whom you look after or give special help to (for example, a sick or handicapped or elderly relative/husband/wife/child/friend, etc.) (SPECIFY ALL HOUSEHOLD MEMBERS)?
Q2: And how about people not living with you, do you provide some regular service or help for any sick, handicapped or elderly relative, friend or neighbour not living with you? (Green, 1988 : 6)

It has been suggested that many respondents who were not providing what is normally understood by the term 'care' would have responded positively to these questions because they were indeed undertaking 'extra' responsibilities. Conversely, many women who were providing substantial levels of care would not have thought of this as an 'extra' responsibility (Arber and Ginn 1990; Parker 1993):

> The phrasing of the OPCS (GHS) questions aims to distinguish 'caring' from 'normal' family care and domestic provisioning work; this may introduce some gender bias, because the latter is performed more often by women. The first screening question refers to 'extra family responsibilities...'. A man might include shopping and cooking for his disabled wife as 'extra family responsibilities', but this may not be the case for a woman caring for her disabled husband. (Arber and Ginn 1990 : 433)

We would argue that, given the different expectations and obligations of men and women within family life, it is inevitable that there will be gender differences in the perception of what constitutes 'having extra responsibilities'. There will be tasks that women too may define as 'extra', but that many men would regard as normal family responsibilities. It is, of course, absurd to suppose that the same responses to these questions might reflect equivalent levels of involvement in specific caring activities. What is being recorded is self-reported care related to carer-assessed dependency. The critical point is not that the question is biased but that it is subjective. There will be enormous variation in how people respond to the question in relation to what they actually do, but all who respond positively are registering the belief that they have 'extra' responsibilities that arise from their 'looking after' someone.

Doubts about the legitimacy of the huge number of carers revealed by Green's analysis of the General Household Survey were raised by Parker (1992), who undertook a secondary analysis of the data. She suggested that accepting the figure of 6 million was 'not helpful' and that a more appropriate figure would be between 1.3 and 1.7 million. By examining findings on caring activities and taking some account of the time spent in caring, she distinguished between *informal care* defined as being heavily involved in personal and physical assistance and *informal help* defined as practical support, often provided 'as part of a network where others take main responsibility' (1992 : 14). Parker and others claimed that the definition of caring had been too broad and 'brought into the net people who performed small peripheral tasks such as giving medicines, writing letters, or sitting in for half an hour' (Redding 1991 : 18). Parker focused attention, therefore, on those providing intensive personal and physical care.

Not surprisingly, Pitkeathley, the director of the Carers National Association, disputed Parker's revised conceptualisation:

> It may be 1.7 or 1.4 million at the heavy end, but on the other hand there are a lot of people caring for someone in another household, for less than 20 hours a week, who have their lives restricted, and who are picking up the burden which the state is not. (Quoted in Redding 1991 : 20)

There is, in this exchange, a certain recognition that 6 million people cannot all be carers who are spending a large proportion of their time providing physical care: that many are people who are 'part of a network', supporting others they see to be more heavily involved, as well as helping those being cared for. By implication, where several people believe themselves each to have taken on extra family responsibilities in playing their part in looking after the same person, all are represented by the survey, not just the one 'primary carer'. Whereas Parker's concern was to assist policy-makers and service agencies to target those primary carers who should be given practical support, Pitkeathley's concern was to sustain the strength of the carers movement and to develop a powerful case for the contribution of all carers to the overall provision of care to be properly recognised.

Regarding the explanation of the unexpectedly high proportion of male carers identified in the General Household Survey, Arber and Ginn (1990) focused attention on 'spouse care'. Their analysis showed that four in ten carers were spouses, mainly 'elderly', and half of these were men. They suggested that the high percentage of males in the General Household Survey was due largely to the contribution of older husbands caring for ill wives. In doing so they also pointed to the ageism implicit in much of the earlier informal care literature:

> The prevailing view of elderly people as a 'social problem' emphasises the 'burden' of elderly people and concentrates on the problems for the rest of society of the increasing number of elderly people in the population. This negative and blinkered vision has almost entirely neglected the provision of care by the elderly themselves. (Arber and Ginn 1990 : 446)

This same point was made by Townsend thirty years earlier: 'In previous surveys the fact that old people perform services for others has had less attention than the fact that others perform services for them' (1957 : 62).

■ Disaggregating carers

With the extension of ICA to all carers, the formation of the National Carers Association and the impressive national statistics from the 1985 survey, the category of 'carer' was secured. A 'generic' approach to research on carers began to be adopted (Twigg 1992). The archetypical question was no longer 'who *provides* care?' but 'who *are* the carers?' Paradoxically, however, this new question meant that the category of 'carers' required disaggregation. Arber and Ginn had started this by challenging the stereotype of the carer as a middle-aged daughter and drawing attention to 'the forgotten male carer'. The implications of this for social workers were developed by Fisher (1994 : 677)

We will have to develop a new appreciation of the caring capacities of men, particularly older husbands. There are circumstances where men accept the obligation to care, undertake intimate personal care, and derive identity and reward from their caring work.

Similarly, Atkin (1992) argued that 'differences need to be recognised if appropriate services are to be developed' and to that end he distinguished between: spouse, parental, filial, sibling, child and non-kin carers. The King's Fund Centre established a carers unit in the late 1980s which specialised in supporting projects focused on work with carers in ethnic minorities.

Meantime the Carers National Association had been campaigning effectively in Parliament. Malcolm Wicks MP, previously director of the influential Family Policy Studies Centre, introduced a Carers' Bill. Against many expectations he was successful and, in 1995, the Carers (Recognition and Services) Act entered the statute book. Under this Act a carer is defined as 'an individual [who] provides or intends to provide a substantial amount of care on a regular basis for the relevant person', the latter being a person (child or adult) whose needs for community care services are being assessed under other legislation. Although, in introducing his Bill, Wicks indicated that he was concerned that it should 'include all carers', he identified three particular groups (House of Commons 1995 : 424). First he referred to 'adults looking after a frail elderly relative', and he accepted that they 'represent the bulk of caring by family carers'. But he then went on to draw attention to two other groups which he sought to include in the legislation: 'parent carers' and 'child carers'. He referred to the latter as 'a newly recognised group' and much of the debate which followed was referenced to these two groups. Although he was concerned to include 'all carers', Wicks also indicated that the policy intention, following the argument of Parker, was to 'target that group of carers who carry the major burden'. So, having begun with a reference to the total estimated number of 6.8 million carers in Britain, he moved on to discuss in more detail the 1.5 million 'who provide care for 20 hours a week or more' and who he described as 'a caring army' (House of Commons 1995 : 426). It is too early to assess the impact of this Act. What this review has done is focus on the way in which the category of 'carer' has emerged over the last twenty years. It began as an operational concept enabling the Equal Opportunities Commission to assess the impact on women of community care policies. It has now become a social identity written into the nation's statutes.

■ Discussion

Robbert (1990) has focused on the part played by researchers, medical practitioners, ordinary people and the media, in defining the characteristics of Alzheimer's disease. She presented a modified version of the sequential model of the social construction of illness, first put forward by Conrad and Schneider (1980). It is not difficult to modify this still further to account for the social construction of 'carers' (Johnson 1994). On the basis of our review of the literature we would tentatively suggest the following:

1. *Recognition.* Certain situations are recognised as not normal and as a cause for concern. Graham (1983 : 14) identifies Leonard Barker and Allen as feminists who raised questions about care and family life in the mid 1970s.
2. *Definition.* The situation is 'discovered', and the discovery is reported in a professional journal or monograph. It is defined and named. The first EOC (1980) is a good example.
3. *Claims making.* Champions and 'moral entrepreneurs' start to make claims for the new discovery and to develop or reorientate interest groups. Finch and Groves (1983) and the early promotional material of the two carers organisations exemplify this stage.
4. *Legitimacy.* Positive reports from, and official recognition by, regulatory and professional bodies (such as the EOC and the British Association of Social Work) follow. The General Household Survey, undertaken by the govern-

ment's Office of Populations, Censuses and Surveys, was a major contribution. Increased funding for research specifically into informal care followed (for example, Bytheway 1987b).

5. *Institutionalisation.* The name and definition become formally recognised as an accepted classification. Agencies are established and developed which provide organised support for local groups, and which issue guidelines to practitioners (such as the King's Fund Centre Carers Unit and the Carers National Association). The future of these projects and the continued employment of those working on them depend on the continued acceptance of the classification.

A model of this kind helps us understand the historical development of the carers movement, but it does not explain why it was so successful. Like Robbert, Gubrium (1986) has also studied the development of the Alzheimer's disease movement in the USA. His analysis demonstrates how it was necessary for the campaigning groups to organise the description of Alzheimer's as a distinct disease entity 'separate from the varied experiences of normal ageing' (Gubrium 1986 : 3). It is not difficult to see the parallel here with the need for the carers groups to make care distinct from normal family life. Gubrium argues that this is achieved by strategically organising the definition and description of the condition. To a significant extent this is accomplished through attention being given to the experiences of individual carers. For example, in introducing his Bill, Wicks recounted that:

> The Minister and I had an opportunity yesterday to meet a small delegation of carers from various parts of the country. They had an opportunity to talk with us about their needs (House of Commons 1995 : 424).

Gubrium brings out how the Alzheimer's movement used both the experience of celebrities (Ronald Reagan being only one of the most recent examples), and the personal testimonies of members of local support groups:

> The cultural apparatus for revealing the disease penetrates and incorporates diverse personal experiences. Those closest to the victim, who are the 'real experts' in the care and management of the disease − the caregivers − are taught or teach each other that they all share the same travail, all in combat with the same enemy. Each comes to know, by one set of interpretive rules or another, that the experiential minutiae of the 36 hour day, as observed and felt, is part of the silent epidemic. Thus Alzheimer's is not only 'over there' in the slogans, crusade, and celebrities, but right at home. (Gubrium 1986 : 209)

Not only was it necessary for the carers movement to develop a popular understanding of the carer's experience which made caring clearly distinct from ordinary family life, but it was also essential that it implicitly denied relevance to the experience of the person receiving care. In order that the government paid attention specifically to the situation of carers, and not just to the need for care, it was necessary for researchers and representatives of carers groups to be silent about the experience of those receiving care. This was all the more critical given the growing concern during the 1980s over the abuse of dependent people, particular children and vulnerable older people. This, significantly, is the one issue upon which the carers movement has been criticised.

Compared with community care policies, there has been little critical discussion of the strategies and actions of the carers movement. A wide range of groups covering a broad political spectrum have supported it and agreed that carers have had a raw deal. The one significant exception to this is the independent living movement. Representing primarily the interests of disabled people, this is driven by three basic principles:

- Those who know best the needs of disabled people, and how to meet those needs, are disabled people.
- The needs of disabled people can best be met by comprehensive programmes which provide a variety of services.
- Disabled people should be fully integrated into their community (Morris 1991 : 172).

It is not difficult to see how these principles conflict with the concept of the carer. This came out into the open in 1990 when Wood began his contribution to a seminar on 'the needs and resources of disabled people' with the simple statement: 'Let us state what disabled people do want by first stating what we don't want. WE DON'T WANT CARE!!!!' (Wood 1991 : 201)

Keith (1990) elaborated this by arguing that what is objectionable about care is the contrast that is drawn between the two parties involved, with the recipient of care often portrayed as passive and almost a non-person.

Morris (1991) was particularly critical of the contribution of feminist researchers to the development of care policies. In particular, Finch (1984) and Dalley (1988) had advocated collectivist, non-community-based policies of care as a way of relieving women of the 'burden' of providing care in the community. Morris rejected their implicit distinction between 'us' (women) and 'them' (disabled or dependent people), and in a particularly powerful passage she tackled the anti-familist stance expressed by Dalley:

> There is no recognition here that disabled people have often been denied the family relationships that she takes for granted. Insult is then added to injury by the assumption that for a disabled person to aspire to warm, caring human relationships within the setting where most non-disabled people look to find such relationships is a form of false consciousness. We are denied not only the rights non-disabled people take for granted, but when we demand these rights we are told that we are wrong to do so. (Morris 1991 : 160)

Keith and Morris have recently returned to the attack over the issue of young carers. They argue that disabled parents resent the interest of both researchers and the media in the idea of 'role reversal' – the child 'parenting the parent'; they challenge the priority being given to services that help to 'ease the burden of care'; and they fear the possible interventions that might follow the assessment of children's needs (Keith and Morris 1995). In particular, they foresee the possible removal of children from the care of their disabled parents.

What is particularly interesting in regard to the arguments being forwarded in this book is how Keith and Morris explain their concerns over this issue in social constructionist terms:

> The research studies of, the campaigning on, and the media interest in 'young carers' have tended to repeat two things which were common in the earlier debate and research on carers generally. They have defined and named a role ('young carers') which, until the children and young people came into contact with researchers or professionals, was not how they described themselves. And secondly, both researchers, campaigners and journalists alike have defined the main policy issue to be that of providing services to 'young carers' which would ease the 'burden of caring'. (Keith and Morris 1995 : 38–9)

From the Equal Opportunities Commission through to the 1995 Act, it is clear that the campaign for carers' rights has been driven by personal accounts of caring which have reinforced the distinctiveness of the carer role, which have neglected the experience of the person receiving care, and which have drawn upon a limited set of key words such as 'restricted' and 'burden'. In this way the descriptive organisation of accounts of the carers experience have fostered the asymmetric and one-to-one nature of the care relationship.

By claiming that disabled people aspire to ordinary caring relationships within a family setting, Morris is pointing to one obvious alternative conceptualisation, one that has a long tradition in family and community sociology (Willmott and Young 1962; Rosser and Harris 1965; Wenger 1984; Finch and Mason 1990, 1992). Research into care, as Jerrome (1996) has demonstrated, has dominated recent work on family relations in later life. Nevertheless, her review points to developments in family research that have avoided 'the reinvention of the wheel' regarding the provision of care. By recasting care within the context of 'ordinary' family life, it is possible to conceive of a different vocabulary which does not appoint one individual to be the 'carer' and one to be receiving care. The efforts of researchers to understand how people become involved in the provision of care, what is entailed, and how effective support might be provided, continues. The multiplicity of roles and relationships associated with care have, however, caused real problems for those researchers required to identify a sample of 'principal carers' (Qureshi and Walker 1989 : 10). Rather than trying to identify populations of 'carers', 'non-carers' and 'cared-for', research and practice might be more effective if it were based on the assumption that all people are involved in a multiplicity of activities relating to care. An alternative concept, that of a 'caring system', emphasises the often reciprocal and interdependent nature of caring relationships. Reflecting this, Daatland (1983 : 2) introduces his paper with the succinct and subtle statement:

This paper deals with the interplay of care as practical tasks and as ways of constructing and reconstructing social relations. We maintain that the division of tasks in care reflects a social organisation, and that the 'who' and 'what' in care are inseparably linked. On this basis we suggest that care be studied as 'care systems'.

In adopting this approach, what is primary is not one particular person but rather the 'system' which provided the care which is needed. Following an earlier study of neighbour care in a sample of streets in Neath, Bytheway (1982) had come to appreciate the critical complexity of care relationships. Given Daatland's theoretical framework, he produced a series of papers based on a study of informal care in the families of a sample of redundant South Wales steelworkers (Bytheway 1987a, 1987b, 1989). A total of 44 families were identified in which, according to common perceptions, care was being provided. Although information on care relations in these families was highly selective and incomplete, it was sufficient to explore the patterning of care within family networks. Perhaps the most significant point is that none of the 44 involved just 2 people in an exclusive care relationship and only 11 included the archetypical one-to-one caring relationship, the principal carer being actively supported by others in the family. Contrasting with these simple care systems, there were 14 instances of three or more people receiving help within the one family and, overlapping with these, 26 instances of 2 or more people providing help for 2 or more receiving it. One of these 26 has been the subject of a detailed case study (Bytheway 1989 : 93–103).

The South Wales study showed clearly how informal care is often a collective response to perceived need. In such circumstances it is dangerous to presume that there is one readily identifiable 'primary carer'. Rather there is a pooling of resources, frequently in a situation of increasing impoverishment. In such situations, the most significant distinction is not between men and women, or between carers and non-carers, or between 'the elderly' and the 'not elderly'. Rather it is between those with paid work (or other equivalent time-consuming commitments) and those without. In areas such as South Wales in which there is a shortage of paid work, there also tends to be greater proportions of older people, disabled people and un-or under-employed people. Unemployed, disabled and retired men, along with women and children, were heavily involved in every kind of care activity.

■ Conclusion

In proposing, in conclusion, that care should be reconceived as part of ordinary family and community life, there is of course an obvious danger that we are thought to be indulging in a certain kind of communitarian nostalgia. To counter this, we would argue that anyone with first-hand experience of care will know that although, for the individual, care implies active involvement in a number of

ically care is provided outside paid working hours and, for this
reason, is often provided by people not in employment: people who are retired,
disabled, of school age or unemployed. The person with first-hand experience of
care will know that care relationships are often mutual, that most people who are
involved are actively involved in both receiving and providing care, albeit
perhaps in very different ways. Lastly it will be widely recognised that while
care is thought of within the framework of family relationships (one incidentally
in which in legal terms the primary person is 'the next of kin': the person who
stands to inherit), the care system often draws heavily upon old friendships and
current patterns of day-to-day neighbouring. This is particularly true for those
people whose family relationships have never been important or have become
tenuous with time.

The carers movement and policy researchers, while bringing to our attention
the real plight of many isolated and unsupported caring individuals, have
obscured to some extent the realities of informal caregiving and, therefore,
appropriate ways of supporting those who provide care in the community.

Chapter 19

Housing and older people

Robert F. Drake

■ Introduction

This chapter has the straightforward purpose of analysing the housing needs of older people, highlighting areas of provision that are particularly problematic, and identifying the actions necessary to bring about improvement. But as a counter-point to this analysis, the recognition of the social construction of both housing needs and housing provision is a constant theme.

> Golden handshakes worth £22.8 millions were divided among 66 company directors in the last financial year, Labour Research said yesterday. The biggest went to Dr Ernst Mario of Glaxo, who left in 1993 but was paid until this June, giving him a total of £1.44 millions. Eleven payoffs were above £500 000 and two were for more than £1 million. (*Independent*, 2 August 1996 : 18)

> Old soldier Jack Brayley aged 76 was just about surviving on £51 a week. The money had to stretch to cover rent, gas, electricity, water and rates bills. He spent about £15 a week on food. He had no television set because he could not afford the licence. 'I'm an invalid and I've been on a low income for years' said Mr. Brayley 'When I didn't have money, I used to stay in, because I don't believe in cadging'. (*South Wales Evening Post* 24 April 1996 : 4)

Except perhaps for the implacable consequences of time itself, the coming of old age may hold few terrors for those elderly people who have made good during their working lives. For others, however – the many as opposed to the few – old age may be as hard a trial as any they have encountered in all their days. Whilst people's own decisions and life chances have some bearing on the circumstances in which they spend their old age, it is also true that the social and physical environment in which older people live has, to a significant degree, been con- structed by others: architects, builders, planners, politicians, welfare workers and so on. The nature and quality of the nation's housing stock, its location, con- struction, state of repair and interior design, all depend at least in part on political decisions and legislation as well as on social assumptions, norms and expecta- tions. Prevailing beliefs about the capacity of older people to live independent lives will influence the amount and type of investment in dwellings intended for their use, and it follows that the kind of housing (and housing finance) available to older people may play a crucial part in determining their ability to remain 'at home' rather than having to face the prospect of life in an institution.

■ Older people's housing

In 1991 there were just in excess of 10 million people in Britain over the age of 60, and the census of that year provided a picture of their accommodation (Table 19.1).

Table 19.1 Elderly people and housing by tenure, 1991

Type of tenure	Number	%
Owner occupiers	6 653 021	65.5
Privately rented	5 56 864	5.5
Rented with a job or business	1 27 349	1.0
Rented from a housing association	3 96 578	4.0
Rented from a local authority, new town or Scottish homes	2 445 980	24.0
Total	10 179 792	100

Source: 1991 Census; *Housing and Availability of Cars*, OPCS (1993).

In addition to houses and flats (including sheltered and warden-controlled dwellings), accommodation is also provided by residential homes and 'long-stay' hospitals. During the 1980's the private and voluntary sector grew dramatically, with an expansion of 400 per cent in nursing home places and 334 per cent in residential homes (Wistow *et al.* 1994), so that by 1994 residential homes, nursing homes and hospital geriatric wards supplied just under half a million beds (Table 19.2). Even so, this figure represents accommodation for only 4.5 per cent of the elderly population, whereas some 95.5 per cent of older people live in their own homes throughout their lives. It is in this context that recent moves towards community care should be seen.

The number of residents will always be a little lower than the number of places available, because of turnover and vacancies. In addition to residential accommodation, there are about half a million sheltered dwellings, most of them owned by local authorities and housing associations (Department of Environment 1990).

What then, are the major housing problems for elderly people, and whom do these most concern? To take the second question first, it is clear that there are at least three directly interested parties: first, older people themselves; second, relatives and carers; and finally, professionals and voluntary workers who are either involved in the provision or enhancement of housing or who seek to help with the consequences of poor housing. The problems with which older people may be faced vary both in type and degree, and may include poor or unfit housing; lack of money; lack of expertise in obtaining resources for (and overseeing) repair work; the impacts of planning decisions and possible lack of coordination between service suppliers and, finally, special difficulties related to rural settings. Another kind of housing problem, homelessness among elderly people, lies beyond the scope of the chapter, but this is not to deny its seriousness, see for example Crane (1993) and, for an international perspective, Keigher (1991).

Table 19.2   Institutions – provision for older people (England), 1994–5

Type of institution	Homes	Places	Residents (65+)
Local authority			
Residential homes (1994)	1 800	68 900	58 900
Voluntary homes (1994)	1 450	45 500	36 200
Private residential homes (1994)	8 580	164 200	138 700
Totals	11 830	278 600	233 800
		Places	
NHS provision (geriatric wards) (1993/4)		38 000	
Nursing homes (1995)		155 214	
Total		193 214	
Institutional and residential provision, 1994/5 (England): c. 471 814 places			

Sources: Dept of Health (1995a, 1995b).

■ Poor housing stock

The 1996 edition of *Social Trends* indicates that less than 1 per cent of households now lack basic amenities such as bath/shower or internal flush toilet and therefore 'central heating is a better indicator of a household's standard of accommodation' (Central Statistical Office 1996 : 181). Not withstanding this improvement in the general position, it remains true that older people often occupy the worst housing stock, though here too there has been some improvement in recent years. In 1986, 18.2 per cent of unfit houses were occupied by single elderly people and 11.4 per cent of unfit houses by elderly couples. By 1991 these figures had fallen to 12.4 per cent and 7.6 per cent respectively (Department of Environment 1993). Even so, as Balchin (1995) points out, although those aged 75 and over constitute just 10 per cent of all households, they occupy 33 per cent of dwellings lacking amenities, and 16 per cent of unfit houses. Notwithstanding recent advances, then, unfit houses still have real impacts on real lives:

> Slipping roof tiles, faulty electrical wiring, damp scullery floors are endemic in much old housing. Our experience is that these kinds of problems are not only dangerous and uncomfortable to live with, but can have a serious effect on people's quality of life. Poor housing leads to intense anxiety and loss of self-respect. House maintenance and repair presents the practical problems of dealing with builders and finding the money. These can be daunting for fit young people on adequate incomes, but are traumatic for elderly people on small pensions, especially if health is also failing. (Harrison and Means, 1990 : iv)

■ Money

As Harrison and Means intimate, a common problem among elderly owner-occupiers is that they may be capital rich, but revenue poor. Most houses are valuable assets, but they are also very costly to keep in good repair. However, in 1993 the (mean) average weekly net income (before housing costs) of old age pensioners was just £148.50, and the median figure was far less at just £98.50. Indeed, some 60 per cent of all pensioners are to be found in the poorest 40 per cent of the population. To put these figures in perspective, the cost of a place in a residential home can exceed £350 per week, and one in a nursing home perhaps £450 per week (Sherman 1995). Concerned that pensioners were having to sell their homes in order to fund their residential care, government ministers drew up proposals for a £150 million scheme to help some 150,000 elderly people facing this dilemma (Sherman, 1995). Residential care apart, no fewer than 1,356,000 elderly householders receive housing benefit, and of these, 673,000 receive income support as well (Department of Health and Social Security 1995).

Clearly, then, very many elderly people may have insufficient money to maintain or repair their homes. Some may be entitled to help from local authorities, and certainly the introduction of renovation grants and minor works grants (for repairs costing up to £1 080) has been a helpful move forward. However the government White Paper *Our Future Homes* has mooted an end to mandatory renovation grants and a move to discretionary awards (Department of Environment 1995). In their present financial circumstances, many local authorities might treat such a change in the law as an opportunity to curb spending.

■ Expertise

Even those older people able to pay for repairs, or entitled to grants, may either have not known about their eligibility for grant aid, or may have been fearful of 'cowboy' builders. The need for good advice and help in renovation work has prompted one of the most innovative developments in voluntary sector activity in the form of home improvement agencies such as 'Care and Repair' or 'Staying Put'. These agencies provide elderly and disabled people with advice on housing options, the need for repairs, practical solutions and sources of finance. They help with form filling, arranging temporary accommodation if necessary, and perhaps most importantly of all, their qualified technical staff recommend good building firms and monitor the quality of building, plumbing and electrical work once it is under way (Casey 1992). There are now some 225 'Care and Repair' schemes in England and Wales.

Nevertheless, improved housing conditions alone cannot guarantee that all older people will have the resources to stay at home. As frailty increases, the need for health and other support services to play a part becomes increasingly pressing. Effective planning is therefore crucial (Meredith 1993).

■ Planning

In setting the scene for community care it is possible that Sir Roy Griffiths underestimated the degree of coordination that might be needed between housing suppliers and social or community services. He recommended that:

The responsibility of public housing authorities (local authority housing authorities, Housing Corporation etc.) should be limited to arranging and sometimes financing and managing the 'bricks and mortar' of housing needed for community care purposes. Social Services authorities should be responsible for arranging the provision of social, personal and domestic services in sheltered housing, and the finance for those services should be provided through social services, not housing budgets. DoH (Griffiths 1988 : 6.10)

While at face value such arrangements seem clear-cut, the need has grown not only for an expansion in support services, but also for far-reaching cooperation between interested authorities. Many authors have expressed disquiet about the omission of a housing perspective from the development of community services for older people. For example, in four case studies conducted in Oxfordshire, Arnold *et al.* (1993) found that official decision-making tended to be both unilateral and makeshift, agencies had a tense relationship one with another, and people were selected to 'fit' into schemes rather than the other way around. Over time, the day-to-day contact between agencies is likely to smooth out many of the procedural difficulties, but budgetary constraints and continuing financial arguments are almost certain to be the bugbear. It is here that the scope for disjunction between the medical, social and housing components of care is most manifest, and gaps are particularly evident when elderly people move from one kind of accommodation to another, especially on their being discharged home from hospital. Schemes to ease such a transition are found, if at all, in the voluntary sector, with all the insecurities of funding and continuity that this status brings (see for example Russell 1989; Jones 1986a). One approach to overcoming such hiatuses has been proposed by Thornton and Tozer (1994), who suggest the need for the close involvement of elderly people in the planning, development and management of services intended to assist them. Crucial decisions about whether an elderly person might continue to live at home, be admitted to sheltered accommodation or require institutional care are often taken in fora where the client has the least powerful position of those involved. Personal wishes may be taken into account, but the condition of the existing accommodation and the availability of ancilliary services are clear factors in such deliberations, so that an individual's influence may be circumscribed (Norman 1987).

In terms of housing rights, then, in order to protect their interests, older people may need advice concerning their entitlements, not only in negotiations with the statutory services, but also where they are subject to insecure forms of tenure, such as flats administered by 'rogue' landlords in the private sector. The deregulation of both tenancies and rents may have left elderly people vulnerable to abuse, and the overarching structures of community care may bear down as well as sustain. As Clarke (1992 : v) has asked: 'how can people choose services that they do not know exist, or how can they be sure a service, available at one point in the financial year, will be available throughout that year?'

■ Special needs in rural areas

Much attention has been devoted to the plight of elderly people living in inner city areas, and particularly those housed in high-rise blocks. However, census data suggest that where the landscape becomes more rural, the proportion of elderly people in the local population increases (Office of Population, Censuses and Surveys 1990). The significance of this phenomenon lies, first, in the fact that unfit housing is particularly concentrated in rural areas, and second, that although there may generally be sufficient sheltered housing for current demand (but see Lund 1996 : 170), there is a particular shortage in rural areas (Pearson *et al.* 1992). Furthermore, a third of all poor housing occupied by elderly people is privately rented, and this kind of tenure accounts for the accommodation of twice as many older people in rural areas than those in urban settings. There is only patchy coverage of rural areas by home improvement agencies and rural councils are less generous than their urban counterparts in the provision of non-mandatory improvement grants (Pearson *et al.* 1992). Council housing provides half the accommodation for people over 75 in rural areas but as a result of the 'Right to Buy' legislation (the Housing Act 1980), rural council stock diminished by a third in the 1980s (Roof 1990).

A picture emerges, then, of a rather isolated older population in rural settings, more likely to occupy unfit or poor dwellings. Other aspects of rural life may exacerbate difficulties caused by substandard accommodation. These include lack of transport, restricted access to social services and primary health care, and lack of access to shops and post offices (Caldock and Wenger 1992; Wenger 1991, 1988; Mason and Taylor 1990).

■ Conclusions

Even if there is no further change in the balance between the number of older people staying at home, those in sheltered accommodation and those living institutional care, simply to maintain and support the *status quo* will cost more in future. This is for three reasons. First, life expectancy is increasing. Second, dependency as measured by use of health and social services increases with age. And third, the number of elderly people will climb steadily from about 10 million now to an estimated 14.3 millions by the year 2031, with the biggest increase taking place in those over the age of 80 (Central Statistical Office 1996 : 39). In some rural counties, such as Powys in Mid-Wales, the number of very elderly people (those over 80) will rise by as much as 40 per cent by 2006 (Welsh Health Planning Forum, 1993) and Grundy (1993, quoted in Balchin, 1995) highlights a potential increase of 50 per cent in the over-85s between 1992 and 2007.

These demographic trends suggest far reaching implications in seeking to raise the level of dependency at which elderly people qualify for nursing or hospital care. Because each additional person who avoids, or is discharged from, the long-stay hospital ward is almost certain to need a higher level of support than has hitherto been the case, the concomitant expansion of community services is likely to be very expensive. Spending on residential and nursing homes has risen from £10 million in 1979 to £2.2 billion now (Sherman 1995). Hospital and local authority spending on elderly people runs at about £11.8 billions per year (Central Statistical Office 1996), and a little under £29 billion is spent on pensions, £3.9 billion on income support, and roughly £6 billion on housing benefit for elderly people (Department of Health and Social Security 1995). These figures do not include other sources of support such as attendance or mobility allowances. While not of itself an argument for limiting ambitions, the timely and realistic recognition of cost implications is, of course, central to any process of community care planning.

As mooted earlier in this chapter, part of the current problem has been caused by past housing policies and the purposes and designs of ordinary housing. Only one-third of one per cent of the domestic housing stock has been built with disabled people in mind, but in terms of housing in the context of community care older people with severe impairments are likely to need extensive aids and adaptations at home, together with higher levels of response or 'on-call' services, to compensate for or replace the level of care normally found in institutional settings. Such additional needs for 'home-based' services would be even more expensive (in both time and money) in rural areas where fewer clients would be spread far more widely. If the burdens on support services such as GPs, home helps, short-stay health services, social work, and housing agencies increase, the existing battles over resource allocations (who pays?) will intensify, and *inter alia*, examples of GPs removing high-cost patients from their lists will multiply.

The rationing of services, the restricted incomes available to the majority of older people, and the dominant 'able-bodied' norms and assumptions that inform housing construction and design, place ever greater demands on (unpaid) carers. the evidence is that a high proportion of carers are themselves either elderly or approaching older age (two-thirds are over 55 and nearly three-quarters are women) and many are just coping as things stand (Carers National Association 1992; Jones 1986b). Within the context of community care, then, there are a number of consequences for housing policy, planning and design. First, housing policies cannot respond to an ageing population without support from other areas of social policy and practice. Second, housing design needs to take the perspective of 'housing for life'. New housing might, for example, be 'aids and adaptations ready', so that owners can fit stair lifts or special baths and so on easily into pre-planned spaces. Ramps and wider doors might become part of standard house designs in order to anticipate wheelchair use. Such moves would have the additional benefit of increasing both mobility and choice for disabled people who are not elderly, as well as those who are.

Finally, as Walker (1980) argued nearly two decades ago, many problems faced by older people are not of their making, having socioeconomic rather than individual origins. Such factors as inadequate pension levels and complex grant application procedures prevent many older people from maintaining their houses as they would wish. These are short-sighted policies, because unfit housing costs more the worse it gets, and demolished houses are lost to future generations altogether. Poor housing leads to poor health, and so costs are incurred not only in the need for extensive programmes of renovation and slum clearance, but also in medicine and social care.

A mistake made repeatedly down the years is the supposition that it is ineffective to invest in services for older people, if for no other reason than that their life expectancy is necessarily short. Those who take this point of view fail to recognise that the elderly population is *permanent*; it is simply made up of different individuals as time goes by. Since older people *always* constitute about a fifth of the population, and since most of us will join that group one day, it makes sense to do as much as possible now, to guarantee our future security and independence then.

Chapter 20

Working with minority ethnic communities

Ken Blakemore

■ Introduction

This chapter focuses upon the way in which dominant assumptions on the composition of 'the community' in Britain are challenged by the presence of many diverse 'communities'. This also presents a challenge for the planning and provision of care if it is to meet the real needs of people from different communities. It will be argued here that many mistaken beliefs which underpin practice can be seen to exist, and these must be addressed in order to meet minority needs.

The concept of community underlying the Griffiths Report (1988) and *Caring for People* (Department of Health 1989) was a bland and featureless construction. Rather than recognising the United Kingdom for what it is – a complex and rapidly changing mosaic of many different kinds of community – 'the' community in Britain was portrayed as a landscape devoid of cultural diversity and the rich ethnic mix that actually exists.

The blandness of official views of community is well illustrated by the single paragraph (2.9) in *Caring for People* devoted to minority ethnic communities:

> The government recognises that people from different backgrounds may have particular care needs and problems. Minority communities may have different concepts of community care and it is important that service providers are sensitive to these variations. Good community care will take account of the circumstances of minority communities and will be planned in consultation with them. (Department of Health 1989: 10–11)

There have been more exciting fire drill or public safety notices than this. However, as Atkin suggests (1996: 144), this statement did demonstrate that the needs of minority groups had been briefly considered at higher levels of policy-making. But early reaction from those closely involved with minority communities and with planning community care was sceptical (see, for instance, Dutt 1990), and arguably the inclusion of only one main paragraph on minority issues in the White Paper smacked of tokenism rather than a considered commitment to minority needs.

On the other hand, *none* of the major social divisions or social groups in need of community care received any detailed consideration in the broad official design of community care policy. To have entered into a sociological audit of the feasibility of community care would have drawn both Griffiths and the subsequent White Paper into deep waters, and would have exposed government assumptions to the harsh realities of gaps in care resources and family support which have come to light since community care policies have begun to be implemented.

■ The significance of minority ethnic communities

Minority communities therefore have a general significance. They illustrate, first, that the concept of community is problematic. We cannot assume, as did offical policy, that there is one single kind of community replicated across the United Kingdom. The existence of minority communities underlines this point. Ethnic diversity also reminds us that what we mean by 'family' cannot be taken for granted. Different cultural values and concepts of family responsibility influence patterns of family care in the various ethnic communities of Britain.

However, the significance of minority ethnic groups is not limited to providing a wider range of examples of 'community', 'family' and 'care'. More important, perhaps, is the value of minority examples in showing *how dominant assumptions about communities are constructed*. It is not simply the given characteristics of particular communities which are of importance, but rather it is these characteristics combined with how policy-makers, community care organisers and professional groups perceive each community that is of key significance.

A reading of *Caring for People*, for instance, gives an impression of resilient community. There is an underlying assumption that state provision of care tends to blunt the willingness of communities to seek their own solutions or to provide care from their own untapped reserves. It was assumed that somehow, at the whistle of a revised community care policy, hitherto underutilised carers would spring from family groups and community institutions to take on new responsibilities. This Micawberish view of the strength of community is very well illustrated, and magnified, in the case of minority communities. Studies of the use of health and social services in minority communities (see, for example, Cameron *et al.* 1989a) report persistent myths among white service providers about the strength of the extended family in minority communities, and views of unconditional support of older and disabled relatives. Badger (1988), discussing the results of the study conducted by Cameron *et al.*, showed that among district nurses working in areas where up to 50 per cent of households are black or Asian, stereotypical views were held about minority families and communities: self-care or the provision of care by relatives was thought to be universal, and there was little or no awareness of differences of migration history, lifestyle or need among minority communities. Low take-up of community nursing services was thought to reflect low demand resulting from a high degree of family support rather than inadequate referral procedures or the failure of health services to respond to unmet need.

These findings suggest that there are two main concerns about community care and and minority ethnic communities: first, there is the question of the *distinctiveness* of minority ethnic communities and thus whether they have 'special needs'. Are the various minorities able to draw upon greater resources of family or informal support? On the other hand, do some of the more vulnerable members of minority communities face a precarious future with little or no family support, and what are the implications for community nursing and other services if this is the case?

Second, issues of distinctiveness and special needs highlight questions about *the design and delivery of mainstream services*. Should mainstream services be adapted to meet any distinctive health or social care needs among older people or disabled people in black, Asian, or other minority communities and, if so, how far and in what ways? What is the evidence on use of various mainstream services, and what problems have been encountered by both service users and service providers in extending community care to minority communities?

Some of the reported shortcomings in mainstream services can be addressed by tackling racist or discriminatory practices in community care and by improving training to give greater awareness of minority 'special' needs. However, there is still a fundamental question to be resolved: do people in minority communities themselves wish to be treated differently?

Another concern, connected to the role of mainstream services working with minority communities, is whether the voluntary sector can successfully mobilise resources for the various communities. This leads to questions about the effectiveness or otherwise of the voluntary sector, both within minority communities (that is, black, Asian and other minority organisations) and in the majority community (for example, Age Concern, MIND). Before looking at these areas of concern, however, it is necessary to consider what is meant by 'minority communities', together with the associated concepts of race and ethnicity to be used in the remainder of this chapter.

■ 'Minority', 'race' and 'ethnicity' in Britain

The minority concept involves three key elements. Two of these are to do with *numbers* and *distribution* in the population:

1. A minority community is outnumbered by a larger majority, but are the various minority communities dwarfed by the majority, or, if considered together, do they represent a sizeable proportion of the population?
2. Minorities may live in concentrated communities and/or be dispersed throughout the majority.
3. A minority is defined by a *power relationship* with the majority. This relationship may be one of equality between minority and majority, or of inferiority and subjugation of the minority or, more unusually, dominance of the majority by a minority (as with apartheid in the former South Africa, where a white minority used state power to control the majority).

The status and position of a minority are determined more by the economic and power resources they control than by numbers or distribution in the population. Some would argue, for instance, that women are sociologically a minority even though they are numerically in the majority. In the USA, the Jewish minority, which is smaller than the black or African American community, enjoys higher social status and generally better occupational positions than the latter group, which is a sizeable minority accounting for almost 1 Americans in 6 (Ogbu 1978). However, the central importance of power does not mean that numbers are unimportant. A tiny or dispersed minority is all the more easily oppressed or assimilated into the majority because its distinctive characteristics and needs can be conveniently ignored. On the other hand, larger or concentrated minority communities can gain power and influence. This can be seen by comparing Britain, where the minority ethnic population is small – approximately 6 per cent of the total – with immigrant societies such as the USA or Australia, where minority groups are much larger and where the mass media, the schools, the health system and all aspects of public life reflect ethnic diversity to a greater extent than in Britain.

Some idea of the numbers involved in the British case can be gained from the accompanying tables. Table 20.1 shows the ethnic make-up of selected parts of the United Kingdom, using the minority groups identified in the 1991 Census as an illustration. Table 20.2 shows where different proportions of each group live. For example, two-thirds (66 per cent) of all 'Black Caribbean' people in the UK live in the South-East.

Table 20.1 Ethnic composition of selected areas of the United Kingdom, 1993 (percentages)[a]

Ethnic group	Inner London	South East	West Midlands	Yorks Humberside	Wales	Scotland
White	75	90	92	96	99	99
Black–Caribbean	7	2	2	0.4	0.1	0.01
Black African	4	1	0.1	0.1	0.09	0.01
Black other	2	0.5	0.2	0.1	0.1	0.05
Indian	3	3	3	1	0.2	0.05
Pakistani	1	1	2	2	0.2	0.2
Bangladeshi	3	0.5	0.2	0.1	0.2	0.4
hinese	1	0.5	0.1	0.1	0.1	0.02
Other Asian	2	0.5	0.1	0.1	0.1	0.09
Other	2	1	0.3	0.1	0.2	0.1
N (000)	2 504	17 208	5 150	4 837	2 837	4 999
Born in Ireland[b]	5	2	2	1	1	1

Source: OPCS 1993a: 134–89 (Tables 6 and 7).
Notes:
[a] Percentages above 1.0 have been rounded
[b] Republic of Ireland and Northern Ireland (*N* = 837464)

Table 20.2   Proportions of each ethnic group[a] in selected areas (as percentages of total in the United Kingdom),[b] 1993

Ethnic Group	Inner London	South East	West Mids	Yorks & Humberside	Wales	Scotland
White	4	30	9	9	5	10
Black Caribbean	36	66	16	4	0.6	0.1
Black African	51	83	2	2	1	1
Black other	28	57	11	6	2	1
Indian	9	53	19	5	0.7	1
Pakistani	6	30	21	20	1	4
Bangladeshi	44	64	12	5	4	0.6
Chinese	18	53	6	5	3	7
Born in Ireland[c]	14	49	11	5	2	6

Notes:
[a] This table excludes 'Other Asian' and 'Other' (cf. Table 20.1).
[b] Percentages above 1.0 have been rounded. Note that rows total more than 100 because the South-East column is inclusive of Inner London.
[c] Refers to combined total of those born in the Republic of Ireland and in Northern Ireland (837,464)
Source: OPCS 1993a: 134–89 (Tables 6 and 7).

Table 20.1 shows that even in areas such as Inner London and the West Midlands, which have among the highest concentrations of minority communities, Britain's minorities are very much in a minority. In total (and including white minority ethnic groups), Britain's minority population is approximately three million – little more than that of Wales, which has a tiny share of the United Kingdom's population (5 per cent).

The South-East is the most ethnically heterogeneous region, though even here only 1 person in 10 belongs to a minority community as defined by the census. Over a third of all Black Caribbean people live in Inner London (see Table 20.2), where they form the largest single minority community, but they still comprise only 7 per cent of Inner London's population. Both Scotland and Wales are virtually all-white countries.

At a more local level, the geographical settlement of minority communities is even more ghettoised than Table 20.1 indicates. In Inner London, for instance, three-quarters of the population is white, but in certain wards or districts the proportion is much higher. In other city wards, minority communities form a 'majority' and the white community is the minority. Similar patterns of inner-city ghettoisation occur in larger cities such as Birmingham, Bristol and Manchester.

These patterns of minority settlement in Britain have two main implications for community care. First, it has been relatively easy for the majority white community to marginalise minorities, both psychologically (as *illustrated by the* position of this chapter in this book) and in terms of policy and service provision. Though British people may see themselves as tolerant of immigrants and newcomers, in reality British history has been marked by official repression of minority cultures and minority religious belief (for example, Catholicism and

Judaism up to the beginning of the nineteenth century). The idea of a *black* minority maintaining its distinctiveness has proved to be particularly problematic for white British people, as illustrated by Fryer's history (1984) of the assimilation of longstanding black communities in Britain. Thus if there is tolerance, it seems to stretch only as far as accepting small minority communities, and only if they show signs of being assimilated into the majority. Intolerance and racism remain significant features of British 'community' life, making it difficult for multicultural communities to develop. This point has been well expressed by Malik, who points out that while young Asian people, for instance, have distinctive cultural backgrounds, they also

> have mores and attitudes barely different from their white peers. Few attend mosque or temple; most eat meat, drink alcohol, have sex. Yet Asians are not fully accepted here. To a generation that feels itself British,the pain of exclusion is felt that much more acutely. What young Asians resent is not the failure of British society to treat them differently but the fact that British society does treat them differently. (Malik 1996 : 21)

Second, another point to make about the pattern of minority settlement in Britain has particularly significance for the planning and delivery of community care. As mentioned above, minority communities are concentrated in certain urban areas, and in certain neighbourhoods within those areas. The needs of black and Asian people have been defined as 'inner city problems' and are accordingly seen as irrelevant to the majority.

However, it is important to stress that *there are members of minority ethnic communities in every area*, including rural and semi-rural districts, and despite the fact that most people in minority communities live in larger cities. In Wales, for instance, black and Asian people form a very small percentage of the total population (see Table 20.1), but in every sizeable Welsh community there are a few dozen people with minority ethnic backgrounds, whether white (Irish, Polish, Italian), black, or South Asian or Chinese. The same point could be made about Scotland, or about the shire counties in England.

While it is possible to develop support systems from within the substantial minority communities in larger urban areas, there may be no such possibility in market towns or rural areas. The disabled or elderly person who belongs to a minority community and who lives in such communities can face an isolated and precarious future unless local people are unusually supportive. They may have no close relatives to provide care, transport or other forms of support when needed, and they can become particularly isolated if they do not speak English and need to communicate in their first language. Though the numbers involved are very small, the unmet need among people in dispersed minorities can therefore become a serious problem.

Thus the question of minority needs cannot be written off as a specialised inner city concern. Addressing hidden minority needs outside the big cities poses serious challenges to organisers of community care: the challenge of developing referral and monitoring systems which are able to pick up minority needs in rural areas where minority communities are thinly dispersed, the challenge of countering prejudice and discrimination in all-white organisations which have little or no experience of minority communities, and the challenge of using local care resources and personnel imaginatively to compensate for a lack of carers and other helpers from the service user's own community.

In inner city and other urban areas, on the other hand, the challenges facing community care policy and provision for minorities are quite different. In these areas it is far more feasible for care resources to be developed by, or in partnership with, minority communities themselves. Shops and other retail outlets, banks, cultural facilities, religious institutions and voluntary sector organisations have grown to meet minority ethnic needs (though this does not mean that everyone's needs in each minority community are well provided for). Also, it is likely that many people in need of care – though again, not all – will have immediate and extended family and other close connections in their surrounding ethnic community. In these respects it is possible to speak of minority ethnic identity as a *resource*: a source of personal identity and meaning, and of social and economic support. It is important not to problematise inner city communities and to recognise their strengths.

However, as mentioned above, there is also a danger of romanticising community and family values among minority ethnic communities. Thus we need to keep an open mind: how far is belonging to a minority ethnic community likely to be supportive and protective, and how far is it unsupportive, restrictive and likely to lead to experiences of being discriminated against?

■ Conceptualising ethnicity and 'race'

Space does not permit a full discussion of these concepts here, though readers will find specialist discussions of 'race', ethnicity and community helpful (see, for instance, Husband 1996). Briefly, it is possible to summarise both ethnicity and 'race' as highly significant ways in which people define themselves and their own communities, and also as labels which are used to define other people and groups. If the accent is upon *ethnic* characteristics or distinctions, then people will be viewing cultural differences as important: making distinctions, for instance, on the basis of how others speak or which language they use, which religion they adhere to, what kinds of food they eat, how they dress, or how they behave in social settings such as at work. Negative discrimination on the basis of others' religion, culture or way of life can occur, and thus ethnicity can have a political dimension involving conflict or political tension, as the dreadful term 'ethnic cleansing' implies. Sometimes, as occurred in Serbia and Bosnia, nationalism and political rivalries can feed upon ethnic divisions, exploiting them to create fear and hatred of other groups.

Unlike ethnic distinctions, *'race'* and racism are based upon people's beliefs about the supposedly innate or inborn traits of different 'racial' groups, rather than upon their ways of life or cultures. A racialised view of the world is one in which stereotypes of white and black people emerge. One 'race' is seen as inherently superior or inferior to the other.

Despite a recent re-emergence of the question of whether there are significant biological or genetic differences between various 'racial' groups, there is no firm evidence to suggest that differences between human beings from different world regions are anything but superficial. Genetic difference among black African peoples, for instance, has been found to be greater than between black African and white European groups. This is not to deny that there are some genetic or inherited factors which predispose some populations to a higher incidence of certain diseases (for instance, sickle cell anaemia among African and Afro-Caribbean people) or which may possibly have an effect in lowering incidence of others, such as heart attack rates among Afro-Caribbeans (Ebrahim *et al.* 1987). However, these differences, though they are of key concern to minority patients and health service users, are relatively isolated phenomena; they cannot provide any scientific justification for racist myths about differences in behaviour, character or intellectual skills among 'racial' groups.

In sum, then, both ethnic and 'racial' divisions are primarily social construc-tions. Racial distinctions are based on highly visible differences of skin colour and physical appearance which are, in themselves, of little consequence. As markers of social status and power, however, they are loaded with enormous significance. Similarly, with ethnic or cultural differences, what matters are the beliefs one group has about the supposed superiority or inferiority of others' religions, diets, or ways of life.

The constructed and arbitrary nature of both 'racial' and ethnic divisions can be illustrated by reference to the categories of ethnic group employed in the census (see Table 20.1). For instance, a glance at terms such as 'Indian', 'Pakis-tani' and so on tells us that these are not ethnic distinctions at all: they are distinctions based on country of origin or national identity. The 'Indian' com-munity is not a single ethnic group, but is composed of a number of ethnic and religious groups such as the Sikh community and the Gujerati (mainly Hindu and Muslim) community.

It is also noticeable that in the census the word 'ethnic' is used to refer to distinctions of 'race': 'whites', for example, are referred to as an 'ethnic' group. A rigid distinction between 'white' and various sub-groups of 'black' (see Tables 20.1 and 20.2) is made, and this has several unfortunate consequences. To begin with, there is no way of finding out from the so-called 'ethnic question' in the census about people of mixed race or mixed descent, even though Afro-Carib-bean and white intermarriage has become common among Afro-Caribbeans aged under 30 and the children of these partnerships represent the fastest-growing minority 'ethnic' group in the United Kingdom today (Nanton 1992).

Second, 'ethnic' subdivisions and categories are reserved for black and other non-white categories, but no ethnic subdivisions of whites have been elicited. This confirms the impression that 'being ethnic' is in some way to do with being black, even though there are marked ethnic differences among the white population. In other words, ethnic distinctions have been *racialised* in the United Kingdom, just as related issues such as immigration have been portrayed in predominantly racial terms. Thus when 'ethnic groups' and 'immigration' are mentioned in Britain, it is usually inferred that black people are under discussion, even though there is white immigration and there are white minority ethnic groups.

In order to complete the picture of minorities in Britain, therefore, it is important to bear in mind the origins of all migrants to the United Kingdom (see Table 20.3). Those with origins in Asian and African countries – in other words, those most likely to be viewed as 'black' minorities – comprise just over half of all those born outside the United Kingdom: 56 per cent are from 'New Commonwealth' countries, Africa and other Asian countries.

Table 20.3 Country or area of birth of all persons born outside the United Kingdom, 1991 (percentages)

New Commonwealth and Pakistan	44.7
Republic of Ireland	16.6
European Community	13.0
Asia (Middle East and Far East) and Turkey	6.8
Remainder of Europe and USSR	5.3
North and South America	4.9
Old Commonwealth	4.7
Africa	3.9
Rest of the world	0.1
Total	100.0
N	3 774 796

Source: OPCS 1993a: 162, Table 7 (country of birth).

The summarised data in Table 20.3 tell us about the origins of first-generation migrants to Britain, but as the 'ethnic question' in the census did not prompt white minority respondents (for instance, people in the Irish, Polish and Cypriot communities) to identify themselves, there is no national picture of how many white minority, British-born, second-or third-generation descendants continue to identify themselves with the ethnic identity of their parents or grandparents.

However, it is safe to say that the Irish community, including British-born children of Irish migrants, forms one of the largest single minority ethnic communities in Britain, just as many of the descendants of Greek and Turkish Cypriot, Polish, and other east European migrants and refugees continue to identify to a degree with their ethnic communities.

■ Minority communities: are they distinctively different in needs and resources?

This is a valid and necessary question but it carries with it the danger of problematising the minorities: they can all too easily be pictured as deviant groups who do not fit a majority norm. As pointed out above, however, there is diversity in the white population and no single type of community, as implied by Griffiths and subsequent policy documents. Therefore any answer to the question 'are minority communities different from the majority?' must depend upon what kind of 'majority' community one is using for comparison: for instance a northern English white working-class community, a Scottish middle-class community, and so on. The other problem with this question is that, if minority communities do have special needs, these arise at least partly from the minority experience of disadvantage. Needs do not emanate from each community as if it were in a social or economic vacuum; some additional or 'special' needs are caused by structural disadvantage and failures of policy and service provision. Cameron *et al.* (1989b : 237), for instance, discuss the disadvantages faced by health carers in black communities. These include greater than average chances of being poor, experiencing unemployment, and of living in housing and in poor urban environments which threaten health. None of these are 'special' needs: they are shared by considerable numbers of white carers in the majority community. The point is that, as a result of racism and other forms of discrimination, people in black and Asian communities tend to experience them more often.

Unemployment rates, for instance, vary between one community and another, but are typically between two and four times greater for black and Asian workers than for whites at similar occupational levels (Blakemore and Drake 1996 : 18); housing conditions are significantly less likely to be satisfactory for black and Asian people, with a higher incidence of overcrowding and problems such as dampness and lack of adequate heating (Atkin and Rollings 1996 : 81). Also, as a result of a number of factors – language differences, not having worked in Britain long enough to complete a full record of National Insurance contributions, reluctance to claim benefits because of the stigma of welfare dependency, and fear of racial discrimination by officials – some older and disabled Asian people experience difficulties in claiming full entitlement to social security benefits (Bhalla and Blakemore 1981; Skellington 1996 : 129–30).

Therefore, if community health services and other kinds of community support are improved to take account of these disadvantages, it is not so much that 'special' needs are being addressed but rather that existing inadequacies and common problems are being recognised. Jackson and Field express this well:

> Discussion of the 'special' or 'additional' needs of Asians can be highly misleading. This is not so much because such needs do not exist as because such terms imply that something extra is to be granted to the disadvantaged This is quite likely to offend ethnic minorities who perceive it as a misrepresentation of the true situation, and offend whites who perceive it as an intention to discriminate against them The main thrust of policy for both the statutory and voluntary sector should be to deliver as effective a service to Asians as is delivered to whites. While this may require special *measures*, such measures will not necessarily be directed at the special or additional *needs* of Asians. (Jackson and Field 1989 : 40; emphasis added).

Inappropriate and insensitive mainstream health and social services are implicated in unmet need among minority communities. The need for better-targeted and more relevant services is discussed below, and has been prompted by a growing number of local research studies which have documented, for instance, a severe lack of interpreting and translation services (Askham *et al.* 1995), or shortages of health and social care staff who are either from users' own communities or thoroughly understand their needs, such as in family support services or respite care (Dobson 1995; Grant 1995).

However, it would be wrong to conclude from these points that minority communities are just like any others except that they are more prone to disadvantage and discrimination, or that they are more likely than majority communities to be ignored by health and social services. Minority communities do have distinctive cultural and social characteristics of their own, together with different kinds of relationship with the majority; not to acknowledge this diversity in Britain would be discriminatory in itself, and the need for multicultural community care would not be an issue.

The problem is, how are we to conceptualise this ethnic diversity to take account of different cultural preferences, religious beliefs and changing ways of life among Britain's minorities? As far as practical intervention by community health workers and other practitioners from 'majority' or white communities is concerned, nothing can substitute for the application of learning about the history, migration experience and changing culture of specific groups to practice-based issues of health, illness and care (for useful practical guides see, for instance, Henley 1983, Mares *et al.* 1985; Qureshi 1989).

However, as a preliminary exercise in understanding minority needs it may be helpful to compare objective findings about minority communities with more subjective, harder-to-pin-down characteristics. The characteristics of a minority community that can be defined more or less objectively are, for instance, family size and residence patterns, demographic structure, patterns of health, illness and dependency. More subjective characteristics include expectations of care in the family, life satisfaction and morale among younger and older people, and cultural aspects of the way people cope with illness and disability. As far as objective characteristics are concerned, there are several key features of minority communities which suggest that at least some of Britain's minorities possess resources and have certain advantages to balance against the disadvantages mentioned above. For example, while overcrowding and inadequate accommodation is a problem, larger family groups among the various Asian communities offer the potential (if not always the reality) of on-the-spot care for older and disabled people in a way that an increasing number of fragmented and dispersed white majority families cannot. A survey of minority families by Askham *et al.*, for instance, found that only 1 older Asian person in 7 lives alone, compared with a third of older Afro-Caribbeans (1995 : 92). Also, surveys in the Midlands showed that a quarter of older Asians in Coventry lived in large households (six or more people) and that even more – almost two-thirds – did so in Birmingham (Blakemore and Boneham 1994 : 82); again, however, older Afro-Caribbean people were found to be living more as the majority elderly population does, mostly either alone or with a spouse or partner.

In addition to family residence patterns, care needs are also shaped by population ageing and the ratio of older people in need of care to those who can provide it. Here again, the minority communities, being in most cases (except white minority communities such as the Irish) much 'younger' than the majority population, have potentially much larger reserves of carers, though we should remember that numbers of older Asian and Afro-Caribbean people will grow rapidly over the next decade (Blakemore and Boneham 1994 : 17).

To more fully understand care needs and the relative position of minority communities we must also put findings about rates of illness and of disability into the equation. Atkin and Rollings (1996 : 75) point to a lack of information on disability and the minority experience of care services, especially as far as learning disability and mental impairment are concerned. There is also a lack of a comprehensive national picture of the incidence of all kinds of disability and illness in minority communities to compare with the majority population.

However, as Atkin and Rollings report, an 'OPCS survey of physical disability (OPCS 1988) showed that when standardised for age the prevalence of disability among Afro-Caribbean and Asian people, compared with that of the white population, was roughly the same' (1996 : 76). The 1991 census revealed that the proportions of people who identified themselves as having a 'limiting long-term illness' were higher among the majority white population (13.4 per cent) than among the Afro-Caribbean (11.5), Pakistani (8.8), Indian (8.7), Bangladeshi (8.7) or Chinese (4.4) communities (OPCS 1993a = 134).

The higher rate of reporting of long-term illness by the majority population is mainly a reflection of the age structures of majority and minority populations. A survey of disability among Gujerati and white people in London confirmed this, but also suggested that even allowing for age there seemed to be a 'somewhat lower household rate' among the Asian sample (Jackson and Field 1989 : 14); the authors suggested that much of this lower rate among Asian families could be explained by under-reporting of minor disabilities. This latter point reminds us of the importance of subjective factors in assessing care needs, and of the dangers of generalisation from supposedly objective findings on incidence of disability and illness.

Though there is no evidence that rates of illness overall are higher among all minority groups combined, when compared with the majority population, this disguises considerable variations in illness, disability and care need *between* different minority communities. Some community surveys (for instance Donaldson 1986; Ebrahim *et al.* 1991) have reported levels of morbidity among older Asian people which are either little different or even somewhat better, in some respects, than in matched white populations. But both of these surveys were of relatively affluent South Asian communities. Other studies (for instance Blakemore 1982; Cruickshank *et al.* 1980; Fenton 1986) have shown much higher incidence of limiting illnesses, and the need to use hospital services, especially where poorer

Asian communities and older Afro-Caribbean people have been included in surveys.

Assessment of need in minority communities is further complicated by social change and the influence of subjective factors such as those mentioned above. More South Asian people may live in larger households and live closer to relatives than people in the white majority, but this broad trend disguises many significant changes of attitude and culture within the minorities (Ahmad 1996). In sum, there are several key reasons for questioning notions of unconditional and beneficial support of older, disabled or chronically ill people by close relatives in the so-called 'extended family' in Asian communities:

> Family life, while usually warm and supportive, can sometimes be oppressive and exploitative for those who carry the burden of care, especially for Asian women who marry into households in which they enjoy little respect or status. Sometimes the stresses upon women in 'traditional' roles are exacerbated by role conflict and by tensions between themselves and their daughters, who 'have often moved away from traditional roles via education, work, and sometimes marriage partners'. (Cameron *et al.* 1989b : 241)

Just as carers experience stress, so may those dependent relatives who feel that they need more social contact or physical help than they are getting. It is possible to be isolated and lonely in a large family even if – or perhaps because – the family lives under one roof. If a widowed or dependent grandmother needs care, for instance, there is usually an expectation that she will live with a son rather than a daughter, and this expectation in Asian communities can set up the well-known pattern of conflict between the son's wife and mother.

Also, as Ahmad (1996) reminds us, subjective feelings of being neglected are sometimes more important than the reality. If traditional expectations are of close daily contact and loving support of older relatives, then any perceived loss of such support can have devastating results on the morale and wellbeing of older people. This is a particularly important point as far as referrals to health and social services are concerned. The entry of a community nurse or social care assistant into some Asian families may be accompanied by strong feelings of resistance, shame and guilt among both the cared-for and the carers, a point which is explained particularly well by McCalman (1990) in a study of carers in three minority communities in London. In some families, any intervention by outsiders was seen as a potential social disgrace, and McCalman highlights the need to build trust and confidence carefully with service users and their families. The extended family is neither unchanging nor universal. As mentioned above, social and geographical mobility is affecting substantial numbers of families in Asian communities, and especially among communities which are becoming more prosperous and middle class than before (Modood 1991). Ahmad (1996) summarises a wide range of evidence which points to the significance of emerging class differences among Asian families, especially as far as filial obligations and ideas about extended and nuclear family living are concerned. Better-off and socially mobile younger Asians are more likely to live independently or as married couples than they were, and are more likely to reject traditional views of arranged marriage (Arlidge 1993).

These trends should not be equated with a change towards a less caring attitude towards older people or disabled people in need of care in Asian communities, nor of a lack of willingness to provide financial or other material forms of support. The point is that a growing proportion of Asian families are subject to the same influences of family fragmentation and separation that have transformed white majority family life in the past two decades, and which make it more difficult than in the past to translate caring attitudes into regular provision of care or on-the-spot support. Even before these trends in Asian communities gathered momentum in recent years, however, a substantial minority of Asian people were living without close relatives nearby. The extended family and multi-generation household were never universal. In Birmingham in 1981, for instance, we found that almost a quarter of older Asians were living with others (for instance, more distant relatives from the same village or district in India or Pakistan) but not with close relatives such as a son, brother or daughter (Bhalla and Blakemore 1981).

In sum, therefore, ideas of pervasive and unconditional support in every Asian family must be jettisoned, even though there are still distinctive differences between the minority communities and the majority. This point, which is highly significant for assumptions about future sources of care in the community, must be underlined as far as other minority communities are concerned: in particular, the Afro-Caribbean community and white minority communities such as the Irish and the various East European communities. The Afro-Caribbean community, for instance, is significantly 'older' than the Asian communities because higher proportions of men and women arrived in Britain at an earlier phase of migration in the 1950s. Older black and disabled people are much more likely to live alone and to lack the support of close relatives than Asians in the same categories.

The Irish migrant community has an even 'older' population structure. While family ties and other links with Ireland may remain close for some Irish people in Britain, there are signs of considerable isolation and psychological stress in the community. These problems of poor health are evidenced by mortality rates which are well above the average for the United Kingdom (McKeigue 1991 : 70–1). Thus as far as 'special' need and community care is concerned, the Irish community is arguably the neediest, yet has the fewest resources in terms of family support of all Britain's minority ethnic communities.

■ Problems with mainstream and voluntary sector services

The diversity of Britain's minority communities makes it difficult to generalise about the level of need for community care services outside the family which are provided by mainstream health and social services, or by voluntary sector organisations. It is certainly not possible to make comfortable assumptions about minority needs being fewer than in the majority community, even in Asian communities which appear to provide more family support than white families do. As pointed out, Asian communities are themselves quite diverse, rapidly changing and socially differentiated by class and other divisions. Even where families provide a lot of care this does not mean that need for extrafamilial services is absent: for instance, need for carer support and advice, help with social security claims in cases of disability, or need for improved access to underused community health services.

How pronounced are problems of underuse of, and poor access to, mainstream and voluntary sector services? In this final section we first review some leading findings on patterns of service use among minority communities and then discuss the implications for the construction of community care: in other words, why do inequalities in access and service use exist?

There is a growing literature on minority communities and health and social services, and this is the product of a number of community studies in a wide range of urban areas in Britain (see, for instance, Ahmad and Aitkin 1996; Askham *et al.* 1995; Bhalla and Blakemore 1981; Blakemore and Boneham 1994; Cameron *et al.* 1989a, 1989b; Jackson and Field 1989; Pharaoh 1995). The findings reflect ethnic and local differences in service use, but have established that there exists a common pattern of racial and ethnic discrimination or disadvantage.

The community care research project in Birmingham by Cameron *et al.* (1989b), for example, showed that Asian clients formed only 7 per cent of users of a range of services (district nursing, health visiting for elderly people, occupational therapy, social work) and 'this seemed much too low given the population structure of central Birmingham' where around 20 per cent of the community live in minority ethnic households (1989b: 232). This study found that, among elderly disabled service users, both sexes in the Asian communities were underrepresented. Disabled Afro-Caribbean and Asian adults were underrepresented in caseloads of health and social service providers, but problems of access and underrepresentation seemed to be more pronounced in community health than in social services. This is an interesting finding, given that registration with GPs is near-universal in the minority communities, as among the majority population, and one would have expected that access to community health services would have been improved by GP contacts. However, as part of the explanation for barriers to community health services, Cameron *et al.* refer to poor referral procedures among GPs and a 'mind-set' among organisers of community nursing about the needs of black and Asian families (for example, ideas about child care needs being a priority rather than any problems in care of older or disabled people); this is an illustration of the way in which socially constructed images or perceptions of minority communities can affect practical outcomes in service provision.

Though some social services may be better used or have fewer problems of access this does not mean, however, that problems are minimal in that sphere of community care – far from it, according to Jackson and Field's (1989) survey of over five hundred Gujerati households in London, which compared use of a number of social services (childcare and youth services as well as services for elderly and disabled people) with a sample of white households in the same areas. They found that under-use of services was more marked for disability than for age. Having identified households in need of care services, they discovered that 43 per cent of eligible white households were receiving services at the time of their survey, compared with only 15 per cent of Asian households. As Asian households are larger, on average, the inequality in use is even greater than that implied by the difference in the numbers of households receiving services.

The inequalities discovered by Jackson and Field apply to services provided to the home (such as home care) rather than to services in the community itself, such as day centres, where use (by about 15 per cent of whites and Asians) was about the same. Older Asians living on their own, or with an elderly partner, were found to receive more help from relatives than their white counterparts, but almost all the help they receive is family care; among whites, community care services substitute for family care, to a greater or lesser extent.

In the Afro-Caribbean community, more is known than in most Asian communities about the range of community health and social services available (Blakemore and Boneham 1994:114). This reflects a number of factors: fewer language barriers between the Afro-Caribbean community and the majority, the relatively high proportion of Afro-Caribbean people who have direct experience of health and social services as employees, and need. In Birmingham, for instance, we found that over a half of older Afro-Caribbean men and almost a third of older black women live alone. Not all of those who live alone are without family support, but an increasing proportion are lonely and isolated, and do need both community facilities (for example social centres, lunch clubs, support groups to help deal with chronic illness) and some domiciliary help.

However, it is often assumed by white service providers that, because Afro-Caribbean people speak English as a first language, there will be fewer barriers to service use than those which affect Asian communities. This assumption is based on a number of misconceptions. First, limited fluency in English is *not* a predictor of underuse of services in Asian communities (Jackson and Field 1989:47). Barriers to service use are much more to do with perceptions of what a service might offer, or fail to offer, combined with expectations among black and Asian people that they will experience some racial discrimination in services geared to the white majority.

By contrast, examples of community services which remove barriers and succeed in meeting minority needs illustrate both what can be done and the limitations of mainstream services. A project to provide respite for black carers, for instance (Dobson 1995), demonstrates how a queue of Afro-Caribbean carers wanting respite services can quickly form. As one informant put it, 'the project was worth funding because it was working with a group of people, that is African and African-Caribbean carers, who have traditionally been invisible and largely ignored' (Dobson 1995:29).

In sum, then, it would be wrong to conclude that underuse of social and health services is simply a matter of ignorance among Asian communities, or of improving publicity about existing services in Afro-Caribbean and other minority ethnic groups. As Jackson and Field suggest, there are strong information networks in minority communities. Once a few members of a community are aware of a service, it will soon be either requested or rejected by others, depending on its suitability or appropriateness to users' needs. Therefore, as Williams (1990) points out, barriers to equal use of community care services lie much more within the organisation and approach of the services themselves than in lack of awareness in minority communities. These organisational barriers do include communication issues, such as reception and telephone services, but also more fundamental points such as the application of equal opportunity policies to staffing, and the employment of more black, Asian and other minority group community nurses, home care workers and other service workers. In rural areas with dispersed minority populations, for instance, the availability of at least a few Afro-Caribbean, Chinese or other minority ethnic care staff would mean that, while such minority employees could deal for the most part with clients and carers in the majority white community, they could also be on hand to improve services for minority users. This point about the need for organisational change, or for changes in the approach and attitude of professional staff such as community nurses, is also of key importance because it is not as though black and Asian people expect to be treated particularly differently from the majority.

Askham *et al.* (1995) survey asked older Asian and Afro-Caribbean respondents whether they thought people from their backgrounds should be treated in a special way when receiving health and social services in general, and whether they thought community nurses should treat them in a special way. None of the Afro-Caribbeans wanted to be treated in a special way; the emphasis was upon equality, and 'common characteristics such as common humanity, being a British citizen, one of God's children, or a tax payer' (1995 : 79). Two-fifths of the Asian respondents did wanted to be treated in a special way, but in the main these preferences boiled down to three things: language and communication issues (being able to talk to someone in one's own language), diet (observing dietary requirements is almost always a matter of religious prescription, not merely preference) and the choice to be treated by a nurse or health practitioner of one's own sex.

Even with regard to Asians' more distinct preferences and needs, however, the emphasis put upon these requirements by Asian respondents themselves was that clients or users should be treated as *individuals* rather than as members of a category. Put that way, so-called 'minority needs' are little different from the need for *any* client or service user to be treated as an individual by professionals and care workers. All older people, disabled people and others who need care in the community have biographies, experiences and preferences which will affect the way they respond to care or, in some cases, to failure to obtain any appropriate services. All service users have ethnic identities, whether they are in the majority white community, or whether they belong to one of the relatively neglected East European white minority communities (see Bowling 1991 for an interesting discussion of the particular needs and difficulties of older Polish and Ukrainian people), or whether they are in an Afro-Caribbean or South Asian community.

■ Conclusion

In this chapter we have seen that minority ethnic communities face several kinds of disadvantage and discrimination as far as community care is concerned. These problems are partly to do with underlying racial discrimination in the health and social services (McNaught 1988). Such attitudes are buttressed, as far as community care is concerned, by socially constructed notions that Asian and other minorities 'look after their own' and do not need as many support services from outside the home as do the majority. If black, Asian and other minority clients do express distinct preferences or needs, these somehow represent 'awkward' demands – the minorities should learn to 'fit in'; their needs are seen as less legitimate than those of majority white service users.

In addition to underlying racism, the problems faced in tackling underuse of community care services by minorities are also a reflection of the way community care has been constructed in Britain. The take-up of community health services continues to be low, although there has been some improvement in the use of day centres and certain social services (Pharaoh and Redmond 1991). According to Pharaoh and Redmond, and later surveys (Askham *et al.* 1995; Pharaoh 1995), there have as yet been only limited attempts to develop community outreach, health liaison and linkworker schemes for, or with, minority communities. They suggest that the causes of this poor level of development are both organisational (the few schemes they found were funded on a short-term basis only, and fell between various health and social service agency stools) and conceptual: there is little awareness in mainstream community health of the needs of disabled and older people in minority communities. Pharaoh and Redmond found that, where ethnic minorities are the focus, the preoccupations of community health nurses and health visitors are with child and maternity health services.

Lack of awareness of the range of minority ethnic health care needs is also worrying because the introduction of a mixed economy of care and changes to the organisation of community care at the 'social' end of the spectrum (provision of mobile meals, home care, and other domiciliary and community services) are also likely to increase some of the disadvantages faced by minority ethnic communities.

As discussed elsewhere in this book, the reorganisation of care in the community has transformed the respective roles of local authorities, now in the main acting as purchasers, and voluntary and independent sector agencies acting as providers. The shift to voluntary sector provision carries with it certain disadvantages for minority ethnic communities, at least in the short term: first, voluntary sector organisations within the various minority communities are relatively patchy and undeveloped (Blakemore 1985) and provide only a small share of the care services used by minority older or disabled people (Jackson and Field 1989). Small and poorly-funded community groups in black, Asian and Chinese communities find it difficult to compete in the 'care market' with larger, white or majority-dominated organisations for contracts with local authorities.

Second, there are as many – if not more – problems of insensitivity to minority needs and problems of racial discrimination in the larger voluntary organisations as in local authority social service departments or health authorities. Atkin (1996 : 147), summarising the problems of the established voluntary sector, notes a neglect of equal opportunity policies in staffing and committee member-ship and widespread lack of awareness of racial and multicultural issues in such areas as training carers or communicating with minority ethnic community groups. However, as Atkin concludes, there is as yet little completed research on the implementation of community care plans or services for minority com-munities, or research 'evaluating the role of black voluntary organisations in the "contract economy"' (1996 : 150). The diversity of Britain's multi-ethnic popula-tion, combined with the rapid social and economic changes alluded to above, make it likely that *some* sections of *some* of Britain's minority communities will continue to develop appropriate social and health care services through their own voluntary and private sector activities. There is a growing number of such initiatives and, though they tend to meet social care and housing needs rather than dovetailing with community health services, they do offer the potential for future cooperation on joint health and social care projects between community health care providers and minority community organisations (see, for instance, Gilbert 1988; Lieberman and Au 1988; Dobson 1995; Grant 1995).

As we have seen, however, it would be wrong to be too optimistic about the self-reliance of minority communities, just as the ability of 'the community' to care has often been overestimated as far as the majority is concerned. Britain's minority communities differ widely in respect of the economic, social and family resources they command, and relatively well-off and well-supported communities coexist with deprived and sometimes very disadvantaged ones. Expecting mi-nority communities to meet all their own community care needs would, in any case, amount to cheating them of mainstream services to which they have contributed by way of taxes and insurance contributions. For that reason Askham *et al.* (1995) identify *specialised* services (mainstream services adapted in various ways for minority communities) as a promising way forward in health and social services, and these would be distinct from either mainstream services as presently structured or the kind of small-scale, often underfunded separate services run by minority voluntary groups. Unless imaginative steps are taken to develop com-munity care services in this way, especially in the community health field, Britain's minority communities will continue to be short-changed by present community care policies.

Part III

Summary

This final part of the book has been concerned with the communities to which community care is to be delivered. It is the final part of the trilogy with which we began:

- Care *in* the community
- Care *by* the community
- Care *for* the community

The contributors in this part have looked at the numerous and various groups which are the recipients of care and have chronicled the wide diversity both within these groups and within society as a whole.

But whether we are looking at services for mentally ill people, for children in need, for older people or for minority ethnic communities, one factor dominates the delivery of care – poverty. This can be defined in three ways: the poverty of language which defines and restricts thinking and the organisation of care delivery, the poverty experienced by a third of the 'citizens' of Britain and the poverty of resources which forms the backdrop to the daily reality of the planning and delivery of care.

The main theme which emerges from this final part, and from the book as a whole, is that care in, by and for the community cannot be delivered in a vacuum. The quality of care given and received is constructed by historical, social, cultural and economic forces which exist in society.

References

Abberley, P. (1987) 'The concept of oppression and the development of a social theory of disability', *Disability, Handicap and Society*, **2** (1), 5–19.

Abbott, P. and Sapsford, R. (1990) 'Health visiting: policing the family', in Abbott, P. and Sapsford, R. (eds) *The Sociology of the Caring Professions*. Basingstoke: Falmer.

Abel-Smith, B. (1964) *The Hospitals 1800–1948*. London: Heinemann.

Abel-Smith, B. and Townsend, P. (1965) *The poet and the poetess*. Bell, London.

Abramson, M. (1989) 'Autonomy vs paternalistic beneficence: practice strategies', *Social Casework* 70, 2, 110–5.

Adams, L. (1991) 'Community development at a national level within the health education authority', in Jones, J. and Tilson, J. (eds.) *Roots and Branches*. Milton Keynes: Open University Press, pp. 133–46.

Addison, P. (1994) *The Road to 1945*. London: Pimlico.

Adler, S., Laney, J. and Packer, M. (1993) *Managing Women*. Buckingham: Open University Press.

Ahmad, W. I. U. (1996) 'Family obligations and social change among Asian communities', in Ahmad, W. I U. and Aitken, K. (eds) *Race and Community Care*. Buckingham: Open University Press, pp. 51–72.

Ahmad, W. I U. and Aitken, K. (eds) (1996) *Race and Community Care*. Buckingham: Open University Press.

American Nurses Association (ANA) (1987) *Standards of Practice for the Primary Health Care Nurse Practitioner* Washington DC: ANA.

Amiel, B. (1994) 'We played a game and the gun won', *Sunday Times*, 22 May 1994.

Amin, K. and Oppenheim, C. (1992) *Poverty in Black and White: deprivation and ethnic minorities*, London: Child Poverty Action Group and Runnymede Trust.

Anderson, B. (1990) *Contracts and the Contract Culture*. London: Age Concern.

Anthony, P.D. (1977) *The Ideology of Work*. London: Tavistock.

Anthony, P.D. (1994) *Managing Culture*. Buckingham: Open University Press.

Anthony, P.D. (1986) *The Foundations of Management*. London: Tavistock.

Anthony, P.D. and Crichton, A. (1969) *Industrial Relations and the Personnel Specialist*. London, Batsford.

Arber, S. and Gilbert, N. (1989) 'Transitions in caring: gender, life course and the care of the elderly', in Bytheway, B., Keil, T., Allatt, P. and Bryman, A. (eds) *Becoming and Being Old*. London: Sage, pp. 72–9.

Arber, and Ginn, J. (1990) 'The meaning of informal care: gender and the contribution of elderly people', *Ageing and Society*, **10** (4), 429–54.

Arber, S. and Ginn, J. (1991) *Gender and Later Life*. London: Sage.

Aries, P. (1962) *Centuries of Childhood*. New York: Vintage Books.

Arlidge, J. (1993) 'Asian men say no to the misery of arranged marriage', *Independent on Sunday, 16 May, p. 6*.

Armstong, L. (1993) 'Mind over matter', *Nursing Times*, **89** (50), 29–30.

Armstrong, D. (1995) 'The rise of surveillance medicine', *Sociology of Health and Illness*, **17**, (3), 393–404.

Arnold, P., Bochel, H. Broadhurst, S. and Page, D. (1993) *Community Care: The Housing Dimension. York: Joseph Rowntree Foundation*.

Ashton, J. (ed.), (1991) *Healthy Cities*, Milton Keynes: Open University Press.

Ashton, J. and Seymour, H. (1992) *The New Public Health*. Milton Keynes: Open University Press.

Ashton, J. and Seymour, H. (1988) *The New Public Health*. Milton Keynes: Open University Press.

Askham, J., Henshaw, L. and Tarpey, M. *Social and Health Authority* (1995) *Services for Elderly People from Black and Minority Ethnic Communities*. London: HMSO.

Atkin, K. (1992) 'Similarities and difference between informal carers', in Twigg, J. (ed), *Carers: Research and Practice*. London: HMSO.

Atkin, K. (1996) 'An opportunity for change: voluntary sector provision in a mixed economy of care', in Ahmad, W. I. U. and Atkin, K. (eds) *Race and Community Care*. Buckingham: Open University Press, pp. 144–60.

Atkin, K. and Rollings, J. 'Looking after their own? Family care-giving among Asian and Afro-Caribbean communities,' in Ahmad, W. I. U. and Atkin, K. (eds) *Race and Community Care*. Buckingham: Open University Press, pp. 73–86.

Audit Commission (1994) *Seen But Not Heard: co-ordinating Community Child Health and Social Services for Children in Need*. HMSO: London.

Badger, F. (1988) 'Put race on the agenda', *Health Service Journal*, **98** (5129), 1426–27.

Bagust, A., Slack, R. and Oakley, J. (1992) *Ward Nursing Quality and Grade Mix*. York Health Economics Consortium. University of York.

Balchin, P. (1995) *Housing Policy: An Introduction*, 3rd edn. London, Routledge.

Baldock, J. (1993) 'Old age', in Dallos, R. and McLaughlin, E. (eds) *Social Problems and the Family*. London: Sage.

Baldock, J. and Ungerson, C. (1994) *Becoming Consumers of Community Care: Households Within the Mixed Economy of Welfare*. York: Joseph Rowntree Foundation.

Baldwin, S. (1994), 'The need for care in later life: social protection of older people and family caregivers', in Baldwin, S. and Falkingham, J. (eds) *Social Security and Social Change*. Hemel Hempstead: Harvester Wheatsheaf.

Baly, M. (1986) *Florence Nightingale and the Nursing Legacy*. London: Croom Helm.

Barker, I. and Peck, E. (eds) (1987) *Power in Strange Places: User Empowerment in Mental Health Services*. London: Good Practices in Mental Health.

Barnes, C. (1990) *Cabbage Syndrome: The Social Construction of Dependence*. Basingstoke: Falmer.

Barnes, C. (1991) *Disabled People in Britain and Discrimination*. London: Hurst.

Barnes, M. (1995) 'Incapacity benefit', *Legal Action*, May 1995.

Barratt Brown, M. (1991) *European Union – Fortress of Democracy*. Nottingham: Spokesman.

Barrett, D. (1992) 'Older peoples' experiences of Community Care', *Social Policy and Administration*, **26** (4) (December), 196–312.

Bartlett, B. (1991) 'Privatisation and quasi-markets', *Studies in Decentralisation and Quasi-markets* No. 7, University of Bristol, SAUS.

Bartlett, W. and Legrand, J. (1993) 'The theory of quasi-markets', in Le Grand, J. and Bartlett, W. (eds) *Quasi Markets and Social Policy*. London: Macmillan.

Barton, L. (ed.) (1989) *Integration: Myth or Reality?* Lewes: Falmer.

Basch, P.F. (1990) *Textbook of International Health*. New York: Oxford University Press.

Beardshaw, V. (1990) *Squaring the Circle, the implementation of caring for people*, London: King's Fund News 13, (1), 1.

Beardshaw, V. and Towell, D. (1990) *Assessment in case management*, London: King's Fund Institute.

Becker, S. and Silburn, R. (1990) *The New Poor Clients*. Nottingham University Benefits Research/Community Care.

Bennett, C. (1994) 'A prophet and porn', *The Guardian* 28 May 1994.

Benzeval, M., Judge, K. and Whitehead, M. (eds) (1995) *Tackling Inequalities in Health; An Agenda for Action*. London: King's Fund.

Beresford, P. and Croft, S. (1993) *Citizen Involvement: A Practical Guide for Change*. London, Macmillan.

Berger, P. and Luckmann, T. (1984) *The Social Construction of Reality: A Treatise in the Sociology of Knowledge*. Harmondsworth: Penguin.

Beveridge, W. (1942) *Social Insurance and Allied Services*. London: HMSO.

Bhalla, A., and Blakemore, K. (1981) *Elders of the Minority Ethnic Groups*. Lozells, Birmingham: AFFOR.

Bhat, A., Carr-Hill, R., and Ohri, S. (1988) *Britain's Black Population: A New Perspective*. Aldershot: Gower, Radical Statistics Group.

Bines, W. (1994) *The Health of Single Homeless People*. Centre for Housing Policy, York University Discussion Paper 9.

Bion, W. (1970) *Attention and Interpretation*. London: Tavistock.

Blakemore, K. (1982) 'Health and Illness among the elderly of minority ethnic groups', *Health Trends*, **14** (3), pp. 68–72.

Blakemore, K. (1985) 'The state, the voluntary sector and new developments in provision for the old of minority racial groups', *Ageing and Society* **5**, 175–90.

Blakemore, K. and Boneham, M. (1994) *Age, Race and Ethnicity*. Buckingham: Open University Press.

Blakemore, K. and Drake, R.F. (1996) *Understanding Equal Opportunity Policies*. London: Prentice-Hall.

Booth, C. (1889–1903) *Life and Labour of the People of London*, 17 volumes. London: Norman.

Barnat, J., Pereira, C., Pilqrum, D. and Williams, F. (eds) *Community Care: A Reader*, London: Macmillan.

Borsay, A. (1986) 'Personal trouble or public issue? Towards a Model of Policy for People with Physical and Mental Disabilities', *Disability, Handicap and Society*, **1**, no. 2, pp. 179–95.

Bosanquet, N. (1984) *Extending Choice for Mentally Handicapped People*. London MIND.

Bourke, J. (1996) *Dismembering the Male: Men's Bodies, Britain and the Great War*. London: Reaktion Books.

Bowlby, J. (1951) *Maternal Care and Mental Health*. Geneva: WHO.

Bowlby, J. (1953) *Children and the Growth of Love*. Harmondsworth: Penguin.

Bowling, B. (1991) 'Ethnic minority elderly people: helping the community to care', *New Community*, **17** (4) 645–52.

Bowling, A. (1994) 'Health Care Returning: The Public's Debate', *British Medical Journal*, **312**, 16 March 1994, 670–4.

Boyd, R. (1993) 'Metaphor and theory change: what is "metaphor" a metaphor for?', in Ortony, A. (ed.) *Metaphor and Thought*, 2nd edn. Cambridge University Press.

Boyd-Orr, J. (1936) *Food, Health and Income*. London: Macmillan.

Bradshaw, J. (1972), 'The taxonomy of social need', in Mclachlan, G. (ed) *Problems and Progress in Medical Care*. Oxford University Press.

Bradshaw, J. (1990) *Child Poverty and Deprivation in the UK*. London: National Children's Bureau.

Brandon, D. (1991) *Consumer Power in Psychiatric Services*. London: Macmillan.

Brenton, M. (1985) *The Voluntary Sector in British Social Services*. London: Longman.

Brisenden, S. (1986) 'Independent living and the medical model of disability', *Disability, Handicap and Society*, **1**, (2), 173–8.

British Paediatric Association (1995) *Health Services for School Age Children*. BPA, London.

Broady, M. (1989) 'The changing state of the voluntary sector in Wales', *Network Wales*, **66**, 4–6.

Brooker, C. and Jayne, D. (1984) 'Time to rethink', *Nursing Times, Community Outlook*. 11 April, 132–4.

Broomberg, J. (1994) 'Managing the health care market in developing countries: prospects and problems', *Health Policy and Planning*, **9**(3), 237–51.

Browse, N. (1996) 'Costs had come down before the reforms', *News Review*, BMA, April.

Bryant, J. H. (ed.) (1988) From Alma Ata to he Year 2000. Geneva, World Health Organisation.

Bryar, R., Fisk, H. (1994) 'An examination of the need for new nursing roles in primary health care', *Journal of Interprofessional Care*, **8**, 1, 73–84.

Buchanan, J.M. (1969) *Cost and Choice: An Inquiry in Economic Theory*. Chicago: Markham.

Burke-Masters, B. (1988) 'A nurse practitioner in a centre for homeless people with alcohol problems', in Bowling, A. and Stilwell, S. (eds) *The Nurse in Family Practice. Practice Nurses and Nurse Practitioners in Primary Health Care*. London: Scutary Press.

Burrow, R. and Loader, B. (1994) *Towards a Post-Fordist Welfare State*. London: Routledge.

Burt, C. (1925) *The Young Delinquent*. London University Press.

Busfield, J. (1986) *Managing Madness*. London: Hutchinson.

Busfield, J. (1992) 'Gender and mental Illness'. *International Journal of Mental Health*, **1** (1–2), 46–66.

Butler, J.R. (1993) 'A case study in the NHS: working for patients', in Taylor-Gooby, P. and Lawson, R. (eds) *Markets and Managers: New Issues in the Delivery of Welfare*. Buckingham: Open University Press.

Butterworth, T. (1989) 'Giving and taking', *Nursing Times* 6 December.

Bytheway, B. (1982) *Street Care*, ARVAC Occasional Paper no. 5.

Bytheway, B. (1987a) 'Male carers: questions of intervention', in Twigg, J. (ed.) *Evaluating Support to Informal Carers*. University of York, Social Policy Research Unit, pp. 66–74.

Bytheway, B. (1987b) *Informal Care System*. Report to Joseph Rowntree Memorial Trust.

Bytheway, B. (1989) 'Poverty, care and age: a case study;, in Bytheway, B., Keil, T., Allatt, P. and Bryman, A (eds) *Becoming and Being Old*. London: Sage, pp. 93–103.

Calas, M.B. and Smircich, L. (1992) 'Re-writing gender into organizational theorizing: directions from feminist perspectives', in Reed, M. and Hughes, M. (eds) *Rethinking Organization: New Directions in Organization Theory and Analysis*. London: Sage.

Calder, A. (1971) *The People's War*. London: Panther.

Caldock, K. and Wenger, G.C. (1992), 'Health and Social Service provision for elderly people: the need for a rural model', in Gilg, A.W. Briggs, D., Dilley, R., Furuseth, O., and McDonald, G. (eds) *Progress in Rural Policy and Planning*, vol. 2. London, Belhaven.

Calnan, M. and Willliams, S. (1995) 'Challenges to professional autonomy in the United Kingdom? The perceptions of general practitioners', *International Journal of Health Services*, **25** (2), 219–41.

Cameron, E., Badger, F. and Evers, H. (1989a) 'District nursing, the disabled and the elderly: where are the black patients?', *Journal of Advanced Nursing*, **14**, 376–82.

Cameron, E., Evers, H., Badger, F. and Atkin, K. (1989b) 'Black old women, disability and health carers', in Jefferys, M. (ed.) *Growing Old in the Twentieth Century*. London: Routledge, pp. 230–48.

Campbell, B. (1993) *Goliath; Britain's Dangerous Places*. London: Methuen.

Campbell, B. (1995) 'Old fogeys and angry young men: a critique of communitarianism', *Soundings*, **1**, 47–65.

Carers National Association. (1992) *Speak Up, Speak Out: Research Amongst Members of the Carers National Association*. London: Carers National Association.

Carr-Hill, R. (1992) *Skill-Mix and the Effectiveness of Nursing Care*. University of York: Centre for Health Economics

Carrell, J. (1996) *Health Visitor*, **69** (June), 210–12.

Casey, J. (1992) *Improving Matters: A Guide to the Development, Management and Running of Home Improvement Agencies*. Nottingham: Care and Repair.

Central Statistical Office (1996) *Social Trends*, London: HMSO.

CETHV (1977) *An Investigation into the Principles of Health Visiting*. London: Council Education and Training of Health Visitors.

Challis, D., Darton, R., Johnson, L. Stone, M. and Traske, K. (1995) *Care Management and Health Care of Older People*. Aldershot, Arena.

Challis, D., Davies, B. (1986) *Case Management in Community Care*. Aldershot Gower.

Charity Commission (1994) *Political Activities and Campaigning by Charities*. London.

Charlesworth, A., Wilkin, D. and Durie, A. (1984) *Carers and Services: A Comparison of Men and Women Caring for Dependent Elderly People*. Manchester: Equal Opportunities Commission.

Chase, E. and Carr-Hill, R. (1994) 'The dangers of managerial perversion: quality assurance in primary health care', *Health Policy and Planning*, **9** (3), 267–78.

Cheetham, J. (1993) 'Social work and community care in the 1990s: pitfalls and potential', in Page, R. and Baldock, J. (eds) *Social Policy Review*, **5**, 155–76.

Chesler, P. (1972) *Women and Madness*. New York: Doubleday.

Child, J. (1969) *British Management Thought: A Critical Analysis*. London: Allen & Unwin.

Clarke, J. (ed.) (1993) *A Crisis in Care? Challenges to Social Work*. London: Sage.

Clarke, M. (1992) *'Summary' Long Term Care for Elderly People*. London: HMSO.

Clarke, S. J. G. (1996) *Social Work as Community Development: A Management Model for Social Change*. Aldershot: Avebury.

Clarke, J., Cochrane, A. and McLaughlin, E. (eds) (1994) *Managing Social Policy*. London: Sage.

Clements, L. (1995) 'Judgement Daze', Community Care, 13–19 July.

Common, R. and Flynn, N. (1992) *Contracting for Care*. York, Joseph Rowntree Foundation.

Clist, L. and Brant, S. (1986) A New Direction for CPN's. *Nursing Times* 1 January, 25–7.

Cockburn, C. (1990) 'Men's power in organizations: "equal opportunities" intervenes, in Hean, J. and Morgan, D. H. J. (eds) *Men, Masculinities and Social Theory*. London, Unwin Hyman.

Cockburn, C. (1991) *In the Way of women: Men's Resistance to Sex Equality in Organisations*. London. Macmillan.

Collinson, D.L., Knights, D. and Collinson, M. (1990) *Managing to Discriminate*. London: Routledge.

Colton, M., Drury, C., and Williams, M. (1995a) *Children in Need*. Aldershot: Avebury.

Colton, M., Drury, C., and Williams, M. (1995b) *Staying Together: Supporting Families Under the Children Act*. Aldershot: Avebury.

Common, R. and Flynn, J. (1992) *Contracting For Care*, York Joseph Rountree Foundation.

Conrad, P. and Schneider, J. (1980) *Deviance and Medicalization: from Baldness to Sickness*. St Louis: Mosby.

Coulter, A (1996) 'Impact on care has been only marginal', *News Review* (BMA), April 22–4.

Cox, D. (1991) 'Health service management – a sociological view: Griffiths and the non negotiated order of the hospital', in Gabe, J. Colnan, M. and Bury, M. (eds) *The Sociology of the Health Service*. London and New York: Routledge.

CPAG (1994) 'JSA White Paper: targeting the "workshy" and cutting benefit', *Welfare Rights Bulletin*, **123** (December) 7–10.

CPAG (1995) 'Incapacity benefit: the countdown begins', *Welfare Rights Bulletin*, **124** (February) 1995, 6–14.

Craig, G. and Glendinning, C. (1990) *Missing the Target* London: Barkingside.

Crane, M. (1993) *Elderly Homeless People Sleeping on the Streets in Inner London: An Exploratory Study*. London: Age Concern Institute of Gerontology.

Croft, S. and Beresford, P. (1990) *From Paternalism to Participation*. London: Open Services Project.

Crossman, R. (1969) *Paying for the Social Services*. London: Fabian Society.

Cruickshank, J., Beevers, D., Osbourne, V., Haynes, R., Corlett, J. and Selby, S. (1980) 'Heart attack, stroke, diabetes and hypertension in West Indians, Asians and whites in Birmingham, England', *British Medical Journal* **281**, (25) (October) 1108.

Culyer, G. (1992) *Economics, Medicine and Health Care*. Hemel Hempstead: Harvester/Wheatsheaf.

Daatland, S.O. (1983) 'Care systems', *Ageing and Society*, **3** (1), 1–21.

Dalley, G. (1988) *Ideologies of Caring: Rethinking Community and Collectivism*. London: Macmillan.

Davey, B. and Popay, J. (eds) (1993). *Dilemmas in Health Care*. Buckingham: Open University Press.

David, M. (1991) 'Putting on an act for children', in M. Maclean and D. Groves (eds) *Women's Issues in Social Policy*. London: Routledge.

Davidson, N. (1987) *A Question of Care: The Changing Face of the National Health Service*. London: Michael Joseph.

Davies, C. (1988) 'The Health Visitor as Mothers' Friend; a woman's place in public health 1900–14'. *Social History of Medicine*, **1** (1), 39–59.

Davies, A. (1994) *Is There A Case for A Care Corporation? The Voluntary Sector and Community Care*. London: Institute for Public Policy Research.

Davin, A. (1978) 'Imperialism and motherhood'. *History Workshop* **5**, 9–65.

Davin, A. (1996) *Growing Up Poor: Home, School and London 1870–1914*. London: Rivers Oram.

Davis Smith, J. (1995) 'The voluntary tradition', in Davis Smith, J. Rochester, C. and Hedley, R. (eds) *An Introduction to the Voluntary Sector*. London: Routledge.

Deakin, N. (1995) 'The perils of partnership: the voluntary secor and the state 1945–1992', in Davis Smith, J. Rochester, C. and Hedley, R. (eds) *An Introduction to the Voluntary Sector*. London: Routledge.

Dean, M. and Bolton, G. (1980) 'The administration of povertyand the development of nursing practice in nineteenth century England', in Davies, C. (ed.) *Re-Writing Nursing History*. London: Croom Helm.

Deming, W.E. (1982) *Out of the Crisis*, Cambridge Mass.: Cambridge University Press.

Dennis, N. (1968) 'The popularity of the neighbourhood community idea', in Pahl, R. (ed.) *Readings in Urban Sociology*. Oxford: Pergammon.

Dennis, N. and Erdos, G. (1993) *Families Without Fatherhood*. London: Institute of Economic Affairs Health and Welfare Unit.

Dennis, N., Henriques, F., Slaughter, C. (1969) *Coal is Our Life: an analysis of a Yorkshire mining community* London: Tavistock.

Department of Environment (1990) *Housing Investment Programme Statistics*. London: HMSO.

Department of Environment (1993) *English House Conditions Survey*, London: HMSO.

Department of Environment (1995) *Our Future Homes: Opportunity, Choice, Responsibility*, CMD. 2901, London: HMSO.

Department of Health (1986) *Neighbourhood Nursing S Focus for Care* Report of the Community Nursing Review (Chair J. Cumberlege) London: HMSO.

Department of Health (1988) *Report of the Inquiry into Child Abuse in Cleveland*, London: HMSO.

Department of Health (1989) *Caring for People: Community Care in the Next Decade and Beyond*, CMND 849, London: HMSO.

Department of Health (1989a) *Working For Patients*, CMND 555 London: HMSO.

Department of Health (1990) *Community Care in the Next Decade and Beyond: Policy Guidance*, London: HMSO.

Department of Health (1991a) *Review Body on Doctors and Dentists Remuneration* 1409, London: HMSO.

Department of Health (1991b) *Review Body on Nursing Staff, Midwives and Health Visitors*, Eighth Report 1410, London: HMSO.

Department of Health (1991c) *Implementing Community Care: Purchaser, Commissioner and Provider Roles*, London: HMSO.

Department of Health (1991d) *The Children Act 1989. Guidance and Regulations Volume 2. Family Support, Day Care and Educational Provision for Young Children*, London: HMSO.

Department of Health (1992) *The Health of the Nation: A Strategy for Health in England*, London: HMSO.

Department of Health (1993) *Targetting Practice: The Contribution of Nurses Midwives and Health Visitors*, London: HMSO.

Department of Health (1993) Social Services Inspectorate, *The Inspection of the Complaints Procedures in Local Authority Social Services Departments*, London: HMSO.

Department of Health (1994) *Implementing Caring for People: the Role of the GP and the Primary Health Care Team*, London: HMSO.

Department of Health (1994a) *Children Act Report 1993*, Cmnd 2584, London: HMSO.

Department of Health (1994b) *Social Service Inspectorate. National Inspection of Services to Disabled Children and their Families*, London: HMSO.

Department of Health (1995) *Partners in Caring: the Fourth Annual Report of the Chief Inspector of Social Services Inspectorate 1994/1995*, London: HMSO.

Department of Health (1995a) *Health and Personal Social Services Statistics for England 1995*, London: HMSO.

Department of Health (1995b) *Private Hospitals Homes and Clinics Registered under Section 23 of the Registered Homes Act 1984* Volume 1, London: HMSO.

Department of Health (1996) *Health of the Young Nation*, London: HMSO.

Department of Health and Social Security (1983) NHS Management Inquiry (Griffiths Report) London: HMSO.

Department of Health and Social Security (1985a) *A Review of Child Care Law*, London: HMSO.

Department of Health and Social Security (1985b) *Social Work Decisions in Child Care. Recent Research Findings and their Implications*, London: HMSO.

Department of Health and Social Security (1988) *Community Care: An Agenda for Action*, The Griffiths Community Care Report, London: HMSO.

Department of Health and Social Security (1995) *Social Security Statistics* 1995, London: HMSO.

Department of Health and Social Security/Scottish Home and Health Department/Welsh Office (1970) *Report of the Working Party on Management Structure in the Local Authority Nursing Services* (The Mayston Report) London: HMSO.

Department of Health and Social Security, Scottish Office, Welsh Office, Northern Ireland Office (1981) *Growing Older*, Cmnd. 8173, London: HMSO.

Department of Health and Social Services Inspectorate (1991) *Care Management and Assessment; Managers' Guide*, London: HMSO.

Department of Health and Social Services Inspectorate (1994) *National Inspection of Services to Disabled Children and Their Families*, London: HMSO.

Department of Health, Welsh Office, Scottish Office (1996) *Choice and Opportunity – The Future*, Cm. 3390, London: HMSO.

Derbyshire Coalition of Disabled People (1985) *Development of the Derbyshire Centre for Integrated Living*. Chesterfield.

Derbyshire Coalition of Disabled People (1989) *Heard About?* Chesterfield.

Dietrich, M. (1994) *Transaction Cost Economies and Beyond: Towards a New Economics of the Firm.* London: Routledge.

Dingwall, R. (1976) 'The social organisation of health visitor training, 3. Health Visiting as an Occupation', *Nursing Times*, **4**, 33–6.

Dingwall, R., Rafferty, A. and Webster, C. (1988) *An Introduction to the Social History of Nursing*. London: Routledge.

Disability Alliance (1991) *A Way Out of Poverty and Disability*. London.

Dixon, K. (1985) 'The Future of a Community Psychiatric Nurse. *CPNJ*. March/April, 30–3. an Identifiable Phlosophy, vol. 5, 2 30–3.

Dobson, R. (1995) 'Reasons to be cheerful: respite for black carers in Nottingham', *Community Care*, 8–14 June, 29.

Donaldson, L. (1986) 'Health and social status of elderly Asians: a community survey', *British Medical Journal* 293, 1079–84.

Donzelot, J. (1980) *The Policing of Families*. London: Hutchinson.

Dowling, W.C. (1973) 'The Missing Link', *Health Visitor*, **46** (10), 337–8.

Dowson, S. (1990) *Who Does What?* London Values Into Action Monograph.

Drake, R.F. (1992) 'A Little Brief authority?' A Sociological Analysis of Consumer Participation in Welsh Voluntary Agencies', PhD Thesis, University of Wales College of Cardiff.

Drake, R.F. (1994) 'The exclusion of disabled people from positions of power in British voluntary organisations', *Disability and Society*, **9**, (4) 461–80.

Drake, R. (1996) 'Charities, authority and disabled people: a qualitative study', *Disability and Society*, **11** (1), 5–23.

Drake, R.F. and Owens, D.J. (1992) 'Consumer involvement and the voluntary sector in Wales : Breakthrough or bandwagon?', *Critical Social Policy*, **33**, 76–86.

Dutt, R. (1990) *Black Community and Community Care*. London: Race Equality Unit, National Institute for Social Work.

Dyke, B. (1984) 'CPNs and primary health care attachment', *Nursing Times*, **80** (8), 55–7.

Ebrahim, S., Smith, C., Giggs, J. (1987) Elderly Immigrants – A Disadvantaged Group? *Age and Ageing*, 16, 4, 249–55.

Ebrahim, S., Patel, N., Coats, M., Greig, C., Gilley, J., Bangham, C. and Stacey, S. (1991) 'Prevalence and severity of morbidity among Gujerati Asian elders: a controlled comparison', *Family Practice*, 8 (1), 57–62.

Eldin, H.K. and Beheshti, H.M. (1981) *Management Science Applications: Computing and Systems Analysis*. New York: North Holland.

Ellis, K. (1993) *Squaring the Circle: User and Carer Participation in Needs Assessment*. York: Joseph Rowntree Foundation/Community Care.

Elston, M.A. (1991) 'The politics of professional power', in Gabe, J., Calnan, M. and Bury, M. (eds), *Medicine in a Changing Health Care Service*, The Sociology of the Health Service. London: Routledge.

Ehrenreich, D. and English, D. (1976) *Complaints and Disorders: The Sexual Politics of Sickness*. London: Writers and Readers Collective.

Enthoven, A. (1985) *Reflections on the Management of the NHS*. London: Nuffied Provincial Hospitals Trust.

EOC (1980) *The Experience of Caring for Elderly and Handicapped Dependants*. Manchester: Equal Opportunities Commission.

Ewles, L. and Simnett, I. (1985) *Promoting Health: a Practical Guide to Health Education*. Chichester: Wiley.

Family Policy Study Centre (1989) *Family Policy Bulletin*, 6. London.

Farnham, D. and Horton, S. (1993a) 'The political economy of public sector change', in Farnham, D. and Horton, S. (eds) (1993) *Managing the New Public Services*. London: Macmillan.

Fenton, S. (1986) *Race, Health and Welfare: Afro Caribbean and South Asian People in Central Bristol*. Department of Sociology: University of Bristol.

Fielding, N. and Gutch, R. (1989) *Contracting In or Out? The Legal Context*. London: National Council of Voluntary Organisations.

Finch, J. (1984) 'Community care – developing non-sexist alternatives', *Critical Social Policy*, **9**, 6–18.

Finch, J. and Groves, D. (1980) 'Community care and the family: a case for equal opportunities', *Journal of Social Policy*, **9** (4), 487–511.

Finch, J. and Groves, D. (eds) (1983) *A Labour of Love: Women, Work and Caring*. London: Routledge & Kegan Paul.

Finch, J. and Mason, J. (1990) 'Filial obligations and kin support for elderly people', *Ageing and Society*, **10** (2), 151–75.

Finch, J. and Mason, J. (1992) *Negotiating Family Responsibilities*. London: Routledge.

Fisher, M. (1994) 'Man-made care: community care and older male carers', *British Journal of Social Work*, **24**, 659–80.

Fletcher, D. (1996) 'New homes for "care in community" patients', *Daily Telegraph*, 21 February, p. 4.

Flynn, N. (1993) *Public Sector Management*. Hemel Hempstead: Harvester Wheatsheaf.

Flynn, N. (1994) 'Control, commitment and contracts', in Clarke, J. Cochrane, A. and McLaughlin, E. (eds) *Managing Social Policy*. London: Sage..

Ford, L. (1993) 'The Initiation, Implementation and Evaluation and the Future of the Nurse Practitioner (1965–1993). A Saga of Social Change', paper presented at the conference: Nurse Practitioners: the UK/USA Experience, London.

Foucault, M. (1967) *Madness and Civilization. A History of Insanity in the Age of Reason.* London: Tavistock Publication.

Foucault, M. (1973) *The Birth of the Clinic.* London: Allen Lane.

Foucault, M. (1980a) 'The eye of power', in Gordon, C. (ed.) *Power and Knowledge, Selected Interviews and Other Writings 1972–1977 by Michael Foucault,* Bughion Harvester Press.

Foucault, M. (1980b) *Power and Knowledge.* Brighton: Harvester Press.

Fox, N. (1993) *Post-Modernism Sociology and Health.* Buckingham: Open University Press.

Frean, A. (1995a) 'Pools firm cuts £8 millions charity aid to fight Lottery', *The Times,* 14 February, p. 5.

Frean, A. (1995b) 'Lottery blamed as cancer charity halts fundraiser', *The Times,* 30 March, p. 2.

Freidson, E. (1970a, 1988) *Profession of Medicine: A Study of the Sociology of Applied Knowledge.* New York: Harper & Row.

Freidson, E. (1970b) *Professional Dominance.* New York: Atherton.

Freire, P. (1972) *Cultural Action for Freedom.* London: Penguin.

French, J. and Raven, B. (1959) 'The bases of social power', in Cartwright, D. (ed.) *Studies in Social Power.* Ann Arbor: University of Michigan.

Frosh, S. (1989) *Psychoanalysis and Psychology: Minding the Gap.* London: Macmillan.

Fry, J. (1993) *Present State and Future Needs in General Practice,* 6th edn. Leicester, MTP Press.

Fryer, P. (1984) *Staying Power: The History of Black People in Britain.* London: Pluto Press.

Fyrth, J. (ed) (1995) *Labour's Promised Land?* London: Lawrence & Wishart.

Galbraith, J.K. (1989) 'Getting the poor off our minds', *Community Care* 23 February, pp. 26–9.

GARI (G. Alan Roeher Institute) (1991), *The Power to Choose.* North York Ontario G. Alan Roeher Institute 50–2.

Gibbon, B. and Luker, K. (1995) 'Uncharted Territory: Masters' Preparation as a Foundation for Nurse Clinicians', *Nurse Education Today,* **15**, 164–9.

Gilbert, J. (1988) 'Excellence in ethnic elderly care', *Social Work Today,* **19** (23), 18–19.

Gilligan, C. (1982) *In a Different Voice: Psychological Theory and Women's Development.* Cambridge, Massachusetts, Harvard University Press.

Gilmore, M., Bruce, N. and Hunt, M. (1974) *The Work of the Nursing Team in General Practice.* London: Council for the Education and Training of Health Visitors.

Gittins, D. (1985) *The Family in Question.* London: Macmillan.

Glazer, N. (1974) *Schools of the Minor Professions.* London: Minerva.

Glendinning, C. (1988) 'Dependency and interdependency: the incomes of informal carers and the impact of social security', in Baldwin, S., Parker, G., and Walker, R. (eds) *Social Security and Community Care.* Aldershot: Avebury.

Glendinning, C. and Millar, J. (eds) (1992) *Women and Poverty in Britain in the 1990s.* Wheatsheaf.

Glennerster, H., Matsaganis, M., Ownes, P., Hancock, S. (1994) *Implementing GP Fundholding: Wild Card or Winning Hand?* Buckingham: Open University Press.

Glennerster, H. and Midgley, J. (eds) (1991) *The Radical Right and the Welfare State: An International Assessment.* Hemel Hempstead: Harvester Wheatsheaf.

Goldberg, D. and Huxley, P. (1980) *Mental Illness in the Community. The Pathway to Psychiatric Care.* Tavistock: London.

Goodman, A. and Webb, S. (1994) *UK Income Distribution 19761–1991,* Social Policy research 50, York: Joseph Rowntree Foundation.

Goodwin, S. (1992) 'Community nursing and the new public health', *Health Visitor,* **65** (3), 78–80.

Gordon, I. (1991) 'Consumer voice growing in Wales', *Openmind,* **49**, 7.

Gordon, L. (1989) *Heroes of Their Own Lives*. London: Virago.

Gott, M. and O'Brien, M. (1990) *The Role of the Nurse in Health Promotion Policies, Perspectives and Practice*. Report of a two year project funded by the Department of Health, London.

Graham, H. (1983) 'A labour of love', in Finch, J., and Groves, D. (eds) *A Labour of Love: Women Work and Caring*. London: Routledge & Kegan Paul.

Gramsci, A. (1971) *Selections from the Prison Notebooks*. London: Lawrence & Wishart.

Grant, L. (1995) *Disability and Debt: The Experience of Disabled People in Debt*. Sheffield Citizens Advice Bureau, Debt Support Unit.

Grant, L. (1995) 'Journey's end: the support needs of black parents', *Community Care* 6–12 July, pp. 26–7.

Greater Manchester Coalition of Disabled People (1989) *Policy and Declaration of Intent*. Manchester.

Green, H. (1988) *General Household Survey 1985: Informal Carers* (seri. GH5, no. 15, suppl. A). London: HMSO.

Green, A. and Barker, C. (1988) 'Priority setting and economic appraisal. Whose priorities, the community or the economist?' *Social Science and Medicine*, **26** (9), 919–29.

Gregg, P. and Wadsworth, J. (1994) *More Work in Fewer Households*, Social Policy Research 61, York Joseph Rowntree Foundation.

Griffiths, Sir R. (1988) *Community Care: Agenda for Action*. London: HMSO.

Grosz, E.A. (1988a) 'In(ter)vention of feminist knowledges', in Caine, B. Grosz, E.A. and De Lepervanche, M. *Crossing Boundaries: Feminisms and the Critique of Knowledges*. Sydney: Allen and Unwin.

Grundy, E. (1993) 'Moves into supported private households among elderly people in England and Wales', *Environment and Planning*, A, 25.

Gubrium, Jaber, F. (1986) *Oldtimers and Alzheimers: The Descriptive Organisation of Senility*. Greenwich, Connecticut: JAI Press.

Gutch, R. (1989) *The Contract Culture: The Challenge for Voluntary Organisations*. London: National Council for Voluntary Organisations.

Hajioff, S. (1996) 'Founding principles of the NHS have gone', *British Medical Association News Review*, 224, 35.

Hall, D.M.B. (1996) *Health for All Children*, 3rd edn. Oxford Medical Publications.

Halsey, A.H. (ed.) (1988) *British Social Trends Since 1900: A Guide to the Changing Structure of Britain*. Macmillan: London.

Hammer, M. (1995) *Re-engineering the Corporation: a manifesto for business revolution*, London: Brierly, Hammer & Champy.

Hamnett, C. (1991) 'A nation of inheritors Housing inheritance wealth and inequality in Britain', *Journal of Social Policy* 20, 2, 509–36.

Hancock, C. (1996) 'Medical staff face extra pressure', *BMA News Review*, April p. 35.

Handy, C. (1976) *Understanding Organisations*. Harmondsworth: Penguin.

Handy, C. (1988) *Understanding Voluntary Organisations*. Harmondsworth: Penguin.

Hannay, D.R. (1980) 'Problems of role identification and confict in multi-disciplinary teams', in Barber, J. and Kratz, C. (eds) *Towards Team Care*. Edinburgh: Churchill Livingstone.

Hardiker, P., Exton, K. and Barker, M. (1991) 'The social policy contexts of prevention in child care', *British Journal of Social Work*, **21** (4), August, 341–60.

Harding, S. and Balarajan, R. (1996) 'Patterns of mortality in second generation Irish living in England and Wales: a longitudinal study', *British Medical Journal*, **7034**, 312, 1389–93.

Harrison, L. and Means, R. (1990) *Housing: The Essential Element in Community Care*. Oxford: Anchor Housing Trust.

Harrison S. Hunter D. Pollitt C. (1990) *The Dynamics of British Health Policy*: London: Unwin Hyman.

Harrison, S. and Pollitt, C. (1994) *Controlling Health Professionals: The Future of Work and Organisation in the NHS*. Buckingham: Philadelphia: Open University Press.

Haskey, J. (1996) 'Mortality among second generation Irish in England and Wales', *British Medical Journal*, **7043**, 312, 1373–1374.

Hasler, F. (1993) 'Developments in the disabled people's movement', in Swain, J., Finkelstein, V., French, S. and Oliver, M. (eds) *Disabling Barriers – Enabling Environments*. London: Sage.

Haycox, A. (1995) *The Costs and Benefits of Community Care*. Aldershot: Avebury.

Hayek, F. (1943) *The Roads to Serfdom*. London: Routledge, Kegan Paul.

Health Visitor (1996) 'Insurers to reap "bonanza"', *Health Visitor*, **69** (5). p. 163.

Hearn, J. and Parkin, W. (1986) *'Sex' at 'Work': The Power and Paradox of Organisation Sexuality*. Brighton: Wheatsheaf.

Hearn, J. (1992) *Men in the Public Eye*. London: Routledge.

Hearn, J. and Morgan, D.H.J. (eds) (1990) *Men, Masculinities and Social Theory*. London: Unwin Hyman.

Hedley, R. and Davey Smith, J. (1992) *Volunteering and Society: Principles and Practice*. London: Bedford Square Press.

Helt, E. and Jellinek, R.C. (1988) 'In the wake of cost cutting, nursing productivity and quality improve', *Nursing Management*, **19** (6), 36–48.

Henderson, P. and Thomas, D.N. (1987) *Skills in Neighbourhood Work*, 2nd edn. London: Allen and Unwin.

Henessy, D.A. (1994) *Changes in Primary Health Care: clinical education*, Oxford: Oxford Health Care Management Institute, Templeton College Oxford.

Henley, A. (1983) *Asians in Britain* (3 volumes). Cambridge: Health Education Council and National Extension College.

Henwood, M. (1995) 'Strained Relations'. *Health Service Journal*, 6 July.

Henwood, M. and Wicks, M. (1984) *Forgotten Army: Family Care and Elderly People*. London: Family Policy Study Centre.

Hevey, D. (1992) *The Creatures Time Forgot*. London: Routledge.

Hills, J. (1990) *The State of Welfare*. Oxford University Press.

Hinshelwood, R. (1991) *A Dictionary of Lenian Thought*. London: Free Association Books.

HMSO (1904) *Report of the Inter-Departmental Committee on Physical Deterioration*, Cmnd. 2175, London: HMSO.

HMSO (1906) *Report of Inter-Departmental Committee on Medical Inspection and Feeding of Children attending Elementary Schools* Cmnd. 2779, London: HMSO.

HMSO (1942) *Social Insurance and Allied Services: Report by Sir William Beveridge*, Cmnd 6404, London: HMSO.

HMSO (1976) Report of the Committee on Child Health Services (1976) *Fit For The Future* (The Court Report) Cmnd. 6684/6684/1, London: HMSO.

HMSO (1978) Report of the Committee of Inquiry into the Education of Handicapped Children and Young People, *Special Educational Needs* (The Warnock report) CMD. 7212, London: HMSO.

HMSO (1989) *Report of the Advisory Group on Nurse Prescribing* (The Crown Report) London: HMSO.

HMSO. (1994) *Civil Rights Disabled Persons Bill*. [Bill 91]. London, HMSO.

HMSO (1995) Report of the Standing Nursing and Midwifery Advisory Committee, *Making It Happen*, London: HMSO.

Hofstede, G. (1994). 'Is there a science of management?', *Management Science*, **40** (1), 4–13.

Hoggart, R. (1957) *The Uses of Literacy*. Harmondsworth: Penguin.

Hoggett, P. (1990) *Modernisation, Political Strategy and the Welfare State: An Organizational Perspective*, Studies in Decentralisation and Quasi-markets, no. 2. Britistol, University of Bristol, SAUS.

Hogreffe, P. (1975) *Tudor Women Commoners and Queens*. Tower State University.

Holman, B. (1988) *Putting Families First: Prevention and Child Care*. London: Macmillan.

Home Office, Department of Health, Department of Education and Science and Welsh Office. (1991) *Working Together Under the Children Act 1989: A Guide to Arrangements for Inter-agency Cooperation for the Protection of Children from Abuse.* London: HMSO.

Honigsbaum, F. (1979) *The Division in British Medicine: A History of the Separation of General Practice from Hospital Care.* London: Kogan Page.

Houghton, P. and Allen, G. (1990) *The Fifth Estate.* Birmingham: European Society of Associations Executives.

House of Commons (1987) *The Law on Child Care and Family Services,* London: HMSO.

House of Commons Health Committee (1993), *Third Report Community Care Funding April 1993.* London: HMSO.

House of Commons (1994) *Civil Rights Disabled Persons (Bill)* Bill 91, London: HMSO.

House of Commons (1995), *Carers (Recognition and Services) Bill* Parliamentary Papers 422–478. London: HMSO.

House of Commons Health Committee (1992) *Maternity Services* Volume 1 (Chair Nicholas Winterton) London: HMSO.

House of Commons Social Services Commission (1984) Second Report *Children in Care,* London: HMSO.

House of Commons Social Service Committee (1990a) *Community Care: Choice for Service Users,* London: HMSO.

House of Commons Social Service Committee (1990b) Eleventh Report *Community Care; Services for People with a Mental Handicap and People with a Mental Illness,* London: HMSO.

Howkins, E. (1995) 'The Political Imperatives in Community Nursing', in Cain, P., Hyde, V. and Howkins, E. (eds) *Community Nursing: Dimensions and Dilemmas.* London: Arnold.

Hoyles, L., Lard, R., Means, R. and Taylor, M. (1994) *Community Care in Transition.* York: Joseph Rowntree Foundation/Community Care.

Hughes, S. (1996) 'Doctors have been forced to be clerks', *BMA News Review,* April, 32–4.

Hugill, B. (1996) 'Breadline Britain', *Observer,* 11 August, p. 18. *Independent,* 7 August, p. 2.

Hunt G. and Wainwright P. (Eds.) (1994) *Expanding The Role of The Nurse.* Oxford: Blackwell Scientific Publications

Hunt, S. and Symonds, A. (1995) *The Social Meaning of Midwifery.* London: Macmillan.

Hunter, D. (1991) 'Managing Medicine. A Response to Crisis'. *Social Science and Medicine* 32.44.8. Vol 32, p. 441–9.

Hunter, D.J. (1994) 'From Tribalism to Corporatism: The Managerial Challenge to Medical Dominance', in Gabe, J., Kelleher, D. and Williams, G. *Challenging Medicine.* London: Routledge.

Husband, C. (1996) 'Defining and containing diversity: community, ethnicity and citizenship', in Ahmad, W. I U. and Atkin, K. (eds) *Race and Community Care.* Buckingham: Open University Press, pp. 29–48.

Hutton, W. (1995) *The State We're In.* London: Jonathan Cape.

HVA/UKSC (1992) *The Principles of Health Visiting: A Re-evaluation.* London: Health Visitors' Association.

HVA/UKSC (1994) *Action for Health.* London: HVA.

Iganski, P. (1992) 'Inequality Street'. *Health Service Journal,* 20 February, 26–7.

Ignatieff, M. (1991) 'Citizenship and moral narcissism', in Andrews, G. (ed.) *Citizenship.* London: Lawrence & Wishart.

Illich, I. (1976) *Limits to Medicine.* London: Marion Boyars.

Illich, I. (1977) 'Disabling professions', in Illich, I., Zola, I.K., McKnight, J., Caplan, J. and Sharkin, H. (eds), *Disabling Professions.* London: Marion Boyars.

Illing, J., Drinkwater, C., Rogerson, T., Forester, D. and Rutherford, P. (1991) 'Evaluation of community psychiatric nursing in general practice', in Booker, C. (ed.) *Community Psychiatric Nursing. A Research Perspective.* London: Chapman & Hall.

Independent (1996a), 12 October.

Independent (1996b), 7 March.

Jackson, H. and Field, S. (1989) *Race, Community Groups and Service Delivery*, Home Office Research Study no. 113. London: HMSO.

Jadeja, S. and Singh, J. (1993) 'Life in a cold climate', *Community Care*, April, 12–13.

Jerrome, D. (1996) 'Continuity and change in the study of family relationships', *Ageing and Society*, **16** (1), 93–104.

Johnson, T.J. (1972) *Professions and Power*. London: Macmillan.

Johnson, N. (1990) *Restructuring the Welfare State: A Decade of Change*. London: Harvester Wheatsheaf.

Johnson, J. (1994) 'Social responses to need', *an Ageing Society* (Unit 10). Milton Keynes: Open University.

Johnson, J. (1996) 'Reforms have turned the NHS into a sweat-shop', *BMA News Review* April.

Jones, D. A. (1986a) *A Study of the Ogwr Hospital Discharge Scheme*. Cardiff: Research Team for the Care of the Elderly.

Jones, D. A. (1986b) *A Survey of Carers of Elderly Dependants Living in the Community*. Cardiff: Research Team for the Care of the Elderly.

Jones, H. (1994) *Health and Society in Twentieth Century Britain*. London: Longman.

Jones, J. (1993) 'GP Fundholding System "Should be Phased Out"', *Guardian*, 30 Sept. p. 12.

Jones, J. and Tilson, J. (eds) (1991) *Roots and Branches*. Buckingham: Open University.

Jordan, B. (1995) 'Are New Right Policies Sustainable? Back to Basics and Public Choice', *Journal of Social Policy*, **24** *(3)*, 363–84.

Jordan, B. and Arnold, J. (1996) 'Poverty' M. Drakeford and M. Vanstone (eds), *Beyond Offending Behaviour*, Aldershot: Arena.

Joseph, K. (1976) *Stranded on the Middle Ground* London: Centre for Policies Studies.

Juran, J. M. (1988) *Juran on Planning for Quality*, New York: Free Press.

Keegan, W. J. Moriarty, S., Duncan, T. (1995) *Marketing* London: Prentice-Hall.

Keigher, S. M. (1991) *Housing Risks and Homelessness Among the Urban Elderly* New York: Haworth.

Keith, L. (1990) 'Caring Partnership', *Community Care*, 22 February.

Keith, L. and Morris, J. (1995) 'Easy targets: a disability rights perspective on the "children as carers" debate', *Critical Social Policy*, issue 44/45.

Kelly, A. (1996) 'The concept of the specialist community nurse', *Journal of Advanced Nursing*, **24**, 42–52.

Kelvin, P. (1969) *The Bases of Social Power*. Aylesbury, Holt, Rinehart & Winston.

Kempson, E. (1996) *Life On A Low Income*. York: Joseph Rowntree Foundation.

Kingdom, J. (1992) *No Such Thing as Society? Individualism and Community*. Buckingham: Philadelphia: Open University Press.

Kitwood, T. (1990) 'The Dialectics of Dementia: With Particular Reference to Alzheimer's Disease', *Ageing and Society*, **10** (2), 177–96.

Klein, R. (1989) *The Politics of the NHS*, 2nd edn. London: Longman.

Kohlberg, L. (1976) Moral stages and moralization: The cognitive developmental approach, in T. Lickona (ed.) *Moral Development and Behaviour: Theory, research and social issues*. New York: Holt, Rinehart & Winston.

Kohlberg, L. (1978) 'Revisions in the theory and practice of moral development', in W. Damon (ed.), *Moral Development New directions For Child Development* 2, 83–8.

Kratz, C. (1980) 'Other members of the primary health care team', in Barber, J. and Kratz, C. (eds) *Towards Team Care*. Edinburgh: Churchill Livingstone.

Kuhn, T.S. (1970) *The Structure of Scientific Revolutions*. Chicago University Press.

Kumar, K. (1978) *Prophecy and Progress*. Harmondsworth: Penguin.

Kunz, C., Jones, R. and Spencer, K. (1989) *Bidding for Change?* Birmingham Settlement and the Community Development Foundation.

Labour Party (1996) *Early Excellence*, Paper 111696, Labour Party London.

Laing, R.D. (1971) *The Politics of the Family and Other Essays*. London: Tavistock.

Lamb, A. (1976) *Primary Health Care Nursing.* London: Ballière Tindall.

Land, H. and Rose, H. (1985) 'Compulsory altruism for some or an altruistic society for all', in Bean, P., Ferris, J. and Whynes, D. (eds) *In Defence of Welfare.* London: Tavistock.

Langley, J. (1976) *Always a Layman* Brighton: Queenspark Books.

Laslett, P. (1989) *A Fresh Map: the Emergence of the Third Age.* London: Weidenfeld & Nicolson.

Le Grand, J. and Robinson, R. (eds) (1984) *Privatisation and the Welfare State.* London: Allen & Unwin.

Leat, D. (1995) 'Funding Matters', Davis Smith, J. *et al.* eds. op. cit.

Leat, D., Smolka, G. and Unell, J. (1981) *Voluntary and Statutory Collaboration: Rhetoric or Reality?* London: Bedford Square Press.

Lee-Potter, J. (1996) 'Reforms have turned off NHS altruism', *BMA News Review*, April, p. 22–24.

Le Grand J. and Bartlett W. (1993), *Quasi-Markets and Social Policy.* London: Macmillan.

Leopoldt, H. (1979) 'Community Psychiatric Nursing', *Nursing Times*, **75** (13), 53–6.

Lewis, J. (1980) *The Politics of Motherhood. Child and Maternal Welfare in England 1900–1939*, London: Croom Helm.

Lewis, J. (1988) *Daughters Who Care.* London: Routledge.

Lewis, J. (1993) 'The Boundary Between Voluntary and Statutory Social Service in the Late Nineteenth and Early Twentieth Century', unpublished paper presented to the Voluntary Action History Society, quoted in Davis Smith, J., Rochester, C. and Hedley, R. (eds) *An Introduction to the voluntary Sector*, London: Routledge, P. 23.

Lewis, J. and Glennerster, H. (1996) *Implementing the New Community Care.* Milton Keynes: Open University.

Lieberman, A. and Au, S. (1988) 'Catering for a minority', *Community Care*, 10 November, 737, 20–2.

Lilley, P. (1993) *Mais Lecture*, 23 June Lava, City University Business School, reported in Financial Times 20 July 1993

Lister, R. (1975) *Social Security.* London: CPAG Poverty Pamphlet.

Lister, R. (1991) 'Women, economic dependency and citizenship', *Journal of Social Policy*, **19** (4), 445–67.

Littlewood, R. and Lipsedge, M. (1982) *Aliens and Alienists: Ethnic Minorities and Psychiatry.* Harmondsworth: Penguin.

Laughlin, M. (1994) 'The poverty of management', *Health Care Analysis*, **2**, 135–9.

Low Pay Unit (1995) *The New Review*, 36, 8.

Lowe, R. (1993) *The Welfare State in Britain Since 1945.* London: Macmillan.

Lund, B. (1996) *Housing Problems and Housing Policy.* London: Longman.

Lynes, T. (1994) 'In sickness and in poverty', *Poverty*, **89**, 10–12.

Mabbott, J. (1992) *Local Authority Funding for Voluntary Organisations.* London: National Council of Voluntary Organisations.

MacAdam, E. (1934) *The New Philanthropy.* London: Allen & Unwin.

Macara, S. (1996) 'Reforms have led to NHS staff despair', *BMA News Review*, April, p.35.

McCalman, J.A. (1990) *The Forgotten People – Carers in Three Minority Ethnic Communities in Southwark.* London: King's Fund Centre/Help the Aged.

McClelland, A. (1996) 'Working girls and working women', *Health Visitor Journal*, **69**, (7), 265–68.

MacDonald, J.J. (1993) *Primary Health Care: Medicine in its Place.* London: Earthscan.

McGonigle, G. and Kirby, J. (1936) *Poverty and Public Health.* London: Gollancz.

McGrath, M. (1989) 'Consumer participation in service planning: the AWS experience', *Journal of Social Policy*, 16, 1, 67–89.

McIver, S. (1991) *Obtaining the Views of Users of Mental Health Services.* London: King's Fund Centre.

McKeigue, P. (1991) 'Patterns of health and disease in the elderly of minority ethnic groups', in Squires, A.J. (ed.) *Multicultural Health Care and Rehabilitation.* London: Edward Arnold, 69–77.

MacKenzie, N. and Mackenzie, J. (1979) *The First Fabians*. London: Quartet.

McKenzie, C., Torkelson, N. and Holt, M. (1989) 'Care and cost: nursing care management improves both', *Nursing Management*, **20** (10), 30–4.

McKinley, J.B. and Arches, J. (1985) 'Towards the proletarianisation of physicians', *International Journal of Health Services*, 5, 2, 161–195

McKeown, T. (1976) *The Role of Medicine: dream mirage or nemesis?* London: Nuffield Provincial Hospitals Trust.

McMahon, R., Barton, E. and Piot, M. (1980) *On Being in Charge: A Guide for Middle-Level Management in Primary Health Care*. Geneva: WHO.

Macmillan, H. (1933) *Reconstruction – A Plan For National Policy*. London: Macmillan.

McMurray, A. (1990) *Community Health Visiting*. Edinburgh: Churchill-Livingstone.

McNaught, A. (1988) *Race and Health Policy*. London: Croom Helm.

Malik, K. (1996) 'We've forgotten equality', *Independent on Sunday*, 23 June, p. 21.

Mann, K. (1992) *The Making of the English 'Underclass'?*, Milton Keynes: Open University.

Mares, P., Henley, A and Baxter, C. (1985) *Health Care in Multiracial Britain*. Cambridge, Health Education Council and National Extension College.

Marshall, T. H. (1950) *Citizenship and Social Class and Other Essays*, Cambridge: Cambridge University Press.

Martin, C. (1994) 'Nurses' role in family health services authorities', *British Journal of Nursing*, 3 (6), 278–82.

Martin, J. and Roberts, C. (1984) *Women and Employment: A Lifetime Perspective*. London: HMSO.

Marwick, A. (1964) 'Middle opinion in the thirties; planning progress and political agreement', *Economic History Review*, April, 285–98.

Marx, K. and Engels, F. (1970) *The German Ideology*. London: Lawrence & Wishart.

Mason, S. and Taylor, R. (1990) *Tackling Deprivation in Rural Areas*. Cirencester: Action with Communities in Rural England (ACRE).

Mayo, M. (1994) *Communities and Caring: The Mixed Economy of Welfare*. London: Macmillan.

Meredith, B. (1993) *The Community Care Handbook*. London: Age Concern England.

Metcalfe, D. (1992) 'The chains of education, experience and culture', *British Medical Journal* **305**, 33–4.

Midgley, J. (1995) *Social Development: The Developmental Perspective in Social Welfare*. London: Sage.

Midwinter, E. (1991) 'The Pensions System: A Hideous Dichotomy' *Community Care*, 16.5.91, 24.

Millar, J. (1995) 'Poor Mothers and Absent Fathers: Support for Lone Parents in Comparative Perspective', paper at Annual Conference of Social Policy Association, University of Liverpool.

Miller, B. (1995), 'Heaviness in the air, *Health Service Journal*', **105**, p 16.

Mills, A.J. and Murgatroyd, S.J. (1991) *Organizational Rules*. Milton Keynes, Open University Press.

MIND (1996) *Increase in Mental Distress and Depression*, Report 21, March, London: MIND.

Ministry of Health (1924) *Maternal Mortality* (by Campbell, J. N.) Report on Public Health and Medical Subjects, 25, London: HMSO.

Ministry of Health (1937) *Report on an Investigation into Maternal Mortality*, Cmnd 5422, London: HMSO.

Ministry of Health, Department of Health Scotland and Department of Education (1956) *An Inquiry into Health Visiting: Report of the Working Party on the Fieldwork Training and Recruiment of Health Visitors* (The Jameson Report) London: HMSO.

Ministry of Health, Scottish Home and Health Department (1966) *Report of the Committee on Senior Nursing, Staff Structure* (Chair B. Salmon) London: HMSO.

Mintzberg, H. (1973) *The Nature of Mangerial Work*, New York and London: Harper & Row.

Mocroft, I. and Thomason, C. (1993) 'The evolution of Community Care and voluntary organisations', in Saxon-Harrold, S. and Kendall, J. (eds) *Researching the Voluntary Sector*. Tonbridge: Charities Aid Foundation.

Modood, T. (1991) 'The Indian economic success: a challenge to some race relations assumptions', *Policy and Politics*, **19** (3), 177–89.

Mohan, J. and Woods, K. (1985) 'Restructuring health care: the social geography of public and private Health care under the British Conservative government', *International Journal of Health Services*, **15** (2), 197–216.

Monks, J. (1996a) 'Political Expediency Supplements Real Need', *BMA News Review*, April, p. 34.

Monks, J. (1996b) 'Staff morale is at an all-time low', *BMA News Review* April, p. 36.

Moody, H. (1992) *Ethics in an Ageing Society*, Baltimore/London: Johns Hopkins University.

Mooney, G. (1994) *Key Issues in Health Economics*. Hemel Hempstead: Harvester Wheatsheaf.

Monkley-Poole, S. (1995) 'The attitudes of British fundholding general practitioners to community psychiatric nursing services', *Journal of Advanced Nursing*, **21**, 238–47.

Morall, P. (1989) 'The professionalisation of the CPN: a review, *CPNJ*, July/August, Vol 9, 4, 14–22.

Morgan, C. and Murgatroyd, S. (1994) *Total Quality Management in the Public Sector*, Buckingham: Open University Press.

Morris, J. (1991) *Pride Against Prejudice*. London: Women's Press

Morris, L. (1994) *Dangerous Classes: The Underclass and Social citizenship*. London: Routledge.

Mowat, C. (1955) *Britain between The Wars*. London: Methuen.

Mulkay, M. (1991) *Sociology of Science: A Sociological Pilgrimage*. Milton Keynes: Open University Press.

Mumford, L. (1945) 'On the future of London'. *Architectural Review*, **97** (577), 3–10.

Murray, C. (1990) *The Emerging British Underclass*. London Institute of Economic Affairs.

Murray, R. (1989) 'Fordism and post-Fordism', in Hall, S. and Jacques, M. (eds) *New Times*. London: Lawrence & Wishart.

Nanton, P. (1992) 'Official statistics and the problem of inappropriate ethnic categorisation', *Policy and Politics*, **20** (4), 277–68.

Nash, W. (1985) *Health at School*. London: Heinemann Nursing.

National Association Citizens Advice Bureaux (1991) *Barriers to benefit: black claimants and social policy*, London: NACAB.

National Association of Probation Officers (1993) 'Probation Caseload: income and employment', *NAPO NEWS* 52, 8–10.

National Council of Voluntary Organisations (1980) *Beyond the Welfare State?* London.

National Health Service Management Executive (1992a) *The Nursing Skill Mix in the District Nursing Service Value for Money Report*, London: HMSO.

National Health Services Management Executive (1992b) *Extension of the Hospital and Community Health Services, Elements of the GP Fundholding Scheme from April 1 1993 Supplementary G Inspectorate*.

National Health Service Management Executive (1992c) *Local Voices. The Views of Local People in Purchasing for Health*, London: NHSME.

National Health Service Executive (1996) *Primary Care – The Future*, Crown Copyright NHSE, London

Naughton, B. (1993) 'The Marketing Imperative', *Nursing Times*, **89** (19), 52–3.

Navarro, V. (1978) *Class Struggle, the State and Medicine*. London: Martin Robertson.

Navarro, V. (1984) 'A critique of the ideological and political positions of the Willy Brandt Report and the WHO Alma Ata Declaration', *Social Sciences and Medicine*, **18**, 467–74.

Nettleton, S. (1995) *The Sociology of Health and Illness*. Cambridge: Polity Press.

Nettleton, S. and Bunton, R. 1995) Sociological critiques of health promotion', in Bunton, R. Nettleton, S. and Burrows, R. (eds) *The Sociology of Health Promotion*. London: Routledge.

Newby, H. (1977) *The Deferential Worker.* Harmondsworth: Penguin.

Newman, J. and Clarke, J. (1994) 'Going about our business? The managerialization of public services', in Clarke, J. Cochrane, A. and McLaughlin, E. (eds) *Managing Social Policy.* London: Sage.

Niskanen, W. A. (1971) *Bureaucracy and Representative Government.* Chicago, Aldine-Atherton.

Nissel, M. and Bonnerjea, I. (1982) *Family Care of the Handicapped Elderly: Who Pays?* London: Policy Studies Institute.

Norman, A. J. (1987) *Rights and Risks. A Discussion on Civil Liberty in Old Age.* London: Centre for Policy on Ageing.

Northern Ireland Council for Voluntary Action (1987) *Reaching for the End of the Rainbow.* Belfast.

Northumbria Probation Services (1994) *Survey of Probation Practice on Poverty Issues.* Northumbria.

Office of Population Censuses and Surveys (1990) *Key Population and Vital Statistics, Local and Health Authority Area Estimates at mid-1988* London: HMSO.

Office of Population Censuses and Surveys (1993) *1991 Census Housing and Availability of Cars,* London: HMSO.

Oakley, A., Hickey, D., and Rigby, A.S. (1994) 'Love or money? social support, class inequality and the health of women and children', *Journal of Public Health,* **4**, 265–73.

Oakley, A. (1984) *The Captured Womb: A History of the Medical Care of Pregnant Women.* Oxford: Blackwell.

Observer (1996), 11 August.

Office for National Statistics (1996) *Ethnicity in the 1991 census volume 2 –The ethnic minority population of Great Britain,* London: HMSO

Ogbu, J. (1978) *Minority Education and Caste.* New York: Academic Press.

Oliver, M. (1990) *The Politics of Disablement.* London: Macmillan.

Oliver M. (1990) *The Politics of Disablement.* London: Macmillan.

Open University Health Education Unit (1991) *Community Development and Health Education.* Milton Keynes: Open University.

Opit, L. (1993) 'Commissioning: an appraisal of a new role', in Tilley, I (ed.) *Managing the Internal Market.* London: Paul Chapman.

Oppenheim, C. (1993) *Poverty: The Facts,* London: Child Poverty Action Group.

Oppenheim C. (1994) *The Welfare State: Putting the Record Straight.* London: CPAG.

Øvretveit, J. (1992) *Health Services Quality.* Oxford: Blackwell Science.

Owen, G. (1983) *Health Visiting.* London: Ballière-Tindall.

Packman, J. and Jordan, B. (1991) 'The children act: looking forward, looking back', *British Journal of Social Work,* 21 (4), **315–28**.

Pahl, R. (1965) *Urbs in Rure.* London: Weidenfeld & Nicolson.

Parker, G. (1992) 'Counting care: numbers and types of informal carers', in Twigg, J. (ed.) *Carers: Research and Practice.* London: HMSO.

Parker, G. (1993) *With This Body.* Buckingham: Open University Press.

Pascall, G. (1986) *Social Policy: A Feminist Analysis.* London: Routledge.

Payne, J. (1984) *Making Partnerships Work: A Case Study of the Implementation of a Joint Funding Pilot Partnership Policy,* Working Paper 34. Bristol: School of Advanced Urban Studies.

Pearce I and Crocker, L. (1943) *The Peckham Experiment.* London: George Allen & Unwin.

Pearson, A., Punton, S. and Durant, I. (1987) *Nursing Beds: An Evaluation of the Effects of Therapeutic Nursing.* Harrow: Scutari Press.

Pearson D., Heathcote, E. and Hodgson, A. (1992) *Growing Old in the Countryside.* London: Help the Aged.

Peck, E. and Smith, H. (1989) 'Safeguarding Service Users', *Health Science Journal,* 7.12.89 1502–4

Pember-Reeves, M. (1979) *Round-About A Pound A Week.* London: Virago.

Peters, T. (1988) *Thriving on Chaos:handbook for a management revolution,* London: Macmillan.

Pharaoh, C. (1995) *Primary Health Care for Elderly People from Black and Minority Ethnic Communities.* London: HMSO.

Pharaoh, C. and Redmond, E. (1991) 'Care for ethnic elders', *Health Service Journal,* 101 (5252), 20–22.

Phillipson, C. (1982) *Capitalism and the Construction of Old Age.* London: Macmillan.

Pilgrim, D. and Rogers, A. (1993) *A Sociology of Mental Health and Illness.* Milton Keynes: Open University.

Plant, R. (1990) 'Citizenship and rights 'in Plant, R. and Barry, N. (eds.) *Citizenship and Rights in Thatcher's Britain: Two Views.* London: IEA Health and Welfare Unit.

Pollitt C. (1990) *Managerialism and the Public Services.* Oxford: Blackwell.

Pollitt C. (1993) 'The struggle for quality: the case of the national health service', *Policy and Politics,* **21**(3), 161–70.

Polanyi, K. (1945) *Origins or Our Time: the great transformation,* London: Gollancz.

Pope, B. (1985) 'Psychiatry in Transition – Implications for Psychiatric Nursing', *CPNJ,* July/Agust, 7–13.

Porter S. (1992) 'Women in a woman's job: the gendered experience of nurses', *Sociology of Health and Illness,* **14**(4), 510–27.

Prescott, P. A. (1993) 'Nursing: an important component of hospital survival under a reformed health care system,' *Nursing Economics,* **11**(4), 192–9.

Prior L. (1993) *The Social Organisation of Mental Illness.* London: Sage.

Puka, B. (1993) 'The liberation of caring: a different voice for Gilligan's "Different Voice",' in Larrabee, M. (ed.) *An Ethic of Care.* New York and London: Routledge.

Quick, A. and Wilkinson, R. (1993) Vol. *Income and Health.* London: Socialist Health Association.

Qureshi, H. and Walker, A. (1989) *The Caring Relationship: Elderly People and Their Families.* Landa: Macmillan.

Quershi, B. (1989) *Transcultural Medicine: Dealing with Patients from Different Cultures.* Lancaster: Kluwer.

Rawls, J. (1972) *A Theory of Justice.* Oxford University Press.

Raynor, P. (1996) 'Probation and the criminal justice system: passengers on a runaway train?', in Drakeford, M. and Vanstone, M. (eds) *Beyond Offending Behaviour.* Aldershot: Arena, pp. 9–20.

Rea, D.M. (1989) 'Working for Patients: changing the patients role', *Critical Social Policy,* **9**(1), 98–108.

Redding, D. (1991) 'Exploding the myth', *Community Care,* 12 December, pp. 18–20.

Reed M. (1989) *The Sociology of Management.* London: Harvester Wheatsheaf.

Report of the Inter-Departmental Committee on Physical Deterioration (1904), CMND. 275, London.

Rifkin, S. and Walt, G. (1986) 'Why health improves: defining the issues concerning comprehensive health care and selective primary health care', *Social Science and Medicine,* **23**, 559–66.

Riley, D. (1984) *War in the Nursery.* London: Virago.

Robbert, R. (1990) 'The Medicalisation of Senile Dementia', paper presented at 2nd International Conference on the Future of Adult Life Leeuwenhorst Netherlands.

Roberts R. (1990) 'The Medicalization of Senile Dementia', paper presented at the 2nd International Conference on the Future of Adult Life, Leeuwenhorst, The Netherlands.

Robert, L. (1976) 'The community psychiatric nurse', *Nursing Times,* 23 December, 2020–1.

Roberts, M. (1991) *Living in a Man-made World: Gender Assumptions in Modern Housing Design.* London: Routledge.

Roberts, R. (1973) *The Classic Slum: Salford Life in the First Quarter of the Century.* Harmondsworth: Penguin.

Roberts, R. (1990) 'The Medicalization of Senile Dementia', paper presented at the 2nd Internation Conference on the Future of Adult Life, Leeuwenhorst, The Netherlands.

Rogers, A. P. Pilgrim (1993) *Experiencing Psychiatry – Users' Views of Services.* London: MIND.

Roof (1990) 'The right to buy: the top 20 council sellers, 1980–1990', London: Roof, September/October 1990.

Rose, S. (ed.) (1982) *Case Management and Social Work Practice*. New York: Longman.

Rose, S. and Black, B. (1985) *Advocacy and Empowerment*, Boston: Routledge & Kegan Paul.

Ross, F. (1990) *Key Issues in District Nursing. New Horizons in Community Care*, Paper 2. UK District Nursing Association, London.

Rosser, C. and Harris, C.C. (1965) *The Family and Social Change*. London: Routledge & Kegan Paul.

Rowe, J. and Lambert, L. (1973). *Children Who Wait*. London: Association of British Adoption and Fostering Agencies.

Rowntree Foundation (1990) *The Contribution of the Social Fund to Relieving Poverty*, Social Policy Research Findings, no. 8. York.

Rowntree B. (1901) *Poverty:A Study of Town Life*. London: Green.

Royal College of Nursing (1992) *Skill Mix and Reprofiling: A Guide for RCN Members*. London: RCN.

Royal College of Nursing, (1993) *Newsletter of the RCN School Nurses Forum*, Summer/Autumn.

Royal College of Nursing London. (1996) *Statement on the Role and Scope of Nurse Practitioner Practice*.

Russel, I. J. (1989) *South Glamorgan Care for the Elderly Hospital Discharge Service. A Pilot Project in the Second European Programme to Combat Poverty: An Evaluation Project Paper*. Cardiff: Social Research Unit, School of Social and Administrative Studies, University of Wales Cardiff.

Salisbury, B., Dickey, J. Crawford, C. (1987) *Service Brokerage (Downs View)* North York, Ontario: G. Alan Roeher Institute.

Saltman, R.B. and Von Otte, R.C. (1992) *Planned Markets and Public Competition* Open University Press.

Salvage, J. (1985) *The Politics of Nursing*. London: Heinemann Nursing.

SANE (1993) *Schizophrenia: The Forgotten Illness*. London: SANE.

Sapsford, R. (1993) 'Understanding people: the growth of an expertise' in Clarke, J. (ed.) *A Crisis in Care? Challenges to Social Work*. London: Sage for Open University.

Saunders, P. (1990) *A Nation of Home Owners*. London: Unwin Hyman.

Saunders, P. (1993) 'Citizenship in a liberal society', in Turner, B. (ed.) *Citizenship and Social Theory*. London: Sage.

Schon, D. (1992) in *Journal of Inter-Professional Care* 6,1, 49–63

Scott, D. and Robinson, H. (1985) 'Community psychiatric nursing: a survey of patients and problems', *Journal College of General Practitioners*, March, 130–2.

Searle, G. (1971) *The Movement for National Efficiency*. Oxford: Blackwell.

Secretary of State for Health (1992) *The Health of the Nation: A Strategy for Health in England*. London: HMSO.

Seed, P. (1973) *The Expansion of Social Work in Britain*. London: Routledge & Kegan Paul.

Seedhouse, D. (1986) *Health. The Foundations for Achievement*. Chichester: Wiley.

Shakespeare, T. (1993) 'Disabled people's self-organisation: a new social movement?' *Disability Handicap & Society*, **8**(3), 249–64.

Shapiro, J. (1996) Global Commissioning by General Practitioners', *British Medical Journal*, **312**, 16 March, 652–3.

Sharpe, D. (1982) 'GP's views of the community psychiatric nurse', *Nursing Times*, 6, October 1664–6.

Shaw, A. (1977) 'CPN Attachment in Group Practice', *Nursing Times, Health Centre*, 24 March, ix–xvi.

Sheard, J. (1995) 'From Lady Bountiful to Active Citizen: volunteering and the voluntary sector', in J. Davis-Smith (eds).

Shepperdson, B. (1987) 'Community Psychiatric Nursing in Gwent', unpublished PhD University of Wales Swansea.

Sherman, J. (1995) 'State aid to cut cost of growing old', *The Times*, 19 October.

Skellington, R. (1996) *'Race' in Britain Today*. London: Sage.

Skidmore, D. and Friend, W. (1984) 'Should CPNs be in the primary health care team?', *Nursing Times, Community Outlook*, 19 September, 310–12.

Smale G. and Tuson, G., Biehal, N. and Marsh, P. (1993) *Empowerment, Assessment, Case Management and the Skilled Worker*. London: National Institute for Social Work.

Smith, H. (1994) 'Liberation of the damned', *The Guardian*, 2 June 1994.

Smith, H. and Morrisey, (1994) 'Ethical Dilemmas for Good Practitioners Under the UK Contract', *Journal of Medical Ethics*, **20**, 175–80.

Smithies, J. and Adams, L. (1993) 'Walking the tightrope: issues in evaluation and community participation for health for all,' in Davies, J.K. and Kelly, M.P. (eds) *Healthy Cities: Research and Practice*. London: Routledge.

Social Services Inspectorate (1991) *Assessment Systems and Community Care*, Section 3, HMSO: London.

Stacey, M. (1988) *The Sociology of Health and Healing*. London: Unwin Hyman.

Stainton, T. (1994) *Autonomy and Social Policy Mental handicap and Community Care*, Aldershot: Avebury.

Stevenson, O. and Parsloe, P. (1993) *Community Care and Empowerment*. York: Joseph Rowntree Foundation.

Stewart, M.J. (1993) *Integrating Social Support in Nursing*. Newbury Park, California: Sage.

Stewart, G. and Stewart, J. (1991) *Relieving Poverty? Use of the Social Fund by Social Work Clients and Other Agencies*. London: Association of Metropolitan Authorities.

Stewart R. (1982) 'Management behaviour: how research has changed the traditional picture' Earl M.J. (ed), *Perspecties in Management*. Oxford: Oxford University Press.

Stillwell, B. (1988a) 'A nurse practitioner in an inner city general practice,' in Bowling? and Stilwell (eds) *The Nurse in Family Practice. Practice Nurses and Nurse Practitioners in Primary Health Care*. London: Scutary Press.

Stilwell B. (1988b) 'Patient's attitudes to the availability of a nurse practitioner in general practice', in Bowling and Stilwell (eds), *The Nurse in Family Practice. Practice Nurses and Nurse Practitioners in Primary Health Care*. London: Scutary Press.

Stillwell B. (1995) 'Developing experts: the nurse in general practice', in Littlewood (ed.), *Current Issues in Community Nursing, Primary Health Care in Practice*. Edinburgh: Churchill-Livingstone.

Stockley, D., Canter, D. and Bishop, D. (1993) *Young People on the Move*. Department of Psychology, University of Surrey.

Strong P. (1979) *The Ceremonial Order of the Clinic*. London: Routledge & Kegan Paul.

Strong, P. and Robinson, J. (1990) *NHS Under New Management*. Milton Keynes: Open University.

Summer, B. (1981) *Working With People: an Introduction to the Caring Professions*. London: Cassell.

Sutherland, A. (1981) *Disabled We Stand*. London: Souvenir Press.

Symonds, A. (1991) 'Angels and Interfering Busy Bodies: the social construction of two occupations', *Sociology of Health and Illness*, **2** (13), 249–64.

Symonds, A. (1996) 'Expectant Mothers are Hospital-Minded: the politicisation of child-birth in the 1930s', *Civilization, Sexuality and Social Life – The Hidden Face of Urban Life*, Budapest Simmelweis University of Medicine and Social Medicine, proceedings of International Conference.

Symonds, A. (1997) 'Ties that bind: Problem with GP attachment', *Health Visitor*, 70, 2, 53–5.

Szasz, T. (1972) *The Myth of Mental Illness*. London: Paladin.

Tew, M. (1995) *Safer Childbirth: A Critical History of Maternity Care*, 2nd edn. London: Chapman & Hall.

Thatcher M. (1975) *Let Our Children Grow Tall*. London: Centre for Policy Studies.

Thomas, D.N. (1995) *Helping Communities to Better Health: The Community Development Approach*. Cardiff: Health Promotion Wales.

Thompson, A. and Dobson R. (1995) 'Death of an ideal', *Community Care*, 6–12 July, 20–1.

Thomson, M: (1992) 'The "Problem" of Mental Deficiency in England and Wales', unpublished PhD thesis, University of Oxford.

Thompson, D. (1993) *Mental Illness: The Fundamental Facts*. London: Mental Health Foundation.

Thornton, P. and Tozer, R. (1994) *Involving Older People in Planning and Evaluating Community Care: A review of Initiatives*. York: Social Policy Research Unit, University of York.

Timmins N. (1995) 'Mencap loses care deal after checks on homes', *Independent*, 28 July, p. 3.

Timmins, N. (1996) *The Five Giants: A Biography of the Welfare State*. London: Fontana.

Timmins, N. and MacKinnon, I. (1995) 'Breakdown of care led to hostel killing', *Independent*, 27 July, p. 1.

Titmuss, R. (1963) *Essays on the Welfare State*. London: Allen & Unwin.

Titmuss R. (1970) *The Gift Relationship*. London: Allen & Unwin.

Titmuss, R. (1979) 'Community: care fact or fiction?' in Titmuss, R. (ed). *Commitment to Welfare*. London: Allen & Unwin.

Tonnies, F. (1957) *Community and Society*. New York: Harper & Row.

Townsend, P. (1957) *The Family Life of Old People*. London: Routledge & Kegan.

Townsend, P. (1962c) *The Last Refuge*. London: Routledge & Kegan Paul.

Townsend P., Davison, N. and Whitehead, M. (eds) (1988) *Inequalities in Health: The Black Report and the Health Divide*. Penguin: Harmondsworth.

Tronbranski, P. (1995) 'Implementation of community care policy in the United Kingdom: will it be achieved?,' *Journal of Advanced Nursing*, **21**, 988–95.

Tronto J. (1993) 'Beyond gender difference to a theory of care', in Larrabee, M. (ed.) *An Ethic of Care*. New York & London: Routledge.

Tuckman, A. (1994) 'The yellow brick road: total quality management and the restructing of organisational culture,' *Organisational Studies*, **15**, (5), 727–51.

Tudor Hart, J. (1994) *Feasible Socialism. The National Health Service Past, Present and Future*. London: Socialist Health Association.

Turner, B.S. (1992) *Regulating Bodies: Essays in Medical Sociology*. London: Routledge.

Turner, T. (1989) Partners in care: How ill they work together? *Nursing Times*, **85** (31), 18.

Turshen, M. (1989) *The Politics of Public Health*, London: Zed Books.

Twigg, J. (1992) 'Introduction' J. Twigg (ed.) *Carers: Research and Practice*, London: HMSO.

Twigg, J. and Atkin, K. (1994) *Carers Perceived: policy and practice in informal care*, Buckingham: Open University Press.

UKCC (1986) *Project 2000: a New Preparation for Practice. London*.

UKCC (1991) *Report on Proposals for the Future of Community Education and Practice* (PREP). London.

UKCC (1992a) *Code of Professional Conduct*, 3rd edn. London.

UKCC (1992b) *The Future of Professional Practice: The Council's Standards for Education and Practice Following Registration*. London.

UKCC (1992c) *The Scope of Professional Practice*. London.

UKCC (1994) *The Future of Professional Practice: The Council's Standards for Education and Practice Following Registration*. London.

UKCC (1995) *Final Report on the Future of Professional Education and Practice*. London.

Ungerson, C. (1988) *Policy is Personal: Sex Gender and Informal Care*. London: Tavistock.

Union of Physically Impaired Against Segregation (UPIAS) (1976) *Fundamental Principles of Disability*. London.

Unsworth, C. (1983). *The Politics of Mental Health Legislation*. Oxford: Clarendon.

Valentine, P. and Capponi, P. (1989) 'Mental health, consumer participation on boards and committees: barriers and strategies', *Canada's Mental Health*, 8–12 June.

Van Every J. (1992) 'Who is the family? The assumptions of British social policy', *Critical Social Policy* **33**, 62–75.

Venn S. (1995) 'Jobseeker's allowance', *Adviser*, 49, May/June, 16–17.

Vincent D. (1991) *Poor Citizens*. Harlow: Longman.

Walby, S. (1992) 'Professionals and Post Fordism. The NHS in Transition', Conference Paper, September. Teeside University.

Walby, S. and Greenwell, J. (1994) 'Managing the NHS' in Clarke, J., Cochrane, A., Mclaughlin, E. (eds). *Managing Social Policy*. Milton Keynes: Open University.

Waldo, D. (ed.) (1971) *Public Administration in a Time of Turbulence*, Scranton: Chandler.

Wales Council for Voluntary Action (1989) 'Policy review: a discussion document of the role and functions of the Wales Council for Voluntary Action', unpublished discussion document. Caerphilly.

Walker, A. (1980) 'The social creation of poverty and dependency in old age', *Journal of Social Policy*, **9**, 49–75.

Watters, C. (1996) Representation and realities: black people, community care and mental illness' in W. Ahmed and K. Atlein (eds), *Race and Community Care*, Buckingham: Open University Press.

Wallerstein, N. (1993) 'Empowerment and health: the theory and practice of community change', *Community Development Journal*, **28**, 218–27.

Webb, S. and Webb, B. (1912) *The Prevention of Destitution*. London: Longman.

Webster, C. (1982) 'The hungry or healthy thirties?', *History Workshop*, **13**, 110–29

Webster, C. (1991) *Aneurin Bevan on the National Health Service*. Oxford: Welcome Unit for History of Medicine.

Webster, C. (ed.) (1993) *Caring For Health: History and Diversity*. Milton Keynes: Open University Press

Welsh Health Planning Forum (1993) *The Challenges for Nursing and Midwifery in the 21st Century* (the Heathrow debate) London: HMSO.

Welsh Office (1991) *Welsh Office Funding of the Voluntary Sector: A Strategic Statement*, Welsh Office Publication.

Welsh Office (1994) *Caring for the Future*, Welsh Office Publication.

Welsh Office (1996) *Improving Access to Evidence and Information: A Clinical Effectiveness Initiative for Wales*, Welsh Office Publication.

Wenger, C. (1984) *The Supportive Network: Coping with Old Age*. London: Allen & Unwin.

Wenger, G. C. (1988) *Old People's Health and Experiences of the Caring Services: Accounts from Rural Communitues in North Wales*. Liverpool University Press.

Wenger, G. C. (1991) 'Informal Care: The Bedrock of Care in the Community', paper given to the Second European Congress of Gerontology, Madrid. Bangor: Centre for Social Policy Research Development.

Werskey, G. (1978) *The Visible College*. London: Allen Lane.

West Wales Health Commission (1993) *Local Strategy for Health 1993–2002*. Carmarthen: Dyfed, East Dyfed and Pembrokeshire Health Authority.

Whelan, C. J. (1993) 'The role of social support in mediating the psychological consequences of economic stress', *Sociology of Health and Illness*, vol. 15(1).

White, E. (1986) 'Factor influencing general practitioners to refer patients to community psychiatric nurses', in Brooking, J. (ed.) *Psychiatric Nursing Research*. Chichester: Wiley.

White, E. (1991) 'Practice nurses and CPNs: changing places?', *Practice Nurse*, February, 4777en;8.

Wilding, P. (1992) 'The British welfare state; Thatcherism's enduring legacy', *Policy and Politics*, 20, 201–12.

Williams, C. (1990) 'Contracting', *Network Wales*, **73**, 14.

Williams, C. M. (1985) Population focused community health nursing and nursing administration: a new synthesis', in McCluskey J.C. and Grace H.K. (eds) *Current Issues in Nursing*. Boston: Blackwell Scientific, 86–101.

Williams, S., Calnan, M., Cant, S. L., Coyle, J. (1993) 'All change in the NHS? Implications of the NHS reforms for primary care prevention', *Sociology of Health and Illness*, 15, 1.

Williams, F. (1994) 'Social relations, welfare and the post-Fordist debate', in Burrows, R. and Loader, B. (eds) *Towards a Post-Fordist Welfare State*. London: Routledge.

Williams, J. (1990) 'Elders from black and minority ethnic communities', in Sinclair, I., Parker, R., Leat, D. and Williams, J. *The Kaleidoscope of Care*. London: National Institute of Social Work/HMSO, pp. 101–34.

Williams R. (1973) *The Country and the City*. London: Chatto & Windus.

Williams, R. (1983) *Keywords: Vocabulary of Culture and Society*. London: Fontana.

Williams, S., Calnan, M., Cont, S.L. and Coyle, J. (1993) 'All Change in the NHS? Implications of the NHS reforms for primary care prevention', *Sociology of Health and Illness*, **15** (1), 43–67.

Williamson, J. (1996) 'Promoting Environmental Health', *British Medical Journal*, 6 April.

Willmott, P. and Young, M. (1957) *Family and Kinship in East London*. London: Routledge & Kegan Paul.

Willmott, P. and Young, M. (1962). *Family and Class in a London Suburb*. London: Routledge & Kegan Paul.

Wilson, E. (1977) *Women and the Welfare State*. London: Tavistock.

Wilson, G. (1995) 'Future developments', in Wilson, E. (ed.), *Community Care: Asking the Users*. London: Chapman & Hall.

Wilson, R. and Wylie, D. (1993) *The Dispossessed*. London: Picador.

Wing, J. and Olsen, R. (1979) *Community Care for the Mentally Disabled*. Oxford University Press.

Wirth, L. (1938) 'Urbanism as a way of life', *American Journal of Sociology*, **44** (1) 1–24.

Wistow, G., Knapp, M., Hardy, B. and Allen, C. (1994) *Social Care in a Mixed Economy*. Buckingham: Open University.

Witz, A. (1992) *Professions and Patriarchy*. London: Routledge.

Wolf, C. Jr (1988) *Markets or Governments: Choosing Between Imperfect Alternatives*. Cambridge, Massachusetts: MIT Press.

Wood, N. (1955) *Communism and British Intellectuals*. London: Routledge.

Wood, R. (1991) 'Care of the disabled people', in Dalley, G. (ed.) *Disability and Social Policy*. London: Policy Studies Institute.

Wright, S. (1985) 'New nurses: new boundaries', *Nursing Practice* 1, 32–9.

Wykes, T. (ed.) (1994) *Violence and Health Care Professionals*, London: Chapman & Hall.

Young A. and Ashton, E. (1956) *British Social Work in the Nineteenth Century*. London: Routledge & Kegan Paul.

Index

308 · *Index*